Psychopharmacology Series 10

Clinical Pharmacology in Psychiatry

Strategies in Psychotropic Drug Development

Edited by
L.F. Gram L.P. Balant
H.Y. Meltzer S.G. Dahl

With 29 Figures

Springer-Verlag
Berlin Heidelberg New York
London Paris Tokyo
Hong Kong Barcelona
Budapest

Prof. Dr. Lars F. Gram
Dept. of Clinical Pharmacology, Odense University,
Winsløwparken 19, 5000 Odense C, Denmark

Dr. Luc P. Balant
I.U.P.G., Unité de Recherche Clinique,
47, Rue du XXXI Décembre, 1207 Genève, Switzerland

Prof. Herbert Y. Meltzer
Department of Psychiatry, Case Western Res. Univ.,
2040 Abington Road, Cleveland, Ohio 44106, U.S.A.

Prof. Svein G. Dahl
Institute of Medicinal Biology, University of Tromsø,
P.O. Box 977, 9037 Tromsø, Norway

Vols. 1 and 2 of this series appeared under the title „Psychopharmacology Supplementum"

ISBN-13:978-3-642-78012-7 e-ISBN-13:978-3-642-78010-3
DOI: 10.1007/978-3-642-78010-3

Softcover reprint of the hardcover 1st edition 1993

Typesetting: Best-set Typesetter Ltd., Hong Kong
25/3130-5 4 3 2 1 0 – Printed on acid-free paper

Preface

This book contains the papers from invited lecturers as well as selected contributions presented at the 6th International Meeting on Clinical Pharmacology in Psychiatry (I.M.C.P.P.) held in Geneva, Switzerland, 5–7 June 1991. At this meeting the basic theme of the previous meetings in this series (Chicago 1979, Tromsø 1980, Odense 1982, Bethesda 1985, Tromsø 1988) was continued, namely, to bridge the gap between experimental development and clinical reality in psychopharmacology.

After more than 25 years of intensive research in biological psychiatry, basic understanding of the biological mechanisms underlying major psychiatric diseases has advanced significantly but is still far from complete. Likewise, the hypotheses underlying the development of new psychotropics have been refined and produced a wide spectrum of novel, yet designed compounds. The crucial condition for all progress in this field is reliable, informative clinical testing of new compounds.

It is our hope that this book, as a continuation of the earlier publications in this series, provides further evidence of the ongoing interaction between preclinical and clinical scientists, who only together can assure progress in this exciting area of research and clinical practice.

Odense, Geneva,
Cleveland, Tromsø

L.F. Gram, L.P. Balant,
H.Y. Meltzer, and S.G. Dahl

Acknowledgements

The 6th International Meeting on Clinical Pharmacology in Psychiatry received generous support from a number of institutions and pharmaceutical companies, which is gratefully acknowledged:

Institutions Universitaires de Psychiatrie de Genève
Department of Clinical Pharmacology, Odense University
Abbot, US
Astra, Sweden
Bristol-Myers Squibb, US
Ciba-Geigy, Denmark, Sweden and Switzerland
Delagrange, France
Eli Lilly, US
Glaxo, UK and US
Janssen, Switzerland
Kabi Pharma, Sweden
Lundbeck, Denmark and Switzerland
Merck, FRG
Merck, Sharp and Dohme, US
Merrell Dow, France and US
Novo Nordisk, Denmark
Organon, The Netherlands, Sweden and Switzerland
Pfizer, US
Pierre Fabre, France
Rhône-Poulenc, France
Roche, Denmark, Sweden and US
Sandoz, Switzerland and US
Sanofi, France
Schering, FRG
Schering-Plough, Sweden and US
SmithKline Beecham, UK
Troponwerke, FRG
Upjohn, UK and US
Wyeth-Ayerst, US

The members of the Organizing Committee were:
A.E. Balant-Gorgia, Switzerland
L.P. Balant, Switzerland
S.G. Dahl, Norway
L.F. Gram, Denmark
H.Y. Meltzer, US

The members of the Scientific Advisory Committee were:
D.E. Casey, US
R. Fog, Denmark
F. Holsboer, FRG
E. Paykel, UK
W.Z. Potter, US
F.-A. Wiesel, Sweden
E. Zarifian, France

We would like to thank:
Symporg SA, Congress Organizers, Geneva, Switzerland, and Henrik Horneberg, Dep. of Clinical Pharmacology, Odense University, for excellent assistance in preparing and arranging the conference.

Contents

List of Contributors

You will find the addresses at the beginning of the respective contribution.

Adham, N. 15
Aimi, J. 26
Andrieux, M. 82
Aulakh, C.S. 52
Balant, L.P. 212, 246
Balant-Gorgia, A.E. 212, 246
Baldessarini, R.J. 138
Bech, P. 190
Bertilsson, L. 230
Besançon, R. 82
Bolwig, T.G. 190
Bouthenet, M.L. 82
Branchek, T. 15
Brøsen, K. 199
Casey, D.E. 101
Ciaranello, R.D. 26
Cohen, B.M. 138
Dahl, M.L. 230
Dahl, S.G. 1
Danish University Andidepressant Group 190
Davis, J.M. 253
Dean, R. 26
Desai, R. 26
Edvardsen, Ø. 1
Ekqvist, B. 230
Farde, L. 94
Garlow, S. 26
Gex-Fabry, M. 246
Giros, B. 82
Göthert, M. 38
Gram, L.F. 163, 190, 199
Hartig, P.R. 15
Heller, M.R. 26
Irwin, R.P. 111
Kane, J.M. 131
Kao, H.-T. 15
Kragh-Sørensen, P. 190
Lannfelt, L. 82
Lesch, K.P. 52
Llerena, A. 230
Macchi, M. 15
Martres, M.P. 82
Meltzer, H.Y. 70
Morilak, D. 26
Murphy, D.L. 52
Nielsen, K.K. 199
Nordström, A.-L. 94
Paykel, E.S. 149
Perel, J.M. 238
Pilon, C. 82
Pollock, B.G. 238
Potter, W.Z. 111
Preskorn, S.H. 174
Reisby, N. 190
Roth, B.L. 26
Schechter, L. 15
Schlicker, E. 38
Schwartz, J.C. 82
Sindrup, S.H. 199
Skjelbo, E. 199
Sokoloff, P. 82
Souil, E. 82
Strosberg, A.D. 9
Sylte, I. 1
Teicher, M.H. 138
Vestergaard, P. 190
Wang, Z. 253
Weinshank, R. 15
Wiesel, F.-A. 124
Zgombick, J. 15

Molecular Modeling of Neurotransmitter Receptors and Ligands

S.G. DAHL, Ø. EDVARDSEN, and I. SYLTE

1 Molecular Structure of Neurotransmitter Receptors

The cloning and sequencing of neurotransmitter receptor molecules has provided new insight into their classification and functioning as well as structural information which may be potentially useful in drug development. X-ray crystallographic diffraction techniques are the most widely used experimental methods for determining three-dimensional protein structures. However, while the amino acid sequences are known for a continuously increasing number of neurotransmitter receptors, there have been no reports on the three-dimensional crystal structure of any such receptor. In the absence of any detailed experimental three-dimensional receptor structure, we have developed models of the dopamine D_2 receptor (Dahl et al. 1991), the serotonin 5-HT_{1A} receptor (Sylte et al., to be published), and the 5-HT_2 receptor (Edvardsen et al. 1992), based on their amino acid sequence. The models were constructed by computer graphics and molecular modeling techniques, and used to examine the mechanisms of drug and neurotransmitter interactions with these receptors.

The dopamine D_2 receptor model was first presented in 1989 (Dahl et al. 1989a,b), at a time when this was the only dopamine receptor which had been cloned. When the D_1 and D_3 receptor sequences were published in 1990, confirming some of the hypotheses behind the D_2 receptor modeling, the paper describing the model (Dahl et al. 1991) was submitted for publication. The D_2 receptor model was based on the structural similarities within the superfamily of G protein coupled neurotransmitter receptors. As indicated in Fig. 1, the peptide chains of all these receptor molecules have seven putative membrane-spanning domains, and the various dopamine, serotonin, α-adrenergic, β-adrenergic, and muscarinic acetylcholine receptors have several conserved amino acid residues in the putative membrane-spanning domains. Site-directed mutagenesis experiments have suggested that aspartic residues in and near transmembrane segments 2 and 3 are required for ligand binding and signal transduction in dopamine D_2 (Neve et al. 1991), β_2-adrenergic (Strader et al. 1988, 1989b; Fraser et al. 1988),

Institute of Medical Biology, University of Tromsø, 9037 Tromsø, Norway

```
                                                                                   I                               II
                                                                                                               x
D1                                      MRTLNTSAMDGTGLVVERDFSVRILTACFLSLLILSTLLGNTLVCAAVIRFRHLRSKVTNFFVISLAVSDLLVAVLVMPWKAVAEIAGF
D2                                MDPLNLSWYDDDLERQNWSRPFNGSEGKADRPHYNYYAMLLTLLIFIIVFGNVLVCMAVSREKALQT.TTNYLIVSLAVADLLVATLVMPWVVYLEVVGE
D3                                MAPLSQIS.....THLNSTCGAENSTGVNRARPHAYYALSYCALILAIIFGNGLVCAAVLRERALQT.TTNYLVVSLAVADLLVATLVMPWVVYLEVTGG
D4                                MGNRSTADADGLLAGRGPAAGASAGASAGLAGQGAAALVGGVLLIGAVLAGNSLVCVSVATERALQT.PTNSFIVSLAAADLLLALLVLPLFVYSEVQGG
D5                             MLPPGSNGTAYPGQFALYQQLAQGNAVGGSAGAPPLGPSQVVTACLLTLLIIWTLLGNVLVCAAIVRSRHLRANMTNVFIVSLAVSDLFVALLVMPWKAVAEVAGY
5HT1a                  MDVLSPGQGNNTTSPPAPFE.........TG..GNTTGI........SDVTVSYQVITSLLLGTLIFCAVLGNACVVAAIALERSLQN.VANYLIGSLAVTDLMVSVLVLPMAALYQVLN.
5HT1c            MVNLGNAVRSLLMHLIGLLVWQFDISISPVAAIVTDTFNSSDGGRLF.....QFPDGVQNWPALSIVVIIIMTIGGNILVIMAVSMEKKLHN.ATNYFLMSLAIADMLVGLLVMPLSLLAILYDY
5HT2  MEILCEDNISLSSIPNSLMQLGDGPRLYHNDFNSRDANTSEASNWTIDAENRTNLSCEGYLPPTCLSILHLQEKNWSALLTTVVIILTIAGNILVIMAVSLEKKLQN.ATNYFLMSLAIADMLLGFLVMPVSMLTILYGY
α1                 MNPDLDTGHNTSAPAQWGELKDANFTGPNQTSSNSTL..P......QLDVTRAISVGLVLGAFILFAIVGNILVILSVACNRHLRT.PTNYFIVNLAIADLLLSFTVLPFSATLEVLGY
α2a                                MGSLQPDAGNASWNGTEAPGGGARATPYSLQVTLTLVCLAGLLMLLTVFGNVLVIIAVFTSRALKA.PQNLFLVSLASADILVATLVIPFSLANEVMGY
α2b                  MASPALAAALAVAAAAGPNASGAGERGSGGVANASGA...SWGPPRGQYSAGAVAGLAAVVGFLIVFTVVGNVLVVIAVLTSRALRA.PQNLFLVSLASADILVATLVMPFSLANELMAY
β1                MGAGVLVLGASEPGNLSSAAPLPDGAATAARLLVPASPPASLLPPASESPEPLSQQWTAGMGLLMALIVLLIVAGNVLVIVAIAKTPRLQT.LTNLFIMSLASADLVMGLLVVPFGATIVVWG.
β2                       MGQPGNGSAFLLAPNGSHA....PDHDVTQ............QRDEVWVVGMGIVMSLIVLAIVFGNVLVITAIAKFERLQT.VTNYFITSLACADLVMGLAVVPFGAAHILM.K
β3                       MAPWPHEN.SSLAPWPDLPT.....LAPNTANTSGLPGVP........WEAALAGALLALAVLATVGGNLLVIVAIAWTPRLQT.MTNVFVTSLAAADLVMGLLVVPPAATLALTG.
M1                                                  MNTSAPPAVSPNITVLAPGKGPWQVAFIGITTGLLSLATVTGNLLVLISFKVNTELKT.VNNYFLLSLACADLIIGTFSMNLYTTYLLMGH
M2                                                 MNNSTNSSNNSLALTSP...YKTFEVVFIVLVAGSLSLVTIIGNILVMVSIKVNRHLQT.VNNYFLFSLACADLIIGVFSMNLYTLYTVIGY
M4                                MANFTPVNGSSGNQSVRLVTSSSHNRYETVEMVFIATVTGSLSLVTVVGNILVMLSIKVNRQLQT.VNNYFLFSLACADLIIGAFSMNLYTVYIIKGY

          III                              IV                                                                  V
       x          x                                                                                       x  x
D1    .WPFGSF.CNIWVAFDIMCSTASILNLCVISVDRYWAISSPFRY..ERKMTPK.AAFILISVAWTLSVLISFIPVQLSWHKAKPTSPSDGNATSLAETID.............NCDSSLSRTYAISSSVISFYIPVAIM
D2    .WKFSRIHCDIFVTLDVMMCTASILNLCAISIDRYTAVAMPMLY..NTRYSSKRRVTVMIAIVWVLSFTISCPL.LFGLNNTDQNE................................C.IIANPAFVVYSSIVSFYVPFIVT
D3    VWNFSRICCDVFVTLDVMMCTASILNLCAISIDRYTAVVMPVHYQHGTGQSSCRRVALMITAVWVLAFAVSCPL.LFGFNTTGDPS.............................ICSISNPDFVIYSSVVSFYVPFGVT
D4    AWLLSPRLCDALMAMDVMLCTASIFNLCAISVDRFVAVAVPLRY...NRQGGSRRQLLLIGATWLLSAAVAAPV.LCGLNDVRGRDPAVCR..............................LEDRDYVVYSSVCSFFLPCPLM
D5    .WPFGAF.CDVWVAFDIMCSTASILNLCVISVDRYWAISRPFRY..KRKMTQR.MALVMVGLAWTLSILISFIPVQLNWHRDQAASWGGLDLPNNLANWTPWEEDFWEPDVNAENCDSSLNRTYAISSSLISFYIPVAIM
5HT1a KWTLGQVTCDLFIALDVLCCTSSILHLCAIALDRYWAITDPIDY.VN...KRTPRPRALISLTWLIGFLISIP.PMLGWRTPEDRSDPD.........................ACTISKDHGYTIYSTFGAFYIPLLLM
5HT1c VWPLPRYLCPVWISLDVLFSTASIMHLCAISLDRYVAIRNP...IEHSRFNSRTKAIMKIAIVWAISIGVSVPIPVIGLRD.E..S...KVFVNNTTCVL...........................NDPNFVLIGSFVAFFIPLTIM
5HT2  RWPLPSKLCAIWIYLDVLFSTASIMHLCAISLDRYVAIQNP...IHHSRFNSRTKAFLKIIAVWTISVGISMPIPVFGLQDD...S...KVFKEGS.CLL..........................ADDNFVLIGSFVAFFIPLTIM
α1    .WVLGRIFCDIWAAVDVLCCTASILSLCAISIDRYIGVRYSLQYPT...LVTRRKAILALLSVWVLSTVISIG.PLLGWKEPAPNDDKE..............................CGVTEEPFYALFSSLGSFYIPLAVI
α2a   .WYFGKTWCEIYLALDVLFCTSSIVHLCAISLDRYWSITQAIEY..NLKRTPRRIKAI.IITCWVISAVISFPPLISIEKKGGGGGPQP............................AEPRCEINDQKWYVISSCIGSFFAPCLIM
α2b   .WYFGQVWCGVYLALDVLFCTSSIVHLCAISLDRYWSVTQAVEY..NLK.RTPRRVKATIVAVWLISAVISFPPLVSLYRQPDG...............................AAYPQCGLNDETWYILSSCIGSFFAPCLIM
β1    RWEYGSFFCELWTSVDVLCVTASIETLCVIALDRYLAITSPFRY..QS.LLTRARARGLVCTVWAISALVSFLPILMHWW.RAESDEARRCY..........................NDPKCCDFVTNRAYAIASSVVSFYVPLCIM
β2    MWTFGNFWCEFWTSIDVLCVTASIETLCVIAVDRYFAITSPFKY..QS.LLTKNKARVIILMVWIVSGLTSF.LPIQMHWYRATHQEAINCY.........................ANETCCDFFTNQAYAIASSIVSFYVPLVIM
β3    HWPLGATGCELWTSVDVLCVTASIETLCALAVDRYLAVTNPLRY..GALVTKRCARTAVVLVWVVSAAVSFAPIMSQWWRVGADAEAQRCH.........................SNPRCCAFASNMPYVLLSSSVSFYLPLLVM
M1    .WALGTLACDLWLALDYVASNASVMNLLLISFDRYFSVTRPLSY..RAKRTPRRAALM.IGLAWLVSFVLWAPAILFWQYLVGERT....VL...........................AGQCYIQFLSQPIITFGTAMAAFYLPVTVM
M2    .WPLGPVVCDLWLALDYVVSNASVMNLLIISFDRYFCVTKPLTY..PVKRTTKMAGMM.IAAAWVLSFILWAPAILFWQFIVGVRTVEDGE...............................CYIQFFSNAAVTFGTAIAAFYLPVIIM
M4    .WPLGAVVCDLWLALDYVVSNASVMNLLIISFDRYFCVTKPLTY..PARRTTKMAGLM.IAAAWVLSFVLWAPAILFWQFVVGKRTVPDNH..............................CFIQFLSNPAVTFGTAIAAFYLPVVIM

- V -                                          VI                                    VII
                                                                                     x
D1    IVTYTRIYRIAQKQIRR    (38)   ...RETKVLKTLSVIMGVFVCCWLPFFILNCILPFCGSGETCQP...FCIDSNTFDVFVWFGWANSSLNPIIY.AFNADFRKAFSTLLGCYRLCPATNNAIE  (87)   446
D2    LLVYIKIYIVLRK....    (117)  SQQKEKKATQMLAIVLGVFIICWLPFFITHILNIHCD.........CNIPPVLYSAFTWLGYVNSAVNPIIYTTFNIEFRKAFMKILHC                       415
D3    VLVYARIYIVLRQ....    (148)  VPLREKKATQMVVIVLGAFIVCWLPFFLTHVLNTHCQA........CHVSPELYRATTWLGYVNSALNPVIYTTFNVEFRKAFLKILSC                       446
D4    LLLYWATFRGL......    (87)   ..GRERKAMRVLPVVVGAFLLCWTPFFVVHITQALCPA........CSVPPRLVSAVTWLGYVNSALNPVIYTVFNAEFRNVFRKALRACC                     387
D5    IVTYTRIYRIAQVQIRR    (31)   ...KETKVLKTLSVIMGVFVCCWLPFFILNCMVPFCSGHPEGPPAGFPCVSETTFDVFVWFGWANSSLNPVIY.AFNADFQKVFAQLLGCSHFCSRT..PVE  (92)   477
5HT1a LVLYGRIFRAARFRIRK    (111)  ....ERKTVKTLGIIMGTFILCWLPFFIVALVLPFCESSC........HMPTLLGAIINWLGYSNSLLNPVIYAYFNKDFQNAFKKIIKCNFCRQ                   421
5HT1c VITYFLTIYVLRRQTLM    (59)   ....EKKASKVLGIVFFVFLIMWCPFFITNILSVLCGKAC.NQ....KLMEKLLNVFVWIGYVCSGINPLVYTLFNKIYRRAFSKYLRCDYKPDKKPPVRQ  (61)   460
5HT2  VITYFLTIKSLQKEATL    (46)   SISNEQKACKVLGIVFFLFVVMWCPFFITNIMAVICKESC.NE....NVIGALLNVFVWIGYLSSAVNPLVYTLFNKTYRSAFSRYIQCQYKENRKPLQLI  (62)   471
α1    LVMYCRVYIVAKRTT..    (54)   ....EKKAAKTLGIVVGMFILCWLPFFIALPLGSLFSTL........KPPDAVFKVVFWLGYFNSCLNPIIYPCSSKEFKRAFMRILGCQCRSGR.RR.RR  (140)  515
α2a   ILVYVRIYQIAKRRTRV    (135)  GQNLEKRFTFVLAVVIGVFVVCWFPFFFTYTLTAVGCS.........VPRTLFKFFFWFGYCNSSLNPVIYTIFNHDFRRAFKKIL...CRGDRKRIV               450
α2b   GLVYARIYRVAKRRTRT    (128)  AQAREKRFTFVLAVVMGVFVLCWFPFFFIYSLYGICREAC..Q....VPGPLFKFFFWIGYCNSSLNPVIYTVFNQDFRPSFKHILFRRRRRGFRQ               461
β1    AFVYLRVFREAQK....    (61)   VALREQKALKTLGIIMGVFTLCWLPFFLANVVKAFHREL........VPDRLFVFFNWLGYANSAFNPIIY.CRSPDFRKAFQGLL.C...CARRAARRR  (76)   477
β2    VFVYSRVFQEAKR....    (35)   FCLKEHKALKTLGIIMGTFTLCWLPFFIVNIVHVIQDNL........IRKEVYILLNWIGYVNSGFNPLIY.CRSPDFRIAFQELL.C..........LR  (70)   413
β3    LFVYARVFVVATR....    (49)   LPLREHRALCTLGLIMGTFTLCWLPFFLANVLRALGGP........SLVPGPAFLALNWLGYANSAFNPLIY.CRSPDFRSAFRRLLC.......RCGRR.  (36)   402
M1    CTLYWRIYRETENRARE    (138)  ....EKKAARTLSAILLAFIVTWTPYNIMVLVSTFCKDC........VPETLWELGYWLCYVNSTINPMCYALCNKAFRDTFRLLLLCR......WDKRR  (19)   437
M2    TVLYWHISRASKSRIKK    (158)  PPSREKKVTRTILAILLAFIITWAPYNVMVLINTFCAPC........IPNTVWTIGYWLCYINSTINPACYALCNATFKKTFKHLLMCHYKNIGATR              463
M4    TVLYIHISLASRSRVHK    (161)  MAARERKVTRTIFAILLAFILTWTPYNVMVLVNTFCQSC........IPDTVWSIGYWLCYVNSTINPACYALCNATFKKTFRHLLLCQYRNIGTAR              475
```

and m_1 muscarinic acetylcholine receptors (Fraser et al. 1989). These residues are conserved in all known sequences of G protein coupled neurotransmitter receptors, including the canine and rat histamine H_2 receptors (Gantz et al. 1991; Ruat et al. 1991). In the modeling of serotonin and dopamine receptors, we assumed that the conserved aspartic residues in helix 2 and helix 3 have similar functions in these receptors and in the β_2-adrenergic and muscarinic m_1 acetylcholine receptors.

A pair of serine residues in transmembrane segment 5, which have been suggested to be involved in agonist binding and activation of β_2-adrenergic receptors (Strader et al. 1989a), are conserved in corresponding positions in the sequences of α_1, β_1- and β_3-adrenergic receptors and in the dopamine receptors, but not in the α_2-adrenergic, serotonin, or muscarinic acetylcholine receptors (Fig. 1), nor in the histamine H_2 receptors.

2 Receptor Modeling

Computer graphics techniques, molecular mechanics energy calculations, and molecular dynamics simulations were used to construct three-dimensional models from the amino acid sequences of the dopamine D_2 (Bunzow et al. 1988), the 5-HT_{1A} (Kobilka et al. 1987; Fargin et al. 1988), and the 5-HT_2 (Julius et al. 1990) receptors. The Assisted Model Building with Energy Refinement (AMBER) force field (Weiner et al. 1984, 1986) was used for molecular mechanics calculations and molecular dynamics simulations, which were done on Sun 4/60 and VAX-8600 computers and on a Cray X/MP-216 supercomputer. The Molecular Interactive Display And Simulation (MIDAS) computer graphics programs (Ferrin et al. 1988) were used for molecular graphics on an Evans and Sutherland PS390 computer graphics system, with a DEC Microvax II as the host machine.

In order to determine which domains of the peptide chains go through the cell membrane, hydropathy indices along the peptide chains were calculated for a series of various G protein-coupled neurotransmitter

◄ **Fig. 1.** Amino acid sequences of various G protein-coupled neurotransmitter receptors, aligned with the Gap computer program of the genetics computer group (GCG) program package (Devereux et al. 1984), using the method of Needleman and Wunsch (1970). Positions of residues which have been suggested from site-directed mutagenesis experiments to be involved in ligand binding and signal transduction are indicated with an *x*. These include an aspartic residue in transmembrane segment 2 of the dopamine D_2 receptor (Neve et al. 1991), aspartic residues in transmembrane segment 2, in transmembrane segment 3, and near transmembrane segment 3 in the β_2-adrenergic (Strader et al. 1988, 1989b; Fraser et al. 1988) and m_1 muscarinic acetylcholine (Fraser et al. 1989) receptor. An asparagine residue in transmembrane segment 7 (Strader et al. 1988; Fraser et al. 1988) and two serine residues in transmembrane segment 5 (Strader et al. 1989a) have been suggested to be involved in agonist binding and activation of β_2-adrenergic receptors

receptors, and average hydropathy indices were calculated from the aligned amino acid sequences (Dahl et al. 1991). Presumably, this enabled more precise prediction of the locations of the seven transmembrane domains in the peptide chains than hydropathy indices calculated from a single receptor sequence. The locations of the transmembrane domains predicted by this method were in excellent agreement with results from experiments with specific antibodies for different domains in β_2-adrenergic receptors (Wang et al. 1989).

In analogy with the solid state structure of bacteriorhodopsin (Henderson et al. 1990), it was presumed that the membrane-spanning segments of G protein-coupled receptors have α-helical secondary structures. Initial models of the seven transmembrane α-helices were constructed from the amino acid sequences with the MIDAS programs and refined by molecular mechanics energy minimization. The transmembrane α-helices were then assembled in an antiparallel, bacteriorhodopsin-like arrangement, with the most polar surface area of each helix forming a central core. This receptor architecture allows access of ligands to a putative binding site involving the conserved aspartic residues near the middle of helix 2 and helix 3.

Models of the loops between helices and the C- and N-terminals were constructed from the amino acid sequences, based on secondary structure predictions by the method of Chou and Fasman (1974a,b). The loops and terminal parts were refined by molecular dynamics simulation and molecular mechanics energy minimization. Figure 2 shows the energy minimized model of the rat dopamine D_2 receptor, with a dopamine molecule at the putative ligand binding site.

3 Ligand–Receptor Interactions

In the dopamine and serotonin receptor models the conserved aspartic acid residue in helix 3 was closer to the synaptic cell membrane surface than the conserved aspartic residue in helix 2. This geometry offers a steric explanation of how the conserved aspartic acid residue in helix 2 may be more essential for agonist binding and signal transduction than for binding of antagonists, as suggested for β_2-adrenergic receptors from site-directed mutagenesis experiments (Strader et al. 1988, 1989b; Fraser et al. 1988).

The three-dimensional models were used to calculate the molecular electrostatic potentials around the receptors. Such electrostatic potentials depend both on the molecular conformation of the protein and on the atomic charges of individual residues (Weiner et al. 1982). In the dopamine and serotonin receptor models the electrostatic potentials were mainly negative on the synaptic side and around the conserved aspartic residues in the central core and positive in the cytoplasmic domains.

The negative electrostatic potentials in the synaptic domains and in the putative ligand binding site in the central core suggest that the protonated

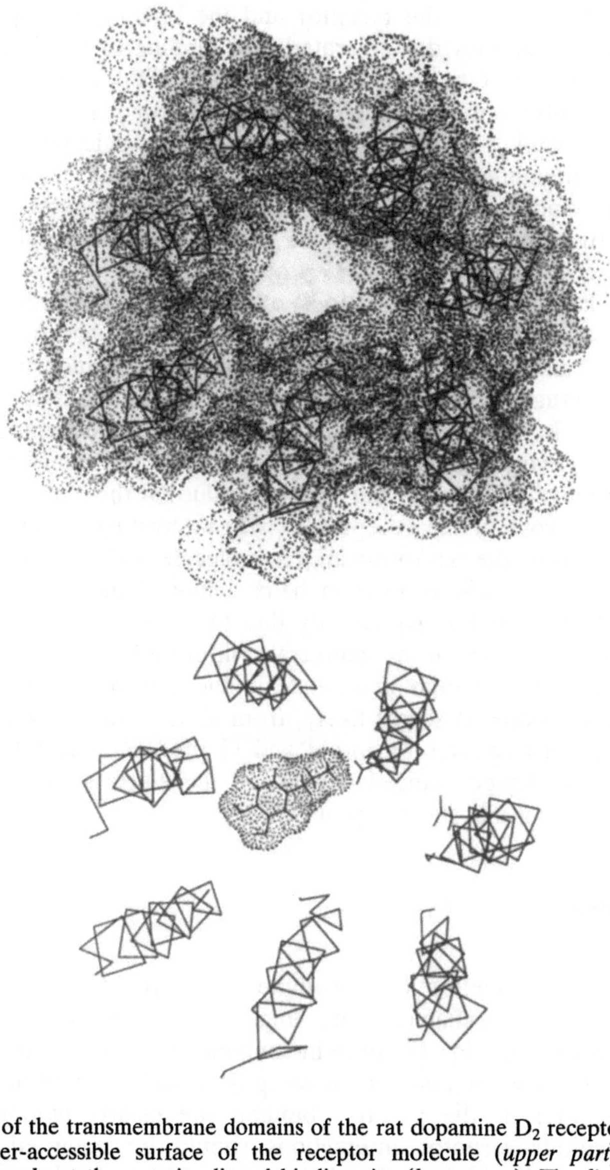

Fig. 2. Model of the transmembrane domains of the rat dopamine D_2 receptor. The *dots* show the water-accessible surface of the receptor molecule (*upper part*) and of a dopamine molecule at the putative ligand binding site (*lower part*). The *lines* show the bonds between α carbon atoms in the peptide chain of the receptor, the side chain of Asp 80 in helix 2 and Asp 114 in helix 3, and all bonds between atoms in dopamine. The amino group in dopamine is close to the carboxylic side chain of Asp 80. (From Dahl et al. 1991)

ligands are attracted to the receptor and the binding site by electrostatic forces. The calculations demonstrated that binding of a protonated ligand increases the electrostatic potentials of the D_2, 5-HT_{1A} and 5-HT_2 receptors, both in the central core near the conserved aspartic residue in helix 2 (Asp 80 in the dopamine D_2 receptor) and in cytoplasmic domains near the intracellular membrane surface. It is possible, therefore, that protonated agonists may induce conformational changes in the receptor, leading to G protein activation, by increasing the electrostatic potentials in domains where the receptor is linked to a G protein.

Molecular dynamics simulations of dopamine (Edvardsen and Dahl 1992), serotonin (Edvardsen and Dahl 1991), and various antipsychotic drugs (Sylte and Dahl 1991a,b; Dahl et al. 1992) demonstrated that the molecules fluctuate rapidly between different conformations as they approach the receptor. In simulations of the neurotransmitter–receptor complexes, the positively charged amino group in the neurotransmitter became oriented towards negatively charged aspartic acid residues at the putative binding site in the central core of the receptor. It was interesting to note that during these simulations, the neurotransmitter molecule and the side chain of the conserved aspartic acid residue in helix 2 moved in a synchronized way (Edvardsen et al. 1992). Apparently due to the strong electrostatic interactions, the movements of the neurotransmitter molecule were accompanied by movements of a similar magnitude in the carboxylic side chain of the aspartic acid residue. It seems likely, from all this, that signal transduction between neurotransmitter receptors and G proteins may take place by a combination of ligand-induced changes in the electrostatic field and conformational changes in the receptor.

4 Conclusions

Our molecular modeling of dopamine and serotonin receptors suggest that electrostatic mechanisms are important for ligand interaction and signal transduction in G protein-coupled neurotransmitter receptors. Molecular dynamics simulations of receptor models with an antagonist or a neurotransmitter at the putative binding site clearly demonstrated that neurotransmitter–receptor interactions should be regarded as dynamic processes, in order to understand the molecular mechanisms. The simulations supported the previously postulated importance of the conserved aspartic residues in helix 2 and helix 3 for ligand interaction and binding. However, our molecular modeling and calculations indicate that several other residues lining the central core of the dopamine and serotonin receptors may also interact with ligands and be of importance for the specificity of ligand recognition and binding.

These calculations were intended to present approximate overall models of the receptors which might provide further insight into the molecular mechanisms of these and other neurotransmitter receptors of the same superfamily. Although probably inaccurate in many details, the models may be used to examine the structural differences between various receptors within a family and to examine molecular receptor mechanisms and possibly explain the affinities of various ligands.

Acknowledgements. This work was supported by grants from the Norwegian Research Council for Science and the Humanities, Troms Fylkeskommune and the L.F. Saugstad Research Foundation.

References

Bunzow JR, Van Tol HHM, Grandy DK, Albert P, Salon J, Christie M, Machida CA, Neve KA, Civelli O (1988) Cloning and expression of a rat D_2 dopamine receptor cDNA. Nature 336:783–787

Chou PY, Fasman GD (1974a) Conformational parameters for amino acids in helical, β-sheet and random coil regions calculated from proteins. Biochemistry 13:211–222

Chou PY, Fasman GD (1974b) Prediction of protein conformation. Biochemistry 13:222–245

Dahl SG, Edvardsen Ø, Heimstad E, Sylte I (1989a) Three dimensional aspects of drug interactions with the dopamine D2 receptor (Abstr 18). European College of Neuro-Psychopharmacology Congress, Gothenburg

Dahl SG, Edvardsen Ø, Heimstad E, Sylte I (1989b) Three dimensional structure of the dopamine D2 receptor (Abstr). In: Stefanis CN, Soldatos CR, Rabavilas AD (eds) Psychiatry today. Excerpta Medica, Amsterdam

Dahl SG, Edvardsen Ø, Sylte I (1991) Molecular dynamics of dopamine at the D_2 receptor. Proc Natl Acad Sci USA 88:8111–8115

Dahl SG, Kollman PA, Rao SN, Singh UC (1992) Structural changes by sulfoxidation of phenothiazine drugs. J Comput Aided Mol Design 6:207–222

Devereux J, Haeberli P, Smithies OA (1984) Comprehensive set of sequence analysis programs for the VAX. Nucleic Acids Res 12:387–395

Edvardsen Ø, Dahl SG (1991) Molecular structure and dynamics of serotonin. Mol Brain Res 9:31–37

Edvardsen Ø, Dahl SG (1992) Molecular dynamics and electrostatic potentials of dopamine. Mol Neuropharmacol 1:165–172

Edvardsen Ø, Sylte I, Dahl SG (1992) Molecular dynamics of serotonin and ritanserin interacting with the 5-HT_2 receptor. Mol Brain Res 14:166–178

Fargin A, Raymond JR, Loshe MJ, Kobilka BK, Caron MG, Lefkowitz RJ (1988) The genomic clone G-21 which resembles a β-adrenergic receptor sequence encodes the 5-HT_{1a} receptor. Nature 335:358–360

Ferrin TE, Huang CC, Jarvis LE, Langridge R (1988) The MIDAS display system. J Mol Graphics 6:13–27

Fraser CM, Chung F-Z, Wang C-D, Venter JC (1988) Site-directed mutagenesis of human β-adrenergic receptors: substitution of aspartic acid-130 by asparagine produces a receptor with high-affinity agonist binding that is uncoupled from adenylate cyclase. Proc Natl Acad Sci USA 85:5478–5482

Fraser CM, Wang C-D, Robinson DA, Gocayne JD, Venter JC (1989) Site-directed mutagenesis of m_1 muscarinic acetylcholine receptors: conserved aspartic acids play important roles in receptor function. Mol Pharmacol 36:840–847

Gantz I, Schäffer M, Delavalle J, Logsdon C, Campbell V, Uhler M, Yamada T (1991) Molecular cloning of a gene encoding the histamine H_2 receptor. Proc Natl Acad Sci USA 88:429–433

Henderson R, Baldwin JM, Ceska TA, Zemlin F, Beckman E, Downing KH (1990) Model for the structure of bacteriorhodopsin based on high-resolution electron cryomicroscopy. J Mol Biol 213:899–929

Julius D, Huang KN, Livelli TJ, Axel R, Jessell TM (1990) The 5HT2 receptor defines a family of structurally distinct but functionally conserved serotonin receptors. Proc Natl Acad Sci USA 87:928–932

Kobilka BK, Frielle T, Collins S, Yang-Feng T, Kobilka TS, Francke U, Lefkowitz RJ, Caron MG (1987) An intronless gene encoding a potential member of the family of receptors coupled to guanine nucleotide regulatory proteins. Nature 329:75–79

Needleman SB, Wunsch CD (1970) General method applicable to the search for similarities in the amino acid sequence of two proteins. J Mol Biol 48:443–453

Neve KA, Tester BA, Henningsen RA, Spanoyannis A, Neve RL (1991) A pivotal role for aspartate-80 in regulation of dopamine D-2 receptor affinity for drugs and inhibition of adenylyl cyclase. Mol Pharmacol 39:733–739

Ruat M, Traiffort E, Arrang J-M, Leurs R, Schwartz J-C (1991) Cloning and tissue expression of a rat histamine H_2 receptor gene. Biochem Biophys Res Commun 179:1470–1478

Strader CD, Sigal IS, Candelore MR, Rands E, Hill WS, Dixon RAF (1988) Conserved aspartic acid residues 79 and 113 of the β-adrenergic receptor have different roles in receptor function. J Biol Chem 263:10267–10271

Strader CD, Candelore MR, Hill WS, Sigal IS, Dixon RAF (1989a) Identification of two serine residues involved in agonist activation of the β-adrenergic receptor. J Biol Chem 264:13572–13578

Strader CD, Candelore MR, Hill WS, Dixon RAF, Sigal IS (1989b) A single amino acid substitution in the β-adrenergic receptor promotes partial agonist activity from antagonists. J Biol Chem 264:16470–16477

Sylte I, Dahl SG (1991a) Molecular structure and dynamics of *cis*(Z)- and *trans*(E)-flupenthixol and clopenthixol. Pharm Res 8:462–470

Sylte I, Dahl SG (1991b) Three dimensional structure and molecular dynamics of *cis*(Z)- and *trans*(E)-chlorprothixene. J Pharm Sci 80:735–740

Wang H, Lipfert L, Malbon CC, Bahouth S (1989) Site-directed anti-peptide antibodies define the topography of the β-adrenergic receptor. J Biol Chem 264:14424–14431

Weiner PK, Langridge RL, Blaney JM, Schaefer R, Kollman PA (1982) Electrostatic potential molecular surfaces. Proc Natl Acad Sci USA 79:3754–3758

Weiner SJ, Kollman PA, Case DA, Singh UC, Ghio C, Alagona G, Profeta S Jr, Weiner P (1984) A new force field for molecular mechanics simulation of nucleic acids and proteins. J Am Chem Soc 106:765–874

Weiner SJ, Kollman PA, Nguyen DT, Case DA (1986) An all atom force field for simulations of proteins and nucleic acids. J Computat Chem 7:230–252

Structure-Function Analysis of the Three β-Adrenergic Catecholamine Receptors

A.D. Strosberg

1 Introduction

The three subtypes of human β-adrenergic receptors (β-ARs) have now been identified and fully characterized at the molecular level. The corresponding genes, two of which (β_1 and β_2) are devoid of introns, have been isolated and sequenced. Structurally, the β-AR proteins display the typical hallmarks of all the other membrane R7G receptors coupled to GTP binding proteins, as represented in Fig. 1. They consist of: (a) a single polypeptide chain, 350–600 residues long, with an extracellular, glycosylated, NH_2-terminal domain, (b) seven hydrophobic, presumably transmembrane segments, interspersed with intra- and extracellular loops of various lengths, and (c) a COOH-terminal intracellular domain often containing several sites for phosphorylation by protein kinases (O'Dowd et al. 1989; Strosberg 1991; Strosberg and Leysen 1991).

To further analyze the pharmacologic properties and structure-function relationships of the individual β-AR subtypes, the genes were introduced into Chinese hamster ovary (CHO) cells, which do not normally express such receptors (Tate et al. 1991). The resulting CHO-β1, CHO-β2, and CHO-β3 cells display typical ligand binding properties and couple to the GTP binding proteins naturally present in these cells. Binding of agonists thus triggers activation of adenylyl cyclase, with K_{act} values close to those described in tissues; this stimulation may be blocked by selective antagonists.

To further study the residues actually involved in ligand binding, the genes encoding the β1- and β2-ARs were also expressed in *Escherichia coli*, in which the resulting receptors displayed binding properties for agonists and antagonists that are observed in tissues or cells containing the same receptors (Marullo et al. 1988, 1989).

We will review here the information obtained to date, comparing the receptor structure and function expressed in cells with the available pharmacologic data obtained in tissues, and propose how a variety of

Laboratoire d'Immuno-Pharmacologie Moléculaire, CNRS UPR 0415 and Université Paris VII, Institut Cochin de Génétique Moléculaire, 22 rue Méchain, 75014 Paris, France

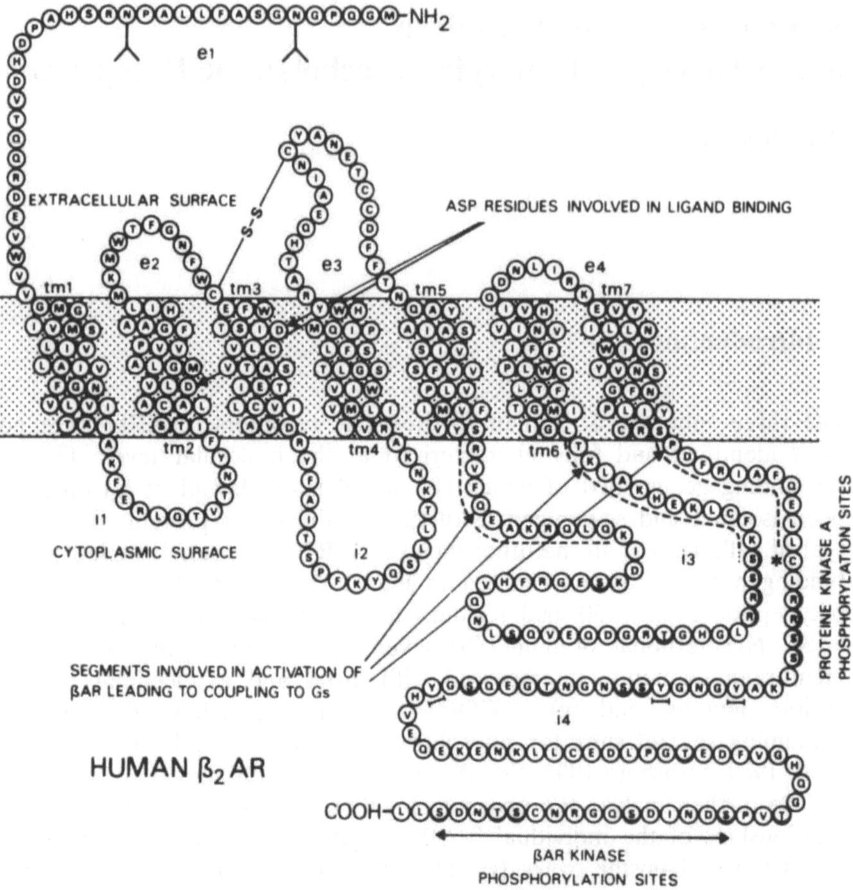

Fig. 1. Primary structure of the human β_2-adrenergic receptor (β_2-AR). The sequences are represented in the one letter code for amino acids. The single polypeptide chain is arranged according to the model for rhodopsin. The disulfide bond, essential for activity, linking Cys^{106} and Cys^{184} is represented by -S-S-. The two N-glycosylation sites in the NH_2-terminal portion of the protein are indicated by *Y*. The palmitoylated Cys^{341} residue in the NH_2-terminal of the i4 loop is indicated by an *asterisk*. Potential Ser and Thr phosphorylation sites are *underlined*. The three Tyr residues found in the i4 of β_2 but not β_1 or β_3AR are indicated by *(−) signs*

mechanisms may actually regulate the individual activity of each of the three β-AR subtypes.

2 β-AR Structures

The three β-ARs are nearly 50% identical in their overall amino acid sequences and 90% identical if one compares only the seven hydrophobic segments which actually participate in ligand binding (reviewed in O'Dowd

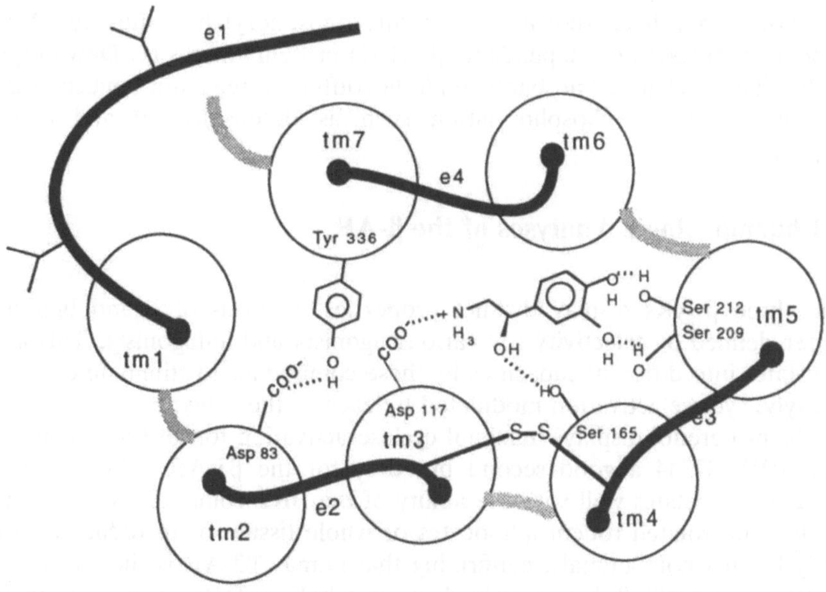

Fig. 2. A composite image of the β_2-adrenergic receptor (β_2-AR) ligand binding region. Proposed interactions in the ligand binding region of the β-AR viewed from the outside of the cell. All seven tm domains are essential for ligand binding. The ligand noradrenaline is shown surrounded by several of the amino acid side chains which were identified, by site-directed or photoaffinity labeling to be involved in agonist binding. These are Asp^{113} in tm3, Ser^{204} and Ser^{205} in tm5, Phe^{290} in tm6 and Tyr^{329} in tm7. The essential disulfide bond (-S-S-) linking Cys^{106} (extracellular e_2 domain) and Cys^{184} (e_3 domain) is also represented. Asp^{79} (tm2), not represented here, is likely to be more important for signal transmission to G_S than for actual ligand binding, in which it is nevertheless involved. Whether all the interactions with the ligand occur simultaneously or sequentially is not known

et al. 1989; Strosberg 1991). Several of the residues involved in the contacts with the ligand are represented in Fig. 2. Asp^{113} (tm3) probably acts as a counter ion for the positively charged group of the catecholamine. Ser^{204}, Ser^{207} (tm5), and Tyr^{329} (tm7), which may form hydrogen bonds with the hydroxyls of the ligand, are conserved in analogous positions in all three β-ARs.

The Asp^{79} residue (tm2) involved in G protein activation and the segments involved in coupling to G_s, located in cytoplasmic loops i2, i3, and i4 (see Fig. 1) in the parts closest to the membrane, are also particularly well conserved, supporting the idea that all three β-ARs may be coupled to the same type of GTP binding G_s protein. Other functionally important residues such as Cys^{106} and Cys^{184}, which probably form a disulfide bond essential for ligand binding, and Cys^{341}, which in hamster β2-AR is palmitoylated, are also conserved in the three subtypes.

There are, however, a few interesting differences between β3-AR and β1- and β2-AR. For instance, the β3-AR displays in i3 and in i4 only a few of the numerous Thr and Ser residues found in β1- and β2-AR, which, for the latter, have been shown to constitute phosphorylation sites by cAMP dependent (PKA) or independent (β-ARK) protein kinases (O'Dowd et al. 1989). These changes probably underlie different regulatory mechanisms known to involve phosphorylation such as desensitization and down-regulation.

3 Pharmacologic Analyses of the β-AR

The three β-ARs display distinct properties in terms of ligand binding, better defined as selectivity for various agonists and antagonists. This also translates into different capacities by these compounds to stimulate or block adenylyl cyclase activation modulated by each of the subtypes.

Isoproterenol displays maximal cyclase activation for all three subtypes with BRL 37344 a good second but only for the β3-AR. This agonistic behavior correlates well with the ability of the BRL compound to stimulate lipolysis in isolated rodent adipocytes or whole tissues or to reduce overall body fat in whole animals, confirming that human β3-AR is the equivalent of the "atypical" β-ARs involved in metabolic effects of noradrenaline described in various animal studies (Zaagsma and Nahorski 1990; Fève et al. 1991).

A large number of β-AR antagonists have been synthesized. While propranolol blocks both β1- and β2-AR, it has little effect on β3-AR. Pindolol and its derivatives cyanopindolol and iodocyanopindolol, which are antagonists for β1 and β2-ARs, are actually agonists for β3-AR; this is also true for oxprenolol and CGP 12177 (Emorine et al. 1989; Fève et al. 1991). The differential behavior towards the three subtypes could well explain the partial agonistic (intrinsic sympathomimetic) activity of these compounds observed in patients.

4 Differential Regulation of the β-ARs

Since the three β-ARs respond to the same natural agonists, adrenaline and noradrenaline, by stimulating adenylyl cyclase, it is likely that exquisitely specific regulatory mechanisms must differentiate their physiological effects. These mechanisms could involve expression of the genes in different tissues at different times during development and under different conditions. At the present time, evidence for several regulatory pathways has already accumulated. β1-AR is the predominant subtype in human heart while the β2-AR is the major form in human lung. β3-AR is mostly expressed in fat cells and is the predominant β-AR present in brown and white adipose tissue. Brown adipose tissue is found in humans only shortly after birth or in pathologic conditions, such as pheochromocytoma, but isolated brown adipocytes seem normally present in white fat depots (Krief et al. 1993).

Implication of the β3-AR in lipolysis control is suggested by the presence of regulatory nucleotide sequences in the promoter region of the gene which are homologous to those found in promoters of genes whose products are involved in fatty acid metabolism.

Glucocorticoids and other effectors modify the ratios of receptors subtypes expressed in the same cells. For example, treatment of 3T-F3-442A adipocytes by dexamethasone suppresses β1- and β3- and up-regulates β2-AR (Fève et al. 1991).

Concentrations of agonists may affect the level of expression of each of the three β-ARs in the same cells f.i. adipocytes. The differential pattern of distribution of phosphorylation sites in i3 and i4 might suggest possible differences in down-regulation susceptibility. The β3-AR may thus represent a postsynaptic receptor whose activity is controlled by norepinephrine released from sympatic nerve endings and could thus maintain basal thermogenic activity even while the two other β-AR subtypes are desensitized.

Acknowledgements. Support for our work comes mostly from grants from the Centre National de la Recherche Scientifique, INSERM, the Ministère de la Recherche et de la Technologie, Université Paris VII, Ligue Nationale contre le Cancer, Fondation pour la Recherche Médicale Française, Association pour la Recherche sur le Cancer and Bristol-Meyers-Squibb Company (USA).

References

Emorine LJ, Marullo S, Briend-Sutren M-M, Patey G, Tate K, Delavier-Klutchko C, Strosberg AD (1989) Molecular characterization of the human β3-adrenergic receptor. Science 245:1118–1121

Fève B, Emorine LJ, Briend-Sutren M-M, Lasnier F, Strosberg AD, Pairault J (1990) Differential regulation of β1- and β2-adrenergic receptor protein and mRNA levels by glucocorticoids during 3T3-F442A adipose differentiation. J Biol Chem 265:16343–16349

Fève B, Emorine LJ, Lasnier F, Blin N, Nahmias C, Baude B, Strosberg AD, Pairault J (1991) Atypical β-adrenergic receptor in 3T3-F442A adipocytes: pharmacological and molecular relationship with the human β3-adrenergic receptor. J Biol Chem

Marullo S, Delavier-Klutchko C, Eshdat Y, Strosberg AD, Emorine LJ (1988) Human β_2-adrenergic receptors expressed in E. coli membranes retain their pharmacological properties. Proc Natl Acad Sci USA 85:7551–7555

Marullo S, Delavier-Klutchko C, Guillet JG, Charbit A, Strosberg AD, Emorine LJ (1989) Expression of human β_1 and β2-adrenergic receptors in E. coli as a new tool for ligand screening. Biotechnology 7:923–927

O'Dowd BF, Lefkowitz RJ, Caron MG (1989) Structure of the adrenergic and related receptors. Annu Rev Neurosci 12:67–83

Strosberg AD (1991) Structure-function relationship of proteins belonging to the family of receptors coupled to GTP binding proteins. Eur J Biochem 196:1–10

Strosberg AD, Leysen JE (1991) Receptor-based assays. Curr Opin Biotechnol 2:30–36

Tate K, Briend-Sutren M-M, Emorine LJ, Delavier-Klutchko C, Marullo S, Strosberg AD (1991) Expression of three human β-adrenergic receptor subtypes in transfected Chinese hamster ovary cells. Eur J Biochem 196:357–361

Zaagsma J, Nahorski SR (1990) Is the adipocyte β-adrenoceptor a prototype for the recently cloned atypical "β_3-adrenoceptor"? Trends Pharmacol Sci 11:3–7

Serotonin Receptor Subtypes

P.R. Hartig, N. Adham, J. Zgombick, M. Macchi, H.-T. Kao,
L. Schechter, T. Branchek, and R. Weinshank

1 Overview of the Serotonin Receptor Family

The fact that nearly all known serotonin receptor subtypes are single subunit proteins, members of the same gene superfamily (the G protein-coupled receptor or 7TM superfamily) and that most are intronless genes has helped accelerate the cloning of this receptor family. The fact that the amino acid sequences of different serotonin receptors are among the least homologous of any single biogenic amine receptor family has had the opposite effect upon our rate of progress. With the recent announcement that a serotonin 5-HT_{1B} receptor gene has been isolated (Adham et al. 1992) genes representing five different pharmacologically defined subtypes – 5-HT_{1A}, 5-HT_{1B}, 5-HT_{1C}, 5-HT_{1D} and 5-HT_2 – have been isolated and characterized. At least four other known or suspected subtypes – 5-HT_3, 5-HT_4, 5-HT_{1E} and 5-HT_{1P} – still remain to be cloned. At least one of these, the 5-HT_3 receptor(s), is a member of the multisubunit ligand-gated ion channel superfamily and likely to be unrelated in structure to the 7TM receptors known at this time.

If we define gene superfamilies as large groups of related genes with similar structures and functions (e.g., the 7TM superfamily), then we could define a receptor family as a group of receptors which respond to the same natural ligand (e.g., cholinergic receptors, serotonergic receptors). Further classification of receptor subtypes into subfamilies can be achieved based upon similarities in amino acid sequences, pharmacological properties, and second messenger coupling. On this basis, four or five different serotonin receptor subfamilies could now be identified (Table 1). The 5-HT_2 subfamily is now an accepted concept as a group containing two closely related receptor subtypes, the 5-HT_2 and 5-HT_{1C} receptors (Hoyer 1988; Hartig 1989; Schmidt and Peroutka 1989). Recent cloning work (reviewed below) has shown that the 5-HT_{1B} pharmacological subtype is a species homologue of the human 5-HT_{1D} receptor, as had been suspected from a variety of functional and pharmacological studies (Hoyer and Middlemiss 1989). In that case, the 5-HT_{1D} and 5-HT_{1B} receptors should be considered to be

Synaptic Pharmaceutical Corporation, 215 College Road, Paramus, NJ 07652, USA

Table 1. Serotonin receptor subfamilies

Superfamily	G Protein-Coupled				Ion channel
Family	Serotonin				
Subfamily	5-HT_{1A}	5-HT_{1D}	5-HT_2	5-HT_4	5-HT_3
Subtypes	5-HT_{1A}	5-HT_{1D} 5-HT_{1B}	5-HT_2 5-HT_{1C}	5-HT_4 5-HT_{1P}?	5-HT_3
Second messenger	Decrease cAMP	Decrease cAMP	PI hydrolysis	Increase cAMP	Gated ion channel

PI, phosphatidylinositol

members of the same receptor subfamily and are probably better reclassified as the same receptor subtype (discussion below). The 5-HT_{1A} receptor exhibits many similarities to the 5-HT_{1D} subtype, but its sequence homology to that subtype (65% in TM regions) is lower than is usually observed for most closely related subtypes, therefore it may deserve to be classified as a separate subfamily. The adenylate cyclase-stimulatory 5-HT_4 receptor forms its own subclass, due to its unique pharmacological properties and cyclase-stimulating activity. The 5-HT_{1E} and 5-HT_{1P} receptors require further study before they can be adequately categorized, although similarities between the 5-HT_{1P} and 5-HT_4 sites suggest that these two receptors may be closely related, and some workers believe they may be different states of the same receptor.

2 Diversity of Receptor Subtypes: The Problem Issues

The entry of molecular biology into the serotonin receptor field has introduced new ways of solving long-standing controversies. Three such issues will be addressed in this brief review, and some remaining issues for future study will be noted. Firstly, the relationship of the 5-HT_{1B} subtype to the 5-HT_{1D} receptor has been a subject of much discussion. This issue can now be directly addressed due to the isolation of a gene encoding a rat 5-HT_{1B} receptor subtype. Secondly, what molecular variations underly species differences in binding properties for the same receptor subtype? Do these differences arise at the gene level where the few observed amino acid changes significantly alter binding properties, or do they arise at the processing level where different mammalian cells process the gene differently and insert it into a different membrane environment? Finally, what is the relationship between agonist and antagonist binding sites for the same receptor subtype? In particular, for the 7TM receptors which cycle through several different states of interaction with G proteins, how do these state changes affect the binding properties of the receptor and thus dictate our approach to drug design?

Table 2. Comparison of 5-HT$_{1B}$ and 5-HT$_{1D}$ receptors

Subtype	Tissue	Functions	Ligands	Species
5-HT$_{1B}$	Substantia nigra, globus pallidus, corpus striatum, neocortex	Decrease cAMP, autoreceptor	5-CT, α-blockers	Rat, mouse
5-HT$_{1D}$	Substantia nigra, globus pallidus, caudate nucleus, neocortex	Decrease cAMP, autoreceptor	5-CT metergoline	human pig calf pigeon

2.1 The 5-HT$_{1B}$ Subtype: Species Homologue or Separate Gene?

Table 2 shows a comparison of the 5-HT$_{1B}$ receptor to the 5-HT$_{1D}$ receptor with regard to several key properties: tissue distribution, species distribution, functional roles, and high-affinity ligands. Both receptor subtypes show similar distribution in the basal ganglia, similar coupling to adenylate cyclase inhibition, and both function as terminal autoreceptors on serotonergic neurons originating in the raphe (Waeber et al. 1990). These two receptors also show reciprocal species distributions, with the 5-HT$_{1B}$ receptor identified in several rodent species, but lacking in all other species (with the possible exception of opposum) according to most investigators, and the 5-HT$_{1D}$ receptor absent in rodents but present in human and a wide range of other tissues (Hoyer and Middlemiss 1989; Waeber et al. 1990). These properties have led several investigators to hypothesize that the 5-HT$_{1B}$ and 5-HT$_{1D}$ receptors represent the rodent and nonrodent homologues of a single gene product (single receptor subtype), having diverged only slightly from a common ancestral gene (Hoyer and Middlemiss 1989; Waeber et al. 1990). Differences in the affinities of certain ligands (notably β-blockers and some ergots) for these two subtypes and reports by some investigators that both subtypes are found in certain tissues (Herrick-Davis and Titeler 1988) suggest a different conclusion: that separate genes encoding two distinct receptor proteins may be involved. The clearest resolution of this issue can be obtained by individually cloning, sequencing, and transfecting the gene representing each of these two pharmacologically defined receptor subtypes.

In an effort to clone the rat 5-HT$_{1B}$ receptor gene, we isolated clones homologous to the human 5-HT$_{1D}$ receptor by screening a rat genomic library at high stringency with a probe derived from the human 5-HT$_{1D}$ receptor coding region (Adham et al. 1992). One strongly hybridizing signal (rs38b) was plaque purified, cloned into a pSVL expression vector, and transiently transfected into COS-7 cells. [^{3}H]5-HT bound in a saturable manner to transfected, but not to mock-transfected cells, displaying a single class of high-affinity binding sites with a dissociation constant of 23 n*M*.

Table 3. Pharmacological characterization of a cloned rat 5-HT_{1B} receptor

Chemical class	Drug	K_i(nM)		
		rs38b	5-HT_{1B}[a]	5-HT_{1D}[a]
Indole derivatives	5-CT	7.3	5.0	2.5
	5-HT	16	25	4.0
	Sumatriptan	465	500	17
	5-MethoxyDMT	3594	1259	32
	DP-5-CT	>10000	>10000	63
	2-CH_3-5-HT	>10000	>10000	398
Alkaloids	Metergoline	129	40	0.79
	Methysergide	1823	1585	4.0
	Rauwolscine	6295	5012	20
Piperazines	Methiothepin	13	50	50
	CGS12066B	110	130	2.9
Others	(−) Propranolol	57	50	3162
	(±) Pindolol	153	398	6310

[a] Hoyer (1989).

[^{125}I]iodocyanopindolol ([^{125}I]ICYP) also bound in a saturable manner to transfected cells, with a dissociation constant of 0.2 nM. Table 3 summarizes the apparent dissociation constants (apparent K_i values) obtained from competition binding studies with [^{125}I]ICYP in comparison to values obtained in similar studies on 5-HT_{1B} and 5-HT_{1D} binding sites in animal tissue preparations. When the values from Table 3 are plotted in log–log correlation plots, a very weak linear correlation coefficient of $r = 0.17$ is obtained in a comparison between the transfected rat clone and the calf caudate 5-HT_{1D} site, whereas a strong correlation coefficient of $r = 0.96$ was obtained for the same compounds against the rat 5-HT_{1B} site. These observations strongly suggest that clone rs38b encodes a serotonin 5-HT_{1B} receptor subtype (Adham et al. 1992).

Preliminary sequence data obtained from clone rs38b suggests that it exhibits an overall amino acid sequence homology of approximately 90% to a human 5-$HT_{1D\beta}$ receptor sequence isolated in our laboratory. Previous studies of monoamine receptors of the 7TM superfamily have shown that highly homologous receptor sequences with very similar pharmacological properties that are isolated from different mammalian species will typically exhibit overall amino acid homologies of approximately 80%–95%. Examples include the human (Fargin et al. 1988) and rat (Albert et al. 1990) 5-HT_{1A} receptors, the human (Kao et al. 1989; Hartig et al. 1990) and rat (Pritchett et al. 1988) 5-HT_2 receptors, and the human (Weinshank et al. 1990) and rat (Zeng et al. 1990) α-2B receptors. In all of these cited examples, the human and rat receptors exhibit very similar pharmacological properties, indicating that they are essentially identical receptor genes that have only diverged minimally since the separation of these two animal species approximately 80 million years ago. These examples of essentially identical receptor genes in two species have been termed "species homologues." The close amino acid sequence relationship between the rat 5-HT_{1B} sequence and the human $5\text{-HT}_{1D\beta}$ sequence is typical of human and rat gene relationships for species homologues. Therefore, it appears that the rat 5-HT_{1B} receptor is an unusual example of pharmacological divergence between homologous rat and human genes, in which significant ligand-binding differences have arisen in the time since these species diverged. The fact that the pharmacological properties of this 5-HT_{1D}/5-HT_{1B} receptor gene in rodents is so divergent from its properties in humans and most other species suggests that rodents may have evolved some unique form of this receptor subtype especially suited to their environmental niche, or to some special adaptation of their nervous systems. At the present time, however, it appears that the 5-HT_{1B} receptor gene that we have characterized represents an unusual species homologue of the $5\text{-HT}_{1D\beta}$ receptor (with unusually divergent pharmacological properties) rather than a separate subtype of serotonin receptor. It remains possible that additional 5-HT_{1D}-like genes will be isolated from the rat genome which code for receptors with different pharmacological properties. The presence of such additional 5-HT_{1D}-like sites has been suggested by several pharmacological and physiological investigations (Charlton et al. 1986; Waeber et al. 1988; Bond et al. 1989; Leonhardt et al. 1989; Schlicker et al. 1989; Sumner and Humphrey 1989; Xiong and Nelson 1989).

2.2 Species Differences: Nature or Nurture?

Species differences in pharmacological binding properties have been observed in human vs rat 5-HT_2 receptor-binding assays, particularly in the case of certain ergot drugs. In this case, it is quite clear that the 5-HT_2 receptors in these two species are species homologues since they share 91% overall sequence homology (Hartig et al. 1990). The question that arises, however, is whether these few amino acid changes are responsible for the pharmacological differences that are observed, or whether the processing of the receptor protein and/or the local membrane environment in different species determines these differences. This is a question of primary importance to molecular neurobiologists and pharmaceutical companies since it may dictate the possible choices of transfection hosts and genes that must be utilized in order to reproduce human pharmacological properties.

One relevant experiment comes from studies on a cDNA clone encoding the human 5-HT_2 receptor. Transfection of this clone into mouse fibroblast cells leads to expression of a serotonin receptor whose binding properties match that of human rather than rat cortical membranes (Table 4) (Hartig et al. 1990). One of the largest rat vs human species differences in drug

Table 4. Serotonin 5-HT_2 receptor binding affinities

Drug	Human clone	Human cortex	Rat cortex[b]
Spiperone	0.22 ± 0.03	0.42	1.5
Ritanserin	1.1 ± 0.16	1.26[b]	7.2
Methysergide	2.62 ± 0.12	2.5[b]	4
Cyproheptadine	2.95 ± 0.10	6.3[b]	1.8
Butaclamol	2.3 ± 0.38	1.21[c]	2.4[a]
Mesulergine	146 ± 5	158[b]	5
5-HT	224 ± 22	174[b]	79
5-CT	7790 ± 50	813[b]	19953

[a] Lyon et al. (1987).
[b] Hoyer et al. (1986).
[c] Schotte (1983).

binding has been observed for mesulergine, which exhibits a 30-fold higher affinity for the rat 5-HT_2 receptor than for either the transfected human 5-HT_2 receptor or for human cortical membranes. This species difference is also seen for the distinctly different chemical structures of spiperone and ritanserin (Hartig et al. 1990, 1992). In both cases, the transfected human receptor exhibits binding affinities in close agreement with human cortical tissue, even though the human gene has been expressed in a rodent, non-neuronal cell line. This observation suggests that it is the amino acid sequence of the receptor (nature) rather than the cellular environment in which the receptor gene is expressed and processed (nurture) that determines the species-specific pharmacological properties of the receptor. Further studies are needed to determine whether this will prove to be a general property of neurotransmitter receptors. For most cases examined so far, it appears that transfection of a human 7TM receptor gene into most available mammalian host cell lines has produced ligand-binding properties in good agreement with previous binding assays in brain tissue preparations. This provides a welcome degree of freedom in the choice of host cells for transfection, which can then be chosen based on ease of transfection, complement of native G proteins, or other desirable criteria.

2.3 Agonist vs Antagonist Binding Sites

It has long been appreciated that G protein-coupled receptors cycle through a complex series of G protein and ligand-binding states that lead to multiple affinity states for agonist ligands. With the availability of transfected cell lines expressing single receptor subtypes, it is now possible to examine the binding states of these receptors in much greater detail. One such study has resolved a long-standing controversy in the serotonin receptor field, namely, whether the serotonergic binding site for the agonist 4-bromo-2,5-dimethoxyphenylisopropylamine (DOB) and other related hallucinogenic

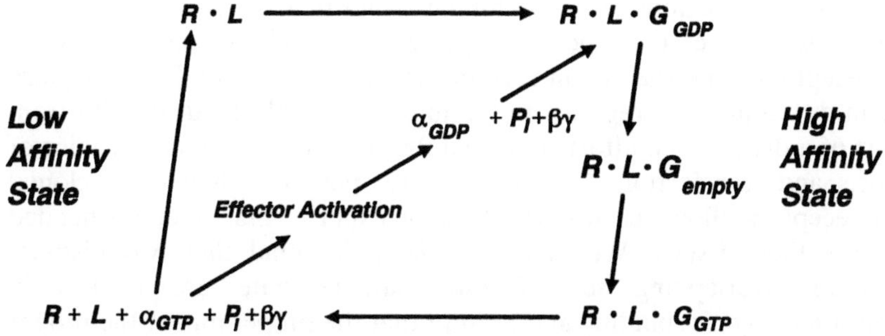

Fig. 1. Hypothetical receptor-activation cycle derived from Freissmuth et al. (1989). Binding of an agonist ligand (*L*) to the receptor (*R*) produces a receptor–ligand complex ($R \cdot L$) which binds a G protein complexed with *GDP*. Agonists induce dissociation of the GDP resulting in a "*G empty*" state, which is the high affinity agonist binding state. "G empty" can then bind *GTP*, which induces dissociation of the complex to an α subunit with GTP bound. This α_{GTP} complex activates effector mechanisms such as adenylate cyclase or phospholipase C until such time (seconds) as the intrinsic GTPase activity of the α subunit hydrolyzes GTP to GDP, starting the cycle over again

amphetamines is the high affinity agonist binding state of the same 5-HT_2 receptor which binds antagonist ligands such as ketanserin, or is a separate, closely related receptor subtype. Both interpretations have gained experimental support (Lyon et al. 1987; Pierce and Peroutka 1989), but the weight of data now appears to strongly support the two site rather than the two receptor interpretation, thanks to two recent studies utilizing transfected human (Branchek et al. 1990) and rat (Teitler et al. 1990) 5-HT_2 receptor clones. Both studies reached the same conclusion through a similar experimental series. Briefly, transfection of a single cDNA clone into host mammalian cells produced two binding sites (for [^{3}H]DOB and [^{3}H]ketanserin) which display related but distinct binding profiles. Addition of guanine nucleotides to these systems produced a reduction in the number of agonist high-affinity binding sites with no change, or a slight increase, in the number of antagonist binding sites. Thus, it appears that [^{3}H]DOB and [^{3}H]ketanserin binding sites are distinct ligand affinity states which exist at different times on the same 5-HT_2 receptor protein as it cycles through various forms of interaction with the G protein complex. A summary of these affinity states, based upon a review article by Freissmuth et al. (1989), is provided in Fig. 1.

Our increasing molecular understanding of this G protein and ligand affinity cycle needs to be better integrated into our investigations of receptor function and into our drug design programs. Since a complex interaction cycle involving two separate proteins and several forms of guanine nucleotides is involved in agonist binding, we need to be sure that the model systems we use as templates for drug design have been carefully chosen and carefully adjusted. They must properly mimic the natural processes occurring in those regions of native human brain that we choose as a target for drug design. Since the types of G proteins, the relative receptor excess (spare receptors), and the amounts of intracellular GDP and GTP may vary widely in different brain regions, this complexity should be dealt with from the start of a drug design effort. Fortunately, the great freedom of choice of cell hosts and transfection densities that are possible when using cloned human receptors allows us just the type of experimental freedom needed to address these issues. We must also keep in mind that two distinct, but partially overlapping, sets of conformational states are involved in antagonist and agonist binding and be sure that the proper mix of the proper states are present in our biological screening models.

A second challenge we face is to adjust our thinking about agonist and antagonist binding sites to reflect our current molecular models for these states. In the past it was often said that antagonists bind to both agonist high-affinity and agonist low-affinity states, and that guanine nucleotides convert agonist high-affinity to agonist low-affinity states. Based on the model shown in Fig. 1, it would seem more accurate to say that antagonists only sample a subset of the interaction states and affinity states that 7TM receptors can pass through when agonists bind to the receptor. Agonists presumably induce a delicately orchestrated series of conformational changes in the receptor–G protein complex, while antagonists merely bind to the receptor without causing the type of conformational change needed to unload GDP from the G protein. Thus, antagonists fail to produce the activated receptor–G protein complex, and only sample a subset of the receptor's possible conformational states. In addition, guanosine 5′-(β,γ-imide) triphosphate, Gpp (NH) p, is now seen to lock the G protein into a form that cannot bind to the receptor–ligand complex, once again preventing the receptor from forming an activated receptor–G protein complex. This new understanding of the receptor–ligand–G protein complex should be especially helpful in guiding us to a better understanding of the physical and chemical properties of agonists that define their intrinsic activities (abilities to function as full or partial agonists).

3 Summary and Future Directions

Although we have progressed quite rapidly towards understanding the molecular basis of serotonin receptor subtypes, several known, and undoubtedly some unknown, serotonin receptor subtypes remain to be cloned. Beyond the simple isolation and characterization of each clone, important issues remain to be resolved. One great challenge will be to determine the physiological role of each receptor subtype and its relationship to human neuropsychiatric diseases. This may well prove to be as difficult a challenge for molecular biologists as it has been for generations of physiologists and pharmacologists. What can, however, be expected with some confidence over the next few years is that sets of cloned human receptors in transfected cell lines will be used to design ligands with higher affinity and specificity for single receptor subtypes than has been previously possible. The fact that many new receptor subtypes are being discovered by gene cloning in every receptor family means that many new agents for manipulation of brain processes should soon become available. Many of these new ligands should prove to be more potent therapeutic agents with fewer side effects, due to their improved human receptor specificities. If this promise is realized, a second renaissance in neuropsychiatric drug design (following the great advances of the 1960s) could well be near at hand.

Receptor cloning is also likely to provide a rapid increase in our understanding of the molecular actions of neurotransmitter receptors. The first three-dimensional models of 7TM receptors and their ligand-binding sites are now beginning to emerge (e.g., Hibert et al. 1991). Refinement and solidification of these models will be one of the most exciting and potentially rewarding challenges in receptor biology for the next few years.

We also need to better understand the reasons for the broad diversity of serotonin receptor subtypes, especially in cases such as the 5-HT_{1C} and 5-HT_2 receptors where their ligand-affinity profiles and second messenger couplings are so similar. What critical difference between these subtypes has caused them to be maintained as separate subtypes over many millions of years of evolution? Since the 5-HT_{1A} and 5-HT_{1D} receptors both couple to adenylate cyclase inhibition, and both function as autoreceptors, what difference exists between them that has made one receptor subtype (5-HT_{1A}) more suited to a role as a somatodendritic autoreceptor, while the other functions as a terminal autoreceptor? Why are serotonin receptors unusual among 7TM receptors in showing such a wide divergence of amino acid sequences, leading to the fact that some receptors (e.g., 5-HT_2 and 5-HT_{1C}) are more closely related to 7TM receptors from different biogenic amine families than they are to other members of their own family (5-HT_{1A} and 5-HT_{1D})? And as mentioned above, what has led to such a large species divergence in pharmacological properties of the 5-HT_{1D}/5-HT_{1B} receptor? Although much attention has been given to the cloning and characterization of serotonin receptor genes, it is clear that imaginative use of these cloned receptors for the investigation of normal and diseased brain processes remains a significant challenge for the near future.

References

Albert PR, Zhou Q-Y, Van Tol HHM, Bunzow JR, Civelli O (1990) Cloning, functional expression and mRNA distribution of the rat 5-$hydroxytryptamine_{1A}$ receptor gene. J Biol Chem 265:5825–5832

Bond RA, Craig DA, Charlton KG, Ornstein AG, Clarke DE (1989) Partial agonist activity of GR43175 at the inhibitory prejunctional 5-$HT_{1\text{-like}}$ receptor in rat kidney. J Auton Pharmacol 9:201–210

Branchek T, Adham N, Macchi M, Kao H-T, Hartig PR (1990) [^{3}H]DOB (4-bromo-2,5-dimethoxyphenylisopropylamine) and [^{3}H]ketanserin label two affinity states of the cloned human 5-HT_2 receptor. Mol Pharmacol 38:604–609

Charlton KG, Bond RA, Clarke DE (1986) An inhibitory prejunctional 5-$HT_{1\text{-like}}$ receptor in the isolate perfused rat kidney. Naunyn Schmiedebergs Arch Pharmacol 332:8–15

Fargin A, Raymond J, Lohse M, Kobilka B, Caron M, Lefkowitz R (1988) The genomic clone G-21 which resembles the β-adrenergic receptor sequence encodes the 5-HT_{1A} receptor. Nature 335:358–360

Freissmuth M, Casey PJ, Gilman AG (1989) G proteins control diverse pathways of transmembrane signaling. FASEB J 3:2125–2131

Hartig PR (1989) Molecular biology of 5-HT receptors. Trends Pharmacol Sci 10:64–69

Hartig PR, Kao H-T, Macchi M, Adham N, Zgombick J, Weinshank R, Branchek T (1990) The molecular biology of serotonin receptors: an overview. Neuropsychopharmacology 3:335–347

Hartig PR, Adham N, Zgombick J, Weinshank R, Branchek T (1992) Molecular biology of the 5-HT_1 receptor subfamily. Drug Dev Res 26:215–224

Herrick-Davis K, Titeler M (1988) Detection and characterization of the serotonin 5-HT_{1D} receptor in rat and human brain. J Neurochem 50:1624–1631

Hibert MF, Trumpp-Kallmeyer S, Bruinvels A, Hoflack J (1991) Three-dimensional models of neurotransmitter G-binding protein-coupled receptors. Mol Pharmacol 40:8–15

Hoyer D (1988) Molecular pharmacology and biology of 5-HT_{1C} receptors. Trends Pharmacol Sci 9:89–94

Hoyer D, Pazos A, Probst A, Palacios JM (1986) Serotonin receptors in the human brain II. Characterization and autoradiographic localization of 5-HT_{1C} and 5-HT_2 recognition sites. Brain Res 376:97–107

Kao H-T, Olsen MA, Hartig PR (1989) Isolation and characterization of a human 5-HT_2 receptor clone. Soc Neurosci Abstr 15:486

Leonhardt S, Herrick-Davis K, Titeler M (1989) Detection of a novel serotonin receptor subtype (5-HT_{1E}) in human brain: interaction with a GTP-binding protein. J Neurochem 53:465–471

Lyon RA, Kavis KH, Titeler M (1987) [^{3}H]DOB (4-bromo-2,5-dimethoxyphenylisopropylamine) labels guanine nucleotide-sensitive state of cortical 5-HT_2 receptors. Mol Pharmacol 31:194–199

Pierce P, Peroutka SJ (1989) Evidence for distinct 5-HT_2 receptor binding site subtypes in cortical membrane preparations. J Neurochem 52:656–658

Pritchett D, Bach A, Wozny A, Taleb O, Dal Taso R, Shih J, Seeburg P (1988) Structure and functional expression of cloned rat serotonin 5-HT_2 receptor. EMBO J 13:4135–4140

Schlicker E, Fink K, Gothert M, Hoyer D, Molderings G, Roschke I, Schoeffter P (1989) The pharmacological properties of the presynaptic serotonin autoreceptor in the pig brain cortex conform to the 5-HT_{1D} subtype. Naunyn Schmiedebergs Arch Pharmacol 340:45–51

Schmidt AW, Peroutka SJ (1989) 5-Hydroxytryptamine receptor "families". FASEB J 3:2242–2249

Schotte A, Maloteaux JM, Laduron PM (1983) Characterization and regional distribution of serotonin S_2-receptors in human brain. Brain Res 276:231–235

Sumner MJ, Humphrey PPA (1989) 5-HT_{1D} binding sites in porcine brain can be subdivided by GR43175. Br J Pharmacol 98:29–31

Teitler M, Leonhardt S, Weisberg EJ, Hoffman BJ (1990) 4-[^{125}I]Iodo-(2,5-dimethoxy)-phenylisopropylamine and [^{3}H]ketanserin labeling of 5-HT_2 receptors in mammalian cells transfected with a rat 5-HT_2 cDNA: evidence for multiple states and not multiple 5-HT_2 receptor subtypes. Mol Pharmacol 38:594–598

Waeber C, Schoeffter P, Palacios JM, Hoyer D (1988) Molecular pharmacology of 5-HT_{1D} recognition sites: radioligand binding studies in human, pig, and calf brain membranes. Naunyn Schmiedebergs Arch Pharmacol 337:595–601

Waeber C, Schoeffter P, Hoyer D, Palacios JM (1990) The serotonin 5-HT_{1D} receptor: a progress review. Neurochem Res 15:567–582
Weinshank RL, Zgombick JM, Macchi M, Adham N, Lichtblau H, Branchek TA, Hartig PR (1990) Cloning, expression and pharmacological characterization of a human α_{2B}-adrenergic receptor. Mol Pharmacol 38:681–688
Xiong WC, Nelson DL (1989) Characterization of a [^{3}H]-5-hydroxytryptamine binding site in rabbit caudate nucleus that differs from the 5-HT_{1A}, 5-HT_{1B}, 5-HT_{1C} and 5-HT_{1D} subtypes. Life Sci 45:1433–1442
Zeng D, Harrison JK, D'Angelo DD, Barber CM, Tucker AL, Lu Z, Lynch KR (1990) Molecular characterization of a rat α_{2B}-adrenergic receptor. Proc Natl Acad Sci USA 87:3102–3106

Developmental Regulation of 5-HT_2 and 5-HT_{1c} Receptor Gene Expression in Rat Brain

R.D. Ciaranello, J. Aimi, R. Dean, R. Desai, S. Garlow, M.R. Heller, D. Morilak, and B.L. Roth[1]

1 Introduction

Serotonin signals in neurons are transduced by a large and rapidly growing family of receptors. To date, four principal types of serotonin receptor have been identified, designated 5-HT_1–5-HT_4. 5-HT_1 receptors have high (nanomolar) affinity for serotonin. Three 5-HT_1 subtypes have been identified by molecular cloning: 5-HT_{1a} (Fargin et al. 1988; Albert et al. 1990), 5-HT_{1c} (Julius et al. 1988), and $5HT_{1d}$. In addition, 5-HT_{1b} and 5-HT_{1e} receptors have been characterized pharmacologically, but their sequences have not yet been deduced from cloned cDNAs. The members of the 5-HT_1 family are all G protein linked receptors; the 5-HT_{1a} (DeVivo and Maayani 1985), 5-HT_{1b} (Ariani et al. 1989), and 5-HT_{1d} (Peroutka 1988) receptors are coupled to adenylyl cyclase inhibitory (G_i) proteins, while the 5-HT_{1c} receptor is coupled to phospholipase C through a Gp protein (Conn et al. 1986).

5-HT_2 receptors have low (micromolar) affinity for serotonin; these, too, are G protein linked receptors which activate phospholipase C via a Gp protein (Roth et al. 1984; Roth and Chaung 1987; Conn and Sanders-Bush 1985). To date, a single member of this family has been identified by molecular cloning (Pritchett et al. 1988; Julius et al. 1990). In contrast, the 5-HT_3 receptor appears to be a Na^+/K^+ channel (Palacios et al. 1990) and therefore is a member of the ligand-gated ion channel superfamily of genes. The 5-HT_4 receptor appears to be an adenylyl cyclase stimulatory receptor (Demuis et al. 1988) and is presumably coupled to this enzyme via a G_s protein.

The family of serotonin receptors has received considerable attention because of its great importance in the pharmacotherapy of psychiatric disorders. In particular, there is significant interest in the use of drugs active

Nancy Pritzker Laboratory of Developmental and Molecular Neurobiology, Lab Surge Building P-104, Department of Psychiatry, Stanford University School of Medicine, Stanford, CA 94305-54285 USA

[1] Present address: Department of Psychiatry, Case Western Reserve University School of Medicine, Cleveland, OH 44106, USA

at the 5-HT_{1a} receptor in the treatment of anxiety and in high potency antagonists of 5-HT_{1c} and/or 5-HT_2 receptors in the treatment of schizophrenia. In addition, several atypical antidepressants bind with high potency at 5-HT_2 receptors.

Our laboratory has been interested in the role serotonergic systems play in brain function and, in particular, how the genes expressing serotonin receptors are expressed and regulated during brain development. We have focused on the 5-HT_{1c} and 5-HT_2 receptors during the initial phases of this work (Roth et al. 1990, 1991) and in this report, we summarize evidence describing the temporal expression of the 5-HT_2 and 5-HT_{1c} receptor genes, propose some hypotheses about the developmental factors controlling gene expression, and present some preliminary data on the structure of the 5-HT_2 receptor gene in rats and on the immunocytochemical localization of 5-HT_2 receptors in rat cerebral cortex.

2 Ontogeny of 5-HT_2 Receptors in Rat Brain

5-HT_2 receptors are moderately abundant in rat cerebral cortex, where they are localized in laminal areas IV and Va (Pazos et al. 1985; Roth et al. 1987). To determine the distribution of 5-HT_2 receptor messenger RNA (mRNA) we prepared a synthetic antisense DNA probe of 51 bases complementary to bases 730–781 of the published 5-HT_2 cDNA sequence (Pritchett et al. 1988). This domain is unique to the 5-HT_2 receptor, which otherwise shares considerable sequence homology, particularly in the transmembrane domains, to the 5-HT_{1c} receptor. In preliminary experiments, we established that there was no cross-hybridization between this probe and the cDNA or the mRNA for the 5-HT_{1c} receptor.

This probe was radiolabeled and used to determine the regional brain distribution of 5-HT_2 receptor mRNA by northern blot analysis. Total RNA was prepared from cingulate gyrus and frontal cortex, choroid plexus, dorsal hippocampus, medulla-pons, striatum and aorta and probed with the 5-HT_2 – specific oligonucleotide. We found 5-HT_2 receptor mRNA to be abundant in cortex, detectable in striatum, and absent in choroid plexus. When the autoradiograms were overexposed to bring up faintly hybridizing bands, 5-HT_2 mRNA was seen in aorta and in hippocampus and medulla-pons.

To determine the developmental profile of 5-HT_2 receptors in brain, we again prepared total RNA from rat brains varying in age from embryonic day 17 (E17) to postnatal day 27 (P27). 5-HT_2 receptor mRNA showed a modest developmental increase between E17 and P2 which was followed by a dramatic burst in receptor gene expression and culminated in the attainment of mRNA levels which were 13-fold greater at P5 than at E17. 5-HT_2 mRNA peaked at P5, then declined to adult levels at P27; these remained about six fold above those seen at E17.

To examine whether the developmental profile of 5-HT_2 mRNA was accompanied by commensurate changes in receptor binding, we carried out radioligand binding studies on cortical membranes at various ages. At most ages, we used [^{3}H]ketanserin in the presence of spiperone to specifically label 5-HT_2 sites. However, receptor binding could only be detected in brains from embryonic rats by incubating with ^{125}I-labeled LSD under site-specific conditions. Using these two ligands, we determined a developmental profile of 5-HT_2 receptor binding. Functional receptor binding increased steadily from E17 (about 10 fmol/mg) to a peak at P12 (about 90 fmol/mg), then declined to adult levels (60 fmol/mg) at P27. These data indicate that the temporal profile of mRNA expression parallels the developmental course of functional receptor binding (Roth et al. 1991).

The dramatic burst in 5-HT_2 mRNA expression followed by a decline to adult levels suggested that this receptor gene was undergoing extensive developmental regulation. The interval in which these changes were taking place has been proposed to be one in which the cortex is undergoing hyperinnervation by serotonergic fibers from the raphe nucleus followed by a period of "pruning back" of these fibers (Lidov and Molliver 1982; D'Amato et al. 1987). This suggested that the presynaptic serotonergic neurons, themselves undergoing developmental modification, might be regulating the expression of 5-HT_2 receptor genes in the postsynaptic cortical target cells.

To study this further, we developed three hypotheses, which were tested in turn: First, serotonin itself regulates the burst in expression of 5-HT_2 mRNA seen between P2 and P5, when receptor mRNA is being maximally expressed. Second, factors (serotonin, other transmitters or neuromodulators) released from ingrowing raphe fibers regulate the expression of 5-HT_2 receptor genes during this period. Third, transcriptional factors responsible for the burst in 5-HT_2 mRNA expression are regulated by developmental cues arising from the cortical target neurons themselves and are independent of presynaptic regulation.

If serotonin modulates the burst of 5-HT_2 receptor gene transcription in the cortex, then it is possible that this signal is transduced by 5-HT_2 receptors themselves. Blockade of 5-HT_2 receptors, then, should alter the temporal appearance of receptor mRNA. To examine this, we treated newborn rats with mianserin, an atypical antidepressant with high potency at 5-HT_2 sites. In other studies, mianserin had been shown to cause a dramatic decline in 5-HT_2 binding (Matsubara and Meltzer 1989). In our hands, treatment of newborn rats with 10 mg/kg mianserin followed by measurement of 5-HT_2 receptor binding on P12 caused a 50%–60% decrease in 5-HT_2 binding but had no effect on receptor mRNA. Treatment with a variety of typical and atypical antidepressants all resulted in declines in 5-HT_2 binding without altering 5-HT_2 receptor mRNA (Roth and Ciaranello 1992). Thus, these data suggest that blockade of 5-HT_2 receptors during the period of maximal 5-HT_2 receptor gene expression does not alter the developmental profile of the receptor mRNA. It is possible, however, that serotonin receptors other than the 5-HT_2 are transducing early serotonergic developmental signals in the cortex, so these data do not entirely eliminate a role for serotonin in regulating 5-HT_2 receptor gene development.

To test this further, and also to determine whether raphe neurons regulate the burst in 5-HT_2 receptor mRNA, we administered 5,7-dihydroxytryptamine, which selectively destroys serotonergic nerve terminals, to newborn rats, then measured 5-HT_2 receptor mRNA at P7, P12, and P27. We achieved a 60% destruction of serotonergic innervation to the cortex, as measured by [^{3}H]paroxetine binding, but this treatment failed to show any effect on 5-HT_2 mRNA. While it is possible that a more extensive degree of lesioning is necessary before mRNA expression is reduced, we take this preliminary data as suggestive that serotonergic fibers are not modulating the developmental burst in 5-HT_2 mRNA.

Testing whether there are developmentally regulated transcriptional factors which are produced by cortical neurons during the peak period of receptor expression requires cloning the 5-HT_2 receptor gene, characterizing its 5′ regulatory elements, and using these to identify DNA binding proteins which act as transcriptional regulators. As the first step in this strategy, we have cloned the 5-HT_2 receptor gene and have obtained some information on its structure.

We cloned the 5-HT_2 receptor gene from a rat genomic library, using synthetic oligonucleotides derived from different regions of the receptor cDNA (Pritchett et al. 1988) as probes. The first oligonucleotide (oligo 1) is a 51 nucleotide long antisense DNA complementary to bases +72–+123 in the published sequence. The second oligonucleotide (oligo 2) is a 30 nucleotide long sense DNA derived from sequences about 600 base pairs (bps) upstream of the region in the cDNA to which oligo 1 is directed. Additional oligonucleotides directed to other portions of the cDNA have been prepared as needed to map the genomic fragments onto the cDNA.

Oligo 1 hybridizes to a 13.7 kilobase (kb) genomic fragment ($5\text{-HT}_2\lambda13$). Surprisingly, oligo 2, which is directed to a region a relatively short distance upstream from oligo 1, does not hybridize to this fragment. Instead, oligo 2 identified a 11.6 kb fragment ($5\text{-HT}_2\lambda1$) to which oligo 1 does not hybridize. Limited restriction endonuclease digestion of these fragments generated several subfragments (10.5, 2.1, and 1.2 kb) whose linkage and orientation we have now worked out. The 10.5 kb fragment contains the entire coding region of the gene, as oligonucleotide probes which include the translation initiation codon and those from the 3′ end of the cDNA hybridize to this clone. Restriction endonuclease digestion of $5\text{-HT}_2\lambda13$ gives four fragments of 6.5, 3.1, 1.2, and 0.8 kb. The 6.5 kb fragment overlaps the 10.5 kb fragment of $5\text{-HT}_2\lambda13$, but this fragment does not hybridize to oligo 2. In addition, polymerase chain reaction (PCR) amplification, using sense primer oligonucleotides derived from transcribed sequences present in the 5′

genomic clone and antisense primers derived from sequences immediately upstream of the translation initiation codon in the 3′ genomic clone, generate appropriate size fragments using cortex first-strand cDNA but fail to amplify any fragment from rat genomic DNA, indicating there must be an intron of substantial size present in the gene in this region. The 3.1 and 1.2 kb genomic fragments hybridize strongly to rat cortical mRNA, indicating these are transcribed parts of the gene. However, the 0.8 kb fragment only faintly hybridizes to rat cortical mRNA, suggesting that much of this portion of the gene is untranscribed. This region could either represent another upstream intron or it could contain the regulatory elements which we seek.

Further characterization of the 0.8 kb fragment of $5\text{-HT}_2\lambda13$ will be necessary before its identity can be established. This will include determining its nucleotide sequence for consensus promoter/enhancer sites and testing it in fusion constructs to reporter genes for ability to stimulate gene expression in transfected cells. If we determine it is a regulatory region, we will then begin using it as a probe to identify DNA binding proteins, since these are the likely transcriptional regulators which are responsible for controlling expression of the gene during its peak developmental period.

In these studies we have used several tools to study discrete steps in 5-HT_2 receptor function. These include nucleic acid probes (oligonucleotides, cDNAs, cRNAs) to study steady-state mRNA levels as a reflection of gene expression and radioligand binding, either to membranes or via in vitro receptor autoradiography, to determine functional receptor binding. However, it is clear from our data with mianserin, in which receptor binding declines dramatically after treatment of rats but mRNA is unaffected, that the receptor protein is subject to regulatory factors distinct from those determining mRNA levels. To dissect these events at a molecular level required preparing an antibody against the 5-HT_2 receptor.

Accordingly, we synthesized oligopeptides representing discrete regions of the 5-HT_2 receptor, coupled these to keyhole limpet hemocyanin, and injected them into rabbits. We obtained antisera directed against each of these conjugates and tested them against the purified antigen for activity. Those which bound purified peptide were selected for further purification using antigen affinity chromatography.

To test the activity of the purified anti-5-HT_2 receptor antibody fraction, we carried out a number of experiments. First, we transfected COS-7 monkey kidney cells with the full-length 5-HT_2 cDNA. These transient transfects exhibit a high degree of 5-HT_2 receptor binding. Figure 1 shows that they also stain positively with anti-5-HT_2 antibody; this staining is particularly intense in the cell membrane where the receptor density is likely to be highest but perinuclear staining is also seen. This is consistent with the high degree of cDNA expression expected from a transiently transfected cell line. Antibody binding can be blocked by preincubation with purified antigen peptide.

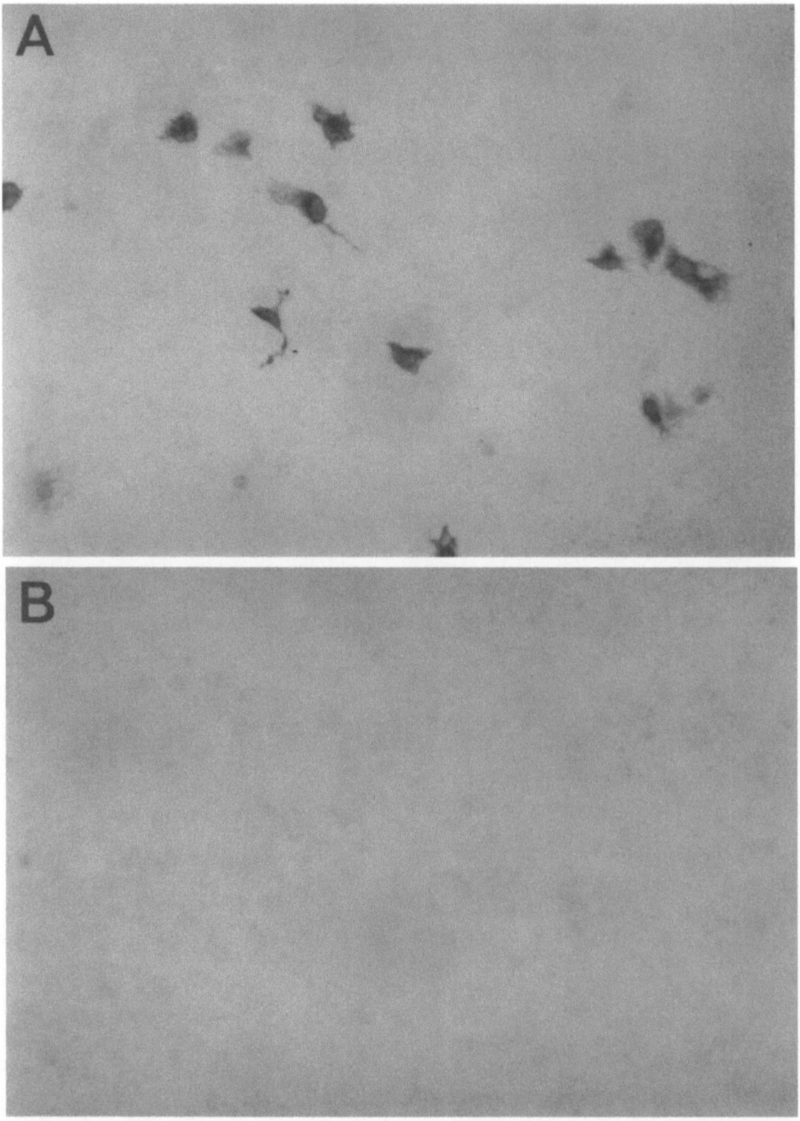

Fig. 1A,B. Demonstration of 5-HT_2 receptor immunoreactivity on transfected COS-7 cells using an anti-5-HT_2 receptor antibody. **A** Transfected COS-7 cells were labeled by the affinity-purified anti-5-HT_2 receptor antibody, visualized by an immunoperoxidase reaction. Note the intense labeling around the perimeter of the cells and in the perinuclear region. Approximately 10%–20% of the cells were immunopositive. Antibody dilution was 1/50. **B** As a control, a second set of transfected cells, run in parallel with those in **A**, were incubated with the same antibody dilution following pre-adsorbtion of the antiserum with 10 μM of the synthetic antigenic peptide. All other conditions were identical. Only faint background staining was observed. Other controls included preimmune serum and use of nontransfected cells. Magnification in both panels: (×200)

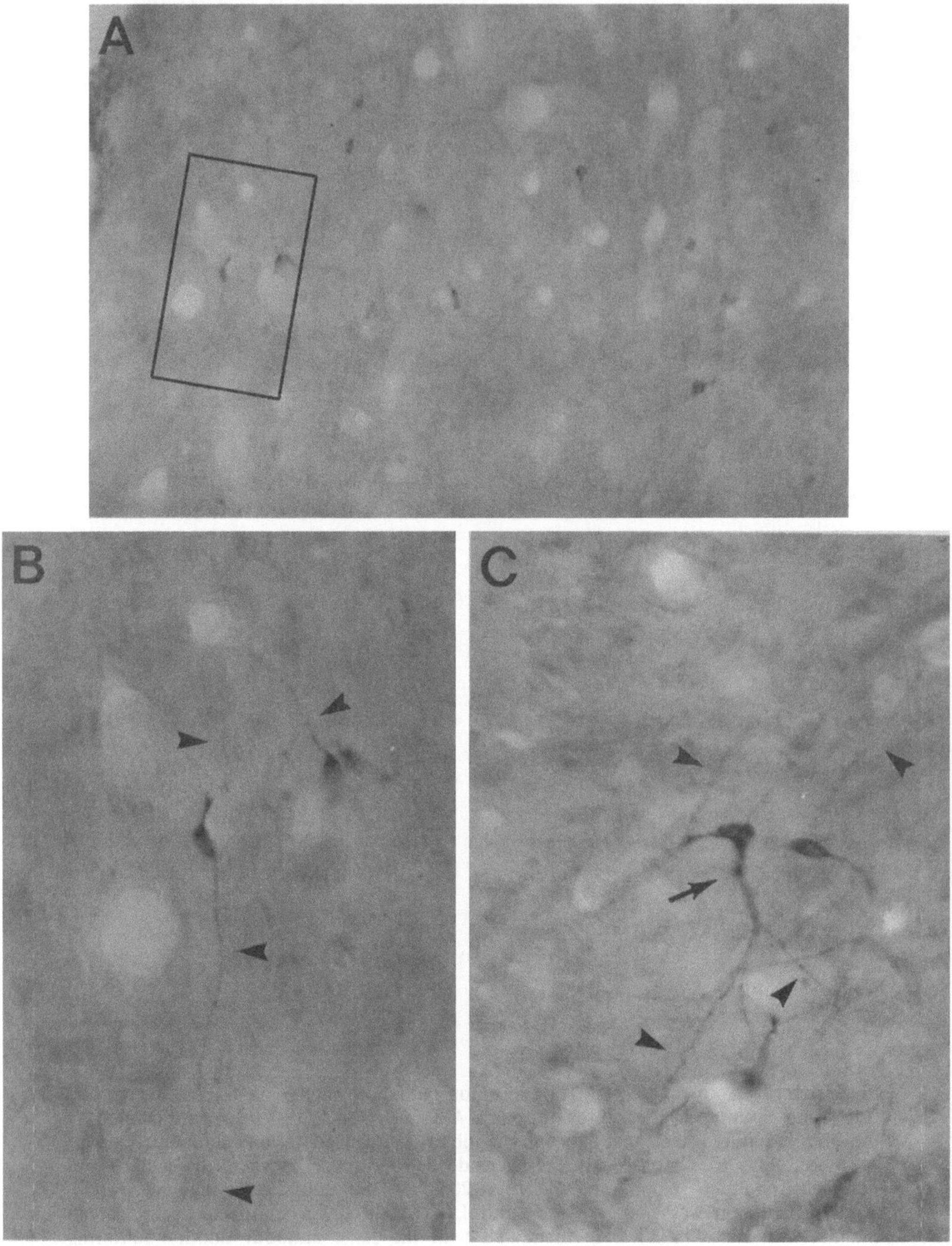
A
B
C

We then used the purified antibody to determine the localization of cortical neurons expressing $5\text{-}HT_2$ receptors. Figure 2 shows typical neurons from the rat ventral forebrain which stain positively for $5\text{-}HT_2$ receptors. In this field, it can be seen that only a small portion of the neurons appear to express $5\text{-}HT_2$ receptors.

3 Ontogeny of $5\text{-}HT_{1c}$ Receptors

We have recently completed a detailed analysis of the development of $5\text{-}HT_{1c}$ receptors in rat brain. In preliminary studies (Roth et al. 1991) we utilized plasmid-derived DNA probes from the full-length cDNA. These studies showed that, in contrast to the $5\text{-}HT_2$ receptor which exhibited a complex developmental profile, the $5\text{-}HT_{1c}$ receptor showed a continued gradual increase in its expression from E17 to P15, when adult levels were attained. Adult levels of $5\text{-}HT_{1c}$ mRNA were about six- to eight fold higher than those measured at E17. Radioligand binding to the $5\text{-}HT_{1c}$ receptor generally mirrored the pattern of mRNA expression, although only a three- to four fold increase in receptor density was seen compared with the larger increase in mRNA. $5\text{-}HT_{1c}$ mRNA was present in extreme abundance in the choroid plexus but could be seen in the striatum, medulla-pons, and ventral hippocampus as well.

We then made a detailed regional study of $5\text{-}HT_{1c}$ receptor gene expression and binding by a combination of in situ hybridization and quantitative receptor autoradiography. Prior to E17, both gene expression and radioligand binding was restricted to the choroid plexus. No significant hybridization was seen in neuronal areas prior to P2, at which some minimal hybridization was detected in caudal regions of CA3 and CA4 of the hippocampus overlying a few pyramidal cells. Additionally, the subthalamic

◀ **Fig. 2A–C.** Demonstration of $5\text{-}HT_2$ receptor immunoreactivity in a subset of rat forebrain neurons. Paraformaldehyde-fixed rat brains were sectioned at 50 μm and processed as free-floating sections. Dilution of the affinity-purified anti-$5\text{-}HT_2$ receptor antibody was 1/50, and positive immunoreactivity was visualized using an immunoperoxidase reaction. **A** A number of immunopositive cells in the ventral forebrain, including the ventral portion of the shell of the nucleus accumbens and the horizontal limb of the nucleus of the diagonal band. The *boxed region* corrresponds to the area shown in **B**. Medial is to the *right*; ventral is *down*. Magnification: ×240. **B** A cluster of bipolar cells in the ventral forebrain showing $5\text{-}HT_2$ receptor immunoreactivity. Note the intense labeling of the cell perimeter, including the long neuronal processes extending away from the cell bodies (*arrowheads*); note also the absence of label in the cell nuclei. Magnification: ×600. **C** A large multipolar cell in the ventral forebrain, just outside the field of view shown in **A**. Again, note the intense perikaryal labeling, which excludes the nuclei, and the extensive network of primary (*arrow*) and secondary branched neuronal processes (a subset indicated by *arrowheads*) that are also positively labeled. Other cells are present out of the plane of focus. Magnification: ×550 nucleus showed faint hybridization. Around P5, a burst of receptor gene expression was noted in hippocampus with intense hybridization over pyramidal cells in the CA3 and CA4 (ventral aspects) layers. The subthalamic nucleus and various thalamic nuclei showed large amounts of hybridization at P5.

By P13, intense hybridization was seen in the olfactory tubercle, cingulate and retrosplenial cortices, thalamic muclei, lateral habenula, nucleus accumbens, and caudate nucleus. Additionally at P13, radioligand binding was detected as well in olfactory tubercle, cortex, nucleus accumbens, and caudate nucleus. The levels of hybridization were roughly equivalent to those seen in the adult.

One of the more interesting points emerging from these studies is that the pattern of 5-HT_{1c} receptor development appears to reflect different modes of regulation in different brain areas. The choroid plexus is of epithelial origin. In our studies, choroid plexus exhibits intense hybridization to 5-HT_{1c} cRNA probes at E17; this remains intense and does not appear to increase further in the adult. In contrast, in the hippocampus, 5-HT_{1c} mRNA is not seen before P2, can be detected at P5, and reaches adult levels at P27. We are now exploring the hypothesis that the 5-HT_{1c} receptor undergoes developmental regulation in neuronal cells and constitutive regulation in epithelial cells. To examine this, we are cloning the 5-HT_{1c} receptor gene and studying its regulatory elements. Furthermore, because it will be an important tool in our studies of regulation of this receptor, we have prepared an antibody against the 5-HT_{1c} receptor. Experiments characterizing the antibody are underway.

4 Conclusions

Molecular biologic approaches offer powerful ways to expand our understanding of how important neurotransmitter receptors work. One of the most significant findings to emerge from recent molecular biologic studies on neurotransmitter receptors is their great number, far more than could have been predicted from subtyping based on pharmacologic specificity alone. For example, at a time when there were thought to be two distinct muscarinic cholinergic receptor subtypes, molecular cloning stategies identified five, then a sixth (Bonner et al. 1987; Bonner 1988). Over the past 15 years arguments have raged to the point of tedium whether there were two, three, or four dopamine receptor subtypes; at this writing five have been identified by molecular cloning, three within the past 6 months (Sokoloff et al. 1990; Van Tol et al. 1991; Sunahara et al. 1991). In both examples, the additional receptor subtypes identified by molecular cloning would not have been detected with the available pharmacologic agents.

Based on the structure of the genes encoding neurotransmitter receptors, it would appear many more receptor subtypes await discovery. This is especially true for the ligand-gated ion channel superfamily of receptors, which consist of multiple protein subunits, each the product of an individual gene. Here, multiple genes, alleles at each gene locus, alternative splicing of complex primary transcripts, and tissue-specific expression of differentially processed mRNA all contribute to a staggering potential for numerical diversity. It is likely that this diversity explains the highly selective response of brain neurons to what are apparently common inputs. Thus a transmitter acting on one cell type in one brain area can have a different effect, both quantitatively and qualitatively, than on another brain neuron in a different location.

Within the G protein coupled receptor superfamily, similar conclusions can be drawn but the potential number of receptor subtypes is probably smaller. This is because the G protein coupled receptors are monomeric proteins; thus the potential number of subtypes of any given receptor is limited by the number of genes encoding each and the complexity of gene structure, which tends to be less than that described for the ligand-gated channel superfamily. However, if one extends this reasoning to include the G proteins, effector enzymes, and protein kinases which lead to functional transduction of a receptor-mediated signal, then it is possible that, at the *output* level, a similar degree of diversity exists in the G protein linked receptor family as in the ligand-gated ion channel family.

The implications of this for pharmaceutical development are enormous. Molecular cloning strategies can yield new receptor subtypes at a pace far faster than new selective ligands for them can be found. In the short term, this situation can be managed by extensive screening of existing chemical libraries using panels of cells expressing cloned receptors, but in the longer term, molecular modeling techniques which analyze receptor tertiary structure on the basis of primary sequence deduced from cloned cDNAs will probably emerge as the strategem of choice in drug development.

These thoughts simply address a different route for what remains the principal path drug development to the present has taken – a targeting on receptors as the principal locus of drug action. What of other strategies?

While much has been learned from molecular biologic approaches about the structure of receptor subtypes, we are just entering the era in which these same strategies are being used to unravel the complexities of receptor regulation. How receptors are controlled – at all levels, from gene transcription to positive and negative feedback mechanisms regulating their response to changes in their synaptic milieu – will probably lead to new targets for selective drug action, representing many, if not all, the steps in the signal transduction cascade. The trick will be to identify those which offer selective targets of drug action.

Anyone who has ever treated psychiatric patients, or any medical patient for that matter, knows the bitter truth that no matter how good a drug might be, there will always be patients who are not helped by it, either because they fail to respond or they experience intolerable side effects. For these individuals, advances in psychiatric therapy do not measure how far we have come, but how far we must yet go. We should not just hope then that new strategies in drug development will simply make existing therapies better, but that they will also increase the number and diversity of therapeutic offerings at our disposal, so that each patient has the greatest opportunity to be helped.

Acknowledgements. This work was supported by a program project grant from the National Institute of Mental Health (MH 39437), and by the Spunk Fund, the Gray Fund, and the endowment to the Nancy Pritzker Laboratory. SG and BLR are recipients of fellowship support from the Dana Research Foundation. RDC is the recipient of a Research Scientist Award from the NIMH (MH 00219).

References

Albert PA, Zhou Q-Y, Van Tol HHM, Bunzow JR, Civelli O (1990) Cloning, functional expression, and mRNA tissue distribution of the rat 5-hydroxytryptamine$_{1A}$ receptor gene. J Biol Chem 265:5825–5832

Ariani K, Hamblin MW, Tan GL, Stratford CA, Ciaranello RD (1989) G protein dependent alterations is [^{125}I]-iodocyanopindolol and cyanopindolol binding at 5HT1b binding sites in rat brain membranes. Neurochem Res 14:835–843

Bonner TI (1988) Cloning and expression of the human and rat M5 muscarinic acetylcholine receptor genes. Neuron 1:403–410

Bonner TI, Buckley NJ, Young AC, Brann MR (1987) Identification of a family of muscarinic acetylcholine receptor genes. Science 237:527–532

Conn PJ, Sanders-Bush E (1985) Serotonin-stimulated phosphoinositide turnover: mediation by the S2 binding site in rat cerebral cortex but not in subcortical regions. J Pharmacol Exp Ther 234:195–203

Conn PJ, Sanders-Bush E, Hoffman BJ, Harting PR (1986) A unique serotonin receptor in choroid plexus is linked to phosphatidylinositol turnover. Proc Natl Acad Sci USA 83:4086–4088

D'Amato RJ, Blue ME, Largent BL, Lynch DR, Ledbetter DJ, Molliver ME, Snyder SH (1987) Ontogeny of the serotonergic projection to rat neocortex: transient expression of a dense innervation to primary sensory areas. Proc Natl Acad Sci USA 84:4322–4326

Demuis A, Bouhelal R, Sebben M, Cory R, Bockaert J (1988) Nonclassical 5-hydroxytryptamine receptor positively coupled with adenylate cyclase in the central nervous system. Mol Pharmacol 34:880–887

DeVivo M, Maayani S (1985) Inhibition of forskolin-stimulated adenylate cyclase activity by 5HT receptor agonists. Eur J Pharmacol 109:231–234

Fargin A, Raymond JR, Lohse MJ, Kobilka BK, Caron MG, Lefkowitz RJ (1988) The genomic clone G-21 which resembles a β-adrenergic receptor sequence encodes the 5HT$_{1a}$ receptor. Nature 335:358–360

Julius D, MacDermott AB, Axel R, Jessel TM (1988) Molecular characterization of a functional cDNA encoding the serotonin 1c receptor. Science 241:558–564

Julius D, Huang KN, Livelli TJ, Axel R, Jessel TM (1990) The 5HT$_2$ receptor defines a family of structurally distinct but functionally conserved serotonin receptors. Proc Natl Acad Sci USA 87:928–932

Lidov HGW, Molliver ME (1982) An immunohistochemical study of serotonin neuron development in the rat: ascending pathways and terminal fields. Brain Res Bull 8:389–430

Matsubara S, Meltzer HY (1989) Effect of typical and atypical antipsychotic drugs on 5-HT2 receptor density in rat cerebral cortex. Life Sci 45:1397–1406

Palacios J, Waeber C, Mengod G, Hoyer D (1990) Visualization of serotonin receptor binding and their messenger RNAs in the mammalian brain: an update. In: Paoletti R, Vanhoutte PM, Brunello N, Maggi FM (eds) Serotonin: from cell biology to pharmacology and therapeutics. Elsevier, Amsterdam, pp 313–388

Pazos A, Cortes A, Palacios JM (1985) Quantitative autoradiographic mapping of serotonin receptors in rat brain. II. Serotonin-2 receptors. Brain Res 34:231–249

Peroutka SJ (1988) 5-Hydroxytryptamine receptor subtypes. In: Cowan WM, Shooter EM, Stevens CF, Thompson RF (eds) Annual review of neuroscience. Annual Reviews, Palo Alto, pp 45–60

Pritchett DB, Bach AW, Wozny M, Taleb O, Dal Toso R, Shih JC, Seeburg PH (1988) Structure and functional expression of cloned rat serotonin 5HT-2 receptor. EMBO J 7:4135–4140

Roth BL, Chaung D-M (1987) Minireview: multiple mechanisms of serotonergic signal transduction. Life Sci 41:1051–1064

Roth BL, Ciaranello RD (1992) Chronic mianserin treatment decreases 5-HT2 receptor binding without altering mRNA levels. Eur J Mol Pharmacol (1992)

Roth BL, Nakaki T, Chaung D-M, Costa E (1984) Aortic recognition sites for serotonin (5HT) are coupled to phospholipase C and modulate phosphoinositide turnover. Neuropharm acology 23:1233–1225

Roth BL, McLean S, Zhu X-Z, Chaung D-M (1987) Characterization of two [^{3}H]-ketanserin recognition sites in rat striatum. J Neurochem 49:1833–1838

Roth BL, Hamblin MW, Ciaranello RD (1990) Regulation of serotonin receptors: methodology and mechanisms. Neuropsychopharmacology 3:427–434

Roth BL, Hamblin MW, Ciaranello RD (1991) Developmental regulation of 5HT2 and 5HT1c mRNA and receptor levels. Dev Brain Res 58:51–58

Sokoloff P, Giros B, Martres M-P, Bouthenet M-L, Schwartz J-C (1990) Molecular cloning and characterization of a novel dopamine receptor (D_3) as a target for neuroleptics. Nature 347:147–151

Sunahara RK, Guan H-C, O'Dowd B, Seeman P, Laurier LG, Ng G, George Sr, Torchia J, Van Tol HM, Niznik HB (1991) Cloning of the gene for a human dopamine D_5 receptor with higher affinity for dopamine than D_1. Nature 350:614–619

Van Tol HHM, Bunzow JR, Guan H-C, Sunahara RK, Seeman P, Niznik HB, Civelli O (1991) Cloning of the gene for a human dopamine D_4 receptor with high affinity for the antipsychotic clozapine. Nature 350:611–614

Relevance of 5-HT Autoreceptors for Psychotropic Drug Action

M. Göthert and E. Schlicker

1 Psychiatric Disorders and Potential Therapeutic Value of Selective Ligands at Pre- and Postsynaptic 5-HT Receptors

Psychiatric disorders such as psychosis, depression, and anxiety have been related to changes in the activity of the serotoninergic system in the brain. Accordingly, drugs influencing this system either have been found to be of therapeutic value in these disorders or they are developed systematically as new classes of psychotropic agents. Evidence for the heterogeneity of serotonin (5-hydroxytryptamine; 5-HT) receptors and recent progress in their classification (reviewed by Bradley et al. 1986; Peroutka 1988; Frazer et al. 1990; Göthert 1990a) have promoted the development of selective agonists and antagonists directed at certain 5-HT receptor classes and subclasses. Some of these drugs are considered as potentially useful for the treatment of psychiatric disorders, for example, 5-HT_{1A} receptor agonists, which act as anxiolytics and antidepressants, and 5-HT_3 receptor antagonists, which appear to possess antipsychotic properties.

5-HT_{1A}, 5-HT_{1B}, 5-HT_{1D}, and 5-HT_3 receptors occur not only in the postsynaptic membrane of nerve cells innervated by serotoninergic neurones but also on the cell bodies, dendrites, and axon terminals of serotoninergic neurones themselves (Fig. 1). Therefore, it is of interest whether these somadendritic and presynaptic 5-HT autoreceptors are relevant for psychotropic drug actions. Here, we discuss this possibility in some detail and point to potential future developments which are conceivable on the basis of pathophysiological considerations. This discussion will be largely hypothetical or even speculative, since the current methodology does not allow a clear-cut decision whether a given response in vivo can be ascribed to a pre- or postsynaptic site of action. Nonetheless, in order to provide a solid basis for such considerations, a brief account of the occurrence, classification, and function of 5-HT autoreceptors is given below. As will be outlined, evidence for the existence of inhibitory autoreceptors belonging to the 5-HT_1 receptor family is strong, but the occurrence by itself of facilitatory 5-HT_3 auto-

Institut für Pharmakologie und Toxikologie, Rheinische Friedrich-Wilhelms-Universität Bonn, Reuterstraße 2b, W-5300 Bonn 1, Federal Republic of Germany

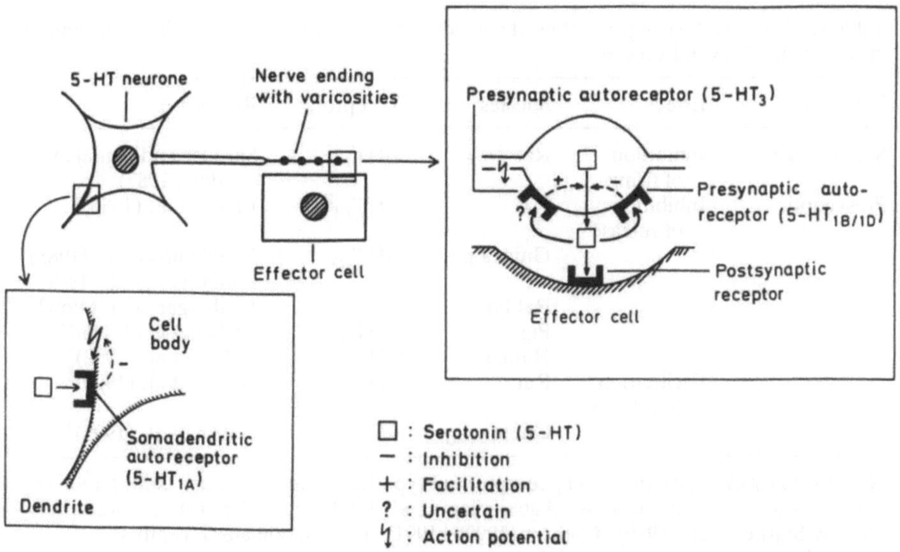

Fig. 1. A 5-HT neurone and its somadendritic and presynaptic 5-HT autoreceptors. The inhibitory presynaptic autoreceptor belongs to the $5\text{-}HT_{1B}$ subtype in the rat and to the $5\text{-}HT_{1D}$ subtype in the guinea pig, pig, rabbit and man. The rather hypothetic (see Table 1 and text) facilitatory presynaptic autoreceptor exhibited the characteristics of the $5\text{-}HT_3$ receptor class. (Adapted from Göthert 1990b)

receptors is very hypothetical (Fig. 1) and, hence, considerations concerning their therapeutic relevance are particularly speculative.

2 Location, Function, and Classification of 5-HT Autoreceptors

Somadendritic 5-HT autoreceptors, which upon stimulation inhibit action potential firing of the respective 5-HT neurones, were identified and characterized in the rat and mouse brain by electrophysiological techniques in vivo and in vitro. In the former type of experiments, the drugs were administered intravenously or locally into the brain by microiontophoresis. The in vitro experiments were carried out in brainstem slice preparations containing the raphe nuclei in which the cell bodies and dendrites of the serotoninergic neurones are located. 5-HT produced an inhibition of spontaneous firing. The effect of 5-HT was mimicked by the selective $5\text{-}HT_{1A}$ receptor agonists 8-OH-DPAT (8-hydroxy-2-(di-*n*-propylamino)-tetralin) and ipsapirone; the inhibitory effect of either drug was antagonized by (−)-propranolol which, besides its known β-adrenoceptor-blocking activity, also possesses antagonistic properties directed against several $5\text{-}HT_1$ receptor subtypes. The conclusion that the somadendritic autoreceptors

Table 1. Pharmacological properties of somadendritic and presynaptic 5-HT autoreceptors in the brain of several species

Location	Effect	Species	Receptors[1]	Reference
Somadendritic	Inhibition of firing	Rat	5-HT_{1A}	Sprouse and Aghajanian (1986, 1987)
Presynaptic	Inhibition of release	Rat	5-HT_{1B}[2]	Engel et al. (1986)[3]
		Guinea pig	5-HT_{1D}	Middlemiss et al. (1988)[4] Limberger et al. (1991)[4]
		Rabbit	5-HT_{1D}	Limberger et al. (1991)[4]
		Pig	5-HT_{1D}	Schlicker et al. (1989)
		Human	5-HT_{1D}	Galzin et al. (1992)[4]
	Facilitation of release	Rat	5-HT_3	Galzin et al. (1990)[4]
		Guinea pig	5-HT_3	Galzin et al. (1990)[4]

[1] Only studies in which the 5-HT_1 receptor subtype was determined are considered. For further studies, see reviews by Aghajanian et al. (1990; somadendritic autoreceptors) and by Starke et al. (1989), Göthert (1990b, 1991) (presynaptic autoreceptors).
[2] According to Limberger et al. (1991), part of the presynaptic autoreceptors in the rat brain cortex may be of the 5-HT_{1D} subtype.
[3] See Starke et al. (1989) for additional references.
[4] The presynaptic location of this receptor has not yet been determined.

belong to the 5-HT_{1A} receptor subclass (Fig. 1; Table 1) was confirmed autoradiographically. Thus, ^{3}H-8-OH-DPAT binding to dorsal raphe nuclei was markedly reduced after destruction of the serotoninergic neurones by the neurotoxin 5,7-dihydroxytryptamine. It has been shown by intracellular recordings that activation of somadendritic 5-HT autoreceptors produces a hyperpolarization which is due to an opening of K^+ channels. The somadendritic 5-HT_{1A} receptors are coupled to a G (e.g., G_i or G_o) protein. Accordingly, the hyperpolarizing effect of 5-HT was almost abolished by pertussis toxin, which inactivates G_i or G_o by ADP-ribosylation.

In most investigations designed to identify and characterize *presynaptic* 5-HT autoreceptors, superfused brain slices or synaptosomes, i.e., isolated pinched off and resealed varicosities of nerve terminals (see Fig. 1), were used. The release of endogenous 5-HT or, in preparations prelabeled with [^{3}H]5-HT, of tritium was evoked by electrical impulses or by high potassium, and the effects of 5-HT receptor ligands on the evoked release were studied. The evoked release of unlabeled or tritiated 5-HT was inhibited by 5-HT or other 5-HT receptor agonists (Table 1, Fig. 1) in brain slices and synaptosomes, whereas certain 5-HT receptor antagonists, given alone, disinhibited (i.e., increased) 5-HT release in brain slices. The operation of such an inhibitory mechanism in synaptosomes provided evidence that the receptors involved are located presynaptically. They were found in several species including humans (Table 1) and in all brain regions (including the limbic structures and the cortex) investigated for this purpose.

These *inhibitory* presynaptic 5-HT autoreceptors may be assumed to play a functional role in the fine regulation of 5-HT release into the synaptic cleft via a short negative feedback loop (Fig. 1). The latter can be interrupted by appropriate 5-HT autoreceptor antagonists, thus facilitating 5-HT release.

The inhibitory presynaptic 5-HT autoreceptors also belong to the 5-HT_1 receptor family, but not to the 5-HT_{1A} subclass. Accordingly, the effect of 5-HT or certain other agonists was blocked by the mixed 5-HT_1/5-HT_2 receptor antagonist metitepine, but not by selective 5-HT_2 or 5-HT_3 receptor antagonists; furthermore the effect of 5-HT was not mimicked by the 5-HT_{1A} receptor agonist ipsapirone. Comparison of the potencies of a series of 5-HT receptor ligands in influencing 5-HT release with their affinities for the different 5-HT binding sites revealed that the pharmacological properties of the inhibitory presynaptic autoreceptors differ among species. The presynaptic autoreceptor in rat brain could be classified as 5-HT_{1B} and in other species including humans as 5-HT_{1D} (Table 1; Fig. 1); in this context it should be noted that the 5-HT_{1B} and 5-HT_{1D} receptors exert the same function in these species. Relatively little is known about the chain of events following activation of the inhibitory presynaptic autoreceptors. Up to now, no clear-cut evidence could be obtained for an involvement of a G protein, adenylate cyclase, or protein kinase C in the modulation of signal transduction induced by action potentials invading the nerve terminal. However, it seems to be clear that the availability of Ca^{2+} for the 5-HT release process is inhibited by autoreceptor activation.

Recently, it has also been suggested that *facilitatory* presynaptic 5-HT autoreceptors may be involved in the regulation of 5-HT release in the brain (Table 1; Fig. 1). This suggestion was based on results obtained in guinea pig and rat brain cortex slices (published in abstract form only). 5-HT and the 5-HT_3 receptor agonist 2-methyl-5-HT increased the electrically evoked [^{3}H]5-HT release in a manner sensitive to blockade by the 5-HT_3 receptor antagonists ondansetron and tropisetron (ICS 205-930; see Table 1). However, it should be emphasized that experiments on synaptosomes have not yet been carried out and that, hence, the location of this receptor on the 5-HT nerve terminal has not yet been proven.

3 Potential Role of Somadendritic 5-HT Autoreceptors in the Anxiolytic and Antidepressant Effect of Mixed Full/Partial 5-HT_{1A} Receptor Agonists

The attempt to develop new anxiolytic drugs interacting with the serotoninergic system in the brain was based on the observation that, besides GABA, 5-HT is crucially involved in the effects of benzodiazepines (Koe 1979). In agreement with this, it was found that serotoninergic neurotransmission is decreased by these drugs (Wise et al. 1972) and that, in line with this observation, their anxiolytic effect is mimicked by an experimentally induced decrease in serotoninergic transmission (Iversen 1984; Chopin and Briley 1987). Limbic structures, e.g., the hippocampus, medial septum, and entorhinal cortex, are well known to be involved in emotional behavior such as anxiety (Gray 1982). Since 5-HT_{1A} receptors occur at high density in these brain structures and since the anxiolytic nonbenzodiazepine drug buspirone (Goldberg and Finnerty 1979) proved to possess high affinity for 5-HT_{1A} recognition sites in addition to dopamine binding sites (Glaser and Traber 1983), it appeared promising to develop drugs acting selectively on the 5-HT_{1A} receptor subclass as new anxiolytics. In fact, drugs with such a selective profile of receptor affinities, e.g., ipsapirone and gepirone (which are closely related to buspirone with respect to their chemical structure, but devoid of affinity for dopamine receptors), could be synthesized (Traber and Glaser 1987). They were effective not only in animal tests predictive for anxiolytic activity in humans (Traber et al. 1984; Traber and Glaser 1987), but also in animal tests suitable to predict an antidepressant effect in humans (Kennett et al. 1987). Accordingly, in clinical trials, they exhibited anxiolytic and antidepressant properties (Amsterdam et al. 1987; Csanalosi et al. 1987).

In view of the fact that the somadendritic 5-HT autoreceptor in the raphe nuclei also belongs to the 5-HT_{1A} subclass, the question arose whether and to what extent these autoreceptors contribute to the psychopharmacological effects of ipsapirone and gepirone. This question can only be answered when considering in more detail the results of biochemical and electrophysiological analyses of their actions at the somadendritic 5-HT_{1A} receptors in the limbic structures. In the two brain areas (raphe nuclei and limbic structures), the drugs under consideration exhibit different intrinsic activities: they are full agonists at the somadendritic 5-HT_{1A} autoreceptors (Sprouse and Aghajanian 1987, 1988; Aghajanian et al. 1990; De Montigny et al. 1990) and only partial agonists at the postsynaptic 5-HT_{1A} receptors (Martin and Mason 1987; Taylor 1990; i.e., their maximum effect at the postsynaptic 5-HT_{1A} receptors is less than that of a full agonist and they possess antagonistic properties against a full agonist).

Since manipulations of the serotoninergic system which enhance 5-HT neurotransmission have been shown to increase *anxiety* (Chopin and Briley 1987), the same system in the brain may be assumed to be "hyperactive" in anxiety of humans. If this prerequisite holds true, the anxiolytic activity of ipsapirone and gepirone may well be explained to a large part by the decrease in activity of the serotoninergic neurones, which is primarily caused by the activation of the somadendritic autoreceptors. If the autoreceptor-mediated inhibitory effect is not sufficient to reduce the serotoninergic activity to a normal level, the antagonistic component of the partial agonists ipsapirone and gepirone at the postsynaptic 5-HT_{1A} receptors in the limbic structures probably comes into play: the postsynaptic effect of the 5-HT released at a still elevated impulse rate from the serotoninergic varicosities in these brain areas may be assumed to be blocked by these compounds. Hence, both the somadendritic autoreceptors in the raphe nuclei and the postsynaptic 5-HT_{1A} receptors in the limbic structures appear to be involved in the anxiolytic effect of drugs such as ipsapirone and gepirone.

Depression in humans has been related to decreased serotoninergic neurotransmission (Coppen 1967; Willner 1985). Under this condition, i.e., decreased release of 5-HT from the serotoninergic neurones, the receptor-stimulating activity of gepirone and ipsapirone predominates at the postsynaptic 5-HT receptors in the limbic system, although these drugs are not full agonists at these receptors (see above). If no additional mechanism (such as that described below) would have to be considered, the agonistic effect of the compounds at the somadendritic 5-HT_{1A} autoreceptors would not contribute to their antidepressant effect.

However, adaptive changes of the 5-HT_{1A} receptors probably come into play after long-term administration of such drugs. Thus, it was found in rats that the decreased firing rate induced by short-term treatment of rats with drugs such as gepirone was followed by a complete recovery within 14 days of continuous treatment (Blier and de Montigny 1987). This adaptation was attributed to a desensitization of the somadendritic autoreceptors. In contrast, no such adaptation occurred with the postsynaptic 5-HT_{1A} receptor on the hippocampal pyramidal neurones. These findings suggest that, after long-term administration of such drugs, the desensitization of the somadendritic 5-HT autoreceptors restores a normal firing activity of the 5-HT neurones; even an overcompensation is conceivable if the firing rate of the 5-HT neurones would be lower than normal in untreated *depressed* patients. Desensitization of somadendritic autoreceptors would lead to a normal release of 5-HT into the synaptic cleft in the limbic structures in which the postsynaptic 5-HT_{1A} receptors have remained normosensitive. The time course of events derived from these considerations may also explain the 2–4 week latency period prior to the therapeutic efficacy of these drugs in depression (Blier and de Montigny 1987): in the first days of treatment, the postsynaptic effect of such drugs may be too weak to compensate for suppression of the firing activity of the 5-HT neurones; after prolonged treatment, the (partial) agonistic activity of these drugs would be superimposed on the effect of a normal amount of 5-HT released from 5-HT neurones which have regained their normal firing activity. Thus, the somadendritic 5-HT autoreceptors may play a role in the antidepressant effect of the mixed full/partial 5-HT_{1A} agonists.

In contrast, if desensitization of the somadendritic autoreceptors actually plays a role, the relative importance of the somadendritic autoreceptors for the *anxiolytic* effect of the mixed full/partial 5-HT_{1A} agonists would be lower than outlined above. However, if the anxiolytic effect would already occur at lower doses than the antidepressant one, it appears possible that the dose necessary for an anxiolytic effect may induce either no or only an incomplete desensitization; thus, a direct autoreceptor-mediated decrease in firing rate of the 5-HT neurones (see above) would be possible.

Taken together, it is clear from the results and considerations compiled here that the somadendritic autoreceptors are basically relevant for the psychotropic effects of the mixed full/partial 5-HT_{1A} agonists, although the relative importance of these receptors remains to be established. It is an advantage of these drugs, when used as anxiolytics, that they do not exert certain side effects typical for benzodiazepines, such as sedation, effects on motor coordination, and dependence. However, it is a disadvantage that these compounds induce their psychotropic effects with a delayed onset, which holds true not only for their antidepressant (Robinson et al. 1989) but also their anxiolytic effect.

4 Potential Role of Presynaptic 5-HT Autoreceptors in the Effects of Psychotropic Drugs and Possible Future Developments

4.1 Effects of Selective and Nonselective 5-HT Uptake Blockers (and Neuroleptic Drugs) on Inhibitory Autoreceptors

Although the evidence supporting a major role for decreased serotoninergic activity in the pathogenesis of depression is equivocal and although this model certainly represents an oversimplification (Boyer and Feighner 1991), it is a fact that selective and nonselective inhibitors of 5-HT reuptake (i.e., classical antidepressant drugs) are suitable to overcome the symptoms of depression. Therefore, it was of interest to investigate whether these drugs exert their psychotropic effect exclusively by 5-HT reuptake inhibition or whether the inhibitory presynaptic 5-HT autoreceptors are also relevant for their antidepressant effect.

4.1.1 Acute (Direct) Effects

It has been suggested on the basis of investigations in rat hypothalamic slices that a functional link exists between the 5-HT uptake mechanism ("5-HT transporter") and the 5-HT autoreceptor (link symbolized in Fig. 2 by the ragged line between the 5-HT transporter and the 5-HT autoreceptor). These experiments revealed that the autoreceptor function was diminished when the 5-HT transporter was blocked (Langer and Moret 1982; Galzin et al. 1985). However, this kind of interaction was not found in other brain areas and species, in which a decreased effect of exogenous 5-HT agonists in activating the autoreceptor was related to an increased concentration of endogenous 5-HT in the receptor biophase when an uptake inhibitor is present: under such a condition of increased autoreceptor activation, exogenous agonists can only produce a slight additional effect

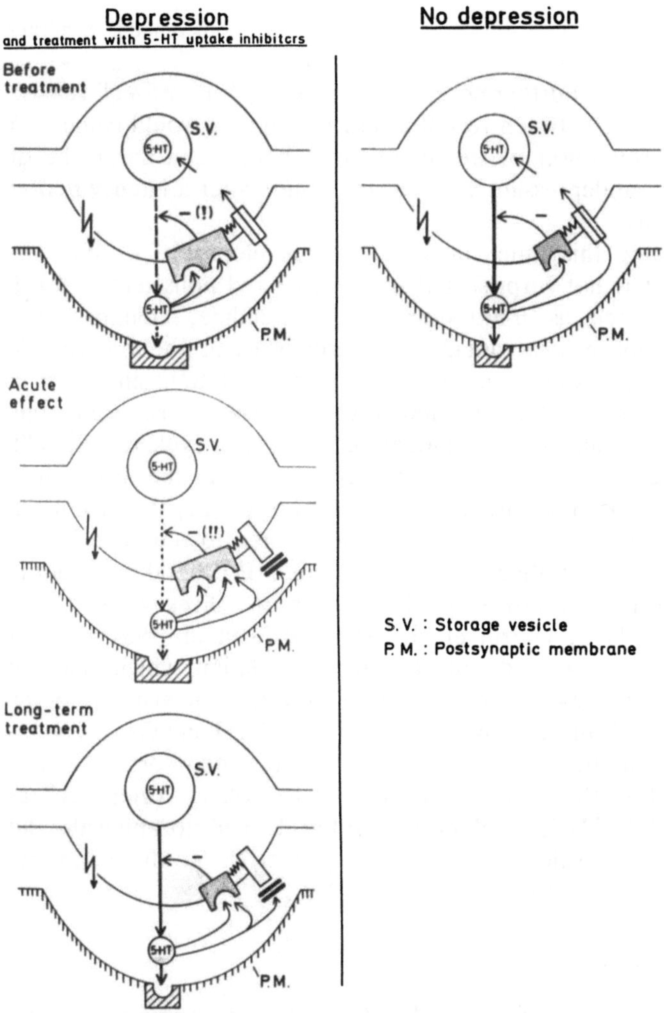

Fig. 2. The function of inhibitory presynaptic 5-HT autoreceptors on a serotoninergic varicosity in the brain under normal conditions (*right panel*) and hypothesized function in depressed patients before and after treatment with selective or nonselective 5-HT uptake inhibitors (*left panel*). *Stippled area* in the membrane of the serotoninergic varicosity, 5-HT autoreceptor; ↯, action potential. *Solid vertical arrows*, normal 5-HT release resulting in normal 5-HT concentration at postsynaptic 5-HT receptors; *broken vertical arrows*, decreased release and decreased 5-HT concentration at postsynaptic 5-HT receptors; *thin solid arrows* (largely within the synaptic cleft), binding of 5-HT to presynaptic autoreceptors and 5-HT uptake by the 5-HT transporter (*rectangle* within the cell membrane). Autoreceptor-mediated inhibition of 5-HT release: −, normal inhibition; −(!) and −(!!), reinforced inhibition. In untreated, depressed patients, autoreceptor function is assumed to be increased, symbolized by the increased *stippled area*, by the two recognition sites for 5-HT and by −(!). Blockade of the transporter by certain antidepressants (‖) first results in an increased concentration of 5-HT at the autoreceptor, leading immediately to further reinforcement of autoreceptor function, symbolized by −(!!). As a result of both effects (uptake blockade and increased autoreceptor function), the 5-HT concentration at postsynaptic receptors remains decreased. After long-term treatment with such antidepressants, a down-regulation of the autoreceptor may occur, resulting in normal serotoninergic synaptic transmission. (Adapted from Göthert 1991)

(Limberger et al. 1990). Furthermore, a relatively increased 5-HT release due to a functional link between receptor and transporter would come into play immediately after onset of treatment, and, hence, can hardly be of importance for the antidepressant effect which occurs after a latency period of at least several days.

When considering this time course of the development of the antidepressant effect, it is not surprising that selective and nonselective 5-HT uptake inhibitors, such as 6-nitroquipazine, zimelidine, clomipramine, and doxepin, did not possess antagonistic properties at the presynaptic 5-HT autoreceptors (Classen et al. 1984; Groß et al. 1987), since such a mechanism would also lead to an immediate increase in serotoninergic neurotransmission (see above). The moderate increase in evoked [^{3}H]5-HT overflow from superfused slices, which was observed with the drugs mentioned, could not be explained by the interruption of the negative feedback loop maintained by the released 5-HT but was related to reuptake inhibition. After acute administration of several other 5-HT uptake inhibitors even no increase in net overflow of [^{3}H]5-HT from the slices was observed (Langer and Moret 1982; Galzin et al. 1985; Groß et al. 1987); this is probably due to the increased autoreceptor stimulation which may be assumed to occur in response to the initial elevation of synaptic 5-HT concentration, induced, in turn, by the inhibition of 5-HT uptake.

In the context of these findings with the uptake inhibitors, it is also of interest to mention that typical and atypical neuroleptic drugs such as levomepromazine, thioridazine, haloperidol, sulpiride, and clozapine also did not possess either agonistic or antagonistic properties at the inhibitory presynaptic 5-HT autoreceptors (Groß et al. 1987).

4.1.2 Adaptive Changes

Depression has been suggested to be related to a "supersensitivity" (due to, e.g., an increased affinity and/or density) of presynaptic 5-HT autoreceptors (Göthert 1991). This may lead to a dimimished 5-HT release and, as a consequence, a decreased 5-HT concentration at the postsynaptic 5-HT receptors (Fig. 2, left panel). As already mentioned, the acute effect of the 5-HT uptake inhibitors probably consists of a transient increase in 5-HT concentration in the biophase of the inhibitory 5-HT autoreceptor, inducing immediately an even more pronounced activation of the 5-HT autoreceptor; as a result, the 5-HT concentration at the postsynaptic 5-HT receptor is not substantially increased by acute administration of such antidepressants (Fig. 2, left panel, center). However, long-term treatment with such drugs may cause a down-regulation of the presynaptic autoreceptors, thus restoring autoreceptor function and the concentration of 5-HT in the biophase of the postsynaptic 5-HT receptors to normal (Fig. 2, left panel, bottom). In agreement with this hypothesis, the responsiveness of the presynaptic 5-HT autoreceptors to 5-HT receptor ligands was found to be

Table 2. Effects of long-term treatment with 5-HT uptake inhibitors on the sensitivity of presynaptic 5-HT autoreceptors in the rat or rabbit brain

Treatment schedule	Effect	Species; brain region; experimental conditions	References
CGP 6085 A[a] 10 mg/kg i.p. plus clorgyline 1 mg/kg i.p. for 15 days	–	Rat cortical synaptosomes; high K^+	Maura and Raiteri (1984)
Citalopram 20 mg/kg i.p. for 14 days	–	Rat hippocampus; electrophysiological technique	Chaput et al. (1986)[b]
Amitriptyline 10 mg/kg i.p. for 21 days	–	Rat hypothalamic slices; electrical impulses	Schoups and De Potter (1988)[b]
Amitriptyline 2 × 10 mg/kg i.p. or clomipramine 10 mg/kg i.p. or imipramine 2 × 10 mg/kg i.p. for 21 days	0	Rabbit hypothalamic slices; electrical impulses	Schoups and De Potter (1988)
Citalopram 10 mg/kg or 50 mg/kg in food pellets for 21 days	–	Rat cortical slices; electrical impulses	Moret and Briley (1990)[b]
Milnacipran[c] 50 mg/kg in food pellets for 21 days	0	Rat cortical slices; electrical impulses	Moret and Briley (1990)

5-HT release in vitro was stimulated either by electrical impulses or by high potassium, or the sensitivity of the presynaptic autoreceptor was determined in vivo by electrophysiological techniques.
–, Decrease of the inhibitory effect of an exogenously added 5-HT receptor agonist or of the facilitatory effect of the 5-HT receptor antagonist metitepine; 0, no alteration.
[a] Chemical name: 4-(5,6-dimethyl-2-benzofuranyl) piperidine.
[b] It is not clear whether the effect of the exogenously added 5-HT receptor ligand was also decreased when the uptake inhibitor was administered acutely.
[c] Previous name: midalcipran or F 2207.

lowered in most (but not all) of the investigations in which animals were pretreated with 5-HT uptake inhibitors for periods of 14–21 days (results and references summarized in Table 2). The time course of these adaptive changes in autoreceptor function would be compatible with the latency period characteristic for the therapeutic effect of uptake inhibitors.

4.2 Relevance of Inhibitory Autoreceptors for the Antidepressant Effect of 5-HT Uptake Inhibitors and Putative Antidepressant Effect of Autoreceptor Antagonists

As outlined in the previous subsections, the presynaptic inhibitory 5-HT autoreceptors are certainly involved to some extent in the overall effect of the 5-HT uptake inhibitors on serotoninergic neurotransmission. Acutely the increased autoreceptor activation may compensate for the effect of 5-HT reuptake inhibition, thus keeping the serotoninergic neurotransmission on the same level as before treatment (Fig. 2, left panel, center); see also Subsect. 4.1.2). If autoreceptor desensitization should occur in depressed patients after long-term administration of 5-HT uptake inhibitors (irrespective of whether or not autoreceptor function is increased in depression), the autoreceptors would in fact be of high relevance for the psychotropic action of these antidepressant drugs, since this mechanism would increase serotoninergic neurotransmission.

If one assumes that an increased serotoninergic neurotransmission relieves certain symptoms of depression, autoreceptor antagonists should be particularly beneficial, since they would probably induce an immediate increase in 5-HT release by interrupting the negative feedback loop in which the inhibitory presynaptic 5-HT autoreceptors are crucially involved (Fig. 1). As mentioned above, this receptor belongs to the 5-HT_{1D} class in humans. Unfortunately, selective 5-HT_{1D} receptor antagonists are not available at the present time. Therefore, development of such compounds (with or without an additional blocking property on the 5-HT transporter) may be a promising strategy to obtain a new class of antidepressant drugs with the advantages of a rapid onset of therapeutic effect and (potentially) a low incidence of cholinergic and cardiovascular side effects.

4.3 Potential Contribution of Blockade of Facilitatory Autoreceptors in the Psychotropic Effect of 5-HT_3 Receptor Antagonists

The recent data suggesting that a positive 5-HT_3 receptor-mediated feedback loop may be operative at the serotoninergic nerve ending (Fig. 1; Table 1; section 2) may also be of interest in the context of psychotropic drug action. Recently, several 5-HT_3 receptor antagonists such as ondansetron, tropisetron, and granisetron have been developed. Such antagonists were effective in several behavioral test systems in animals predictive of anxiolytic and antipsychotic effects in humans (Kilpatrick et al. 1990). However, since even the presynaptic location of the 5-HT_3 receptor involved in the facilitation of 5-HT release is not yet clear, any detailed considerations about their potential involvement in those purported psychotropic effects are too speculative at present time.

Acknowledgement. The expert secretarial help of Mrs. R. Korneli is gratefully acknowledged.

References

Aghajanian GK, Sprouse JS, Sheldon P, Rasmussen K (1990) Electrophysiology of the central serotonin system: receptor subtypes and transducer mechanisms. Ann NY Acad Sci 600:93–103

Amsterdam JD, Berwish N, Potter L, Rickels K (1987) Open trial of gepirone in the treatment of major depressive disorder. Curr Ther Res 41:185–193

Blier P, de Montigny C (1987) Modification of 5-HT neuron properties by sustained administration of the 5-HT_{1A} agonist gepirone: electrophysiological studies in the rat brain. Synapse 1:470–480

Boyer WF, Feighner JP (1991) The serotonin hypothesis: necessary but not sufficient. In: Feighner JP, Boyer WF (eds) Selective serotonin re-uptake inhibitors. Wiley, Chichester, pp 71–80 (Perspectives in psychiatry, vol 1)

Bradley PB, Engel G, Feniuk W, Fozard JR, Humphrey PPA, Middlemiss DN, Mylecharane EJ, Richardson BP, Saxena PR (1986) Proposals for the classification and nomenclature of functional receptors for 5-hydroxytryptamine. Neuropharmacology 25:563–576

Chaput Y, de Montigny C, Blier P (1986) Effects of a selective 5-HT reuptake blocker, citalopram, on the sensitivity of 5-HT autoreceptors: electrophysiological studies in the rat brain. Naunyn Schmiedebergs Arch Pharmacol 333:342–348

Chopin P, Briley M (1987) Animal models of anxiety: The effects of compounds that modify 5-HT neurotransmission. Trends Pharmacol Sci 8:383–388

Classen K, Göthert M, Schlicker E (1984) Effects of DU 24565 (6-nitroquipazine) on serotoninergic and noradrenergic neurones of the rat brain and comparison with the effects of quipazine. Naunyn Schmiedebergs Arch Pharmacol 326:198–202

Coppen A (1967) The biochemistry of affective disorders. Br J Psychiatry 113:1237–1264

Csanalosi J, Schweizer E, Case WG, Rickels K (1987) Gepirone in anxiety: a pilot study. J Clin Psychopharmacol 7:31–33

De Montigny C, Blier P, Chaput Y (1990) Electrophysiological investigation of the effects of antidepressant treatments on serotonin receptors. In: Paoletti R, Vanhoutte PM, Brunello N, Maggi FM (eds) Serotonin. From cell biology to pharmacology and therapeutics. Kluwer, Dordrecht, pp 499–515

Engel G, Göthert M, Hoyer D, Schlicker E, Hillenbrand K (1986) Identity of inhibitory presynaptic 5-hydroxytryptamine (5-HT) autoreceptors in the rat brain cortex with 5-HT_{1B} binding sites. Naunyn Schmiedebergs Arch Pharmacol 332:1–7

Frazer A, Maayani S, Wolfe BB (1990) Subtypes of receptors for serotonin. Annu Rev Pharmacol Toxicol 30:307–348

Galzin AM, Moret C, Verzier B, Langer SZ (1985) Interaction between tricyclic and nontricyclic 5-hydroxytryptamine uptake inhibitors and the presynaptic 5-hydroxytryptamine inhibitory autoreceptors in the rat hypothalamus. J Pharmacol Exp Ther 235:200–211

Galzin AM, Poncet V, Langer SZ (1990) 5-HT_3 receptor agonists enhance the electrically evoked release of $[^3H]$-5-HT in guinea-pig frontal cortex slices. Br J Pharmacol 100:307P

Galzin AM, Poirier MF, Lista A, Chodkiewicz JP, Blier P, Ramdine R, Loo H, Roux FX, Redondo A, Langer SZ (1992) Characterization of the 5-hydroxytryptamine receptor modulating the release of 5-$[^3H]$hydroxytryptamine in slices of the human neocortex. J Neurochem 59:1293–1301

Glaser T, Traber J (1983) Buspirone: action on serotonin receptors in calf hippocampus. Eur J Pharmacol 88:137–138

Goldberg HL, Finnerty RJ (1979) The comparative efficacy of buspirone and diazepam in the treatment of anxiety. Am J Psychiatry 136:1184–1187

Göthert M (1990a) Pharmacological, biochemical and molecular classification schemes of serotonin (5-HT) receptors with special reference to the 5-HT_2 class. In: Göthert M (ed) Serotonin and 5-HT_2 receptor blockade in the cardiovascular system. Fischer, Stuttgart, pp 3–15

Göthert M (1990b) Presynaptic serotonin receptors in the central nervous system. Ann NY Acad Sci 604:102–112

Göthert M (1991) Presynaptic effects of 5-HT. In: Stone TW (ed) Aspects of synaptic transmission, vol 1. Taylor and Francis, London, pp 314–329

Gray JA (ed) (1982) The neuropsychology of anxiety. Oxford University Press, New York
Groß G, Hante K, Göthert M (1987) Effect of antidepressant and neuroleptic drugs on the electrically evoked release of serotonin from rat cerebral cortex. Psychopharmacology (Berl) 91:175–181
Iversen SD (1984) 5-HT and anxiety. Neuropharmacology 23:1553–1560
Kennett GA, Dourish CT, Curzon G (1987) Antidepressant-like action of 5-HT_{1A} agonists and conventional antidepressants in an animal model of depression. Eur J Pharmacol 134:265–274
Kilpatrick GJ, Bunce KT, Tyers MB (1990) 5-HT_3 receptors. Med Res Rev 10:441–475
Koe BK (1979) Biochemical effects of antianxiety drugs on brain monoamines. In: Fielding S, Lal H (eds) Anxiolytics. Futura, New York, pp 173–195
Langer SZ, Moret C (1982) Citalopram antagonizes the stimulation by lysergic acid diethylamide of presynaptic inhibitory serotonin autoreceptors in the rat hypothalamus. J Pharmacol Exp Ther 222:220–226
Limberger N, Starke K, Singer EA (1990) Serotonin uptake blockers influence serotonin autoreceptors by increasing the biophase concentration of serotonin and not through a "molecular link". Naunyn Schmiedebergs Arch Pharmacol 342:363–370
Limberger N, Deicher R, Starke K (1991) Species differences in presynaptic serotonin autoreceptors: mainly 5-HT_{1B} but possibly in addition 5-HT_{1D} in the rat, 5-HT_{1D} in the rabbit and guinea-pig brain cortex. Naunyn Schmiedebergs Arch Pharmacol 343:353–364
Martin KF, Mason R (1987) Isapirone is a partial agonist at 5-hydroxytryptamine (5-HT_{1A}) receptors in the rat hippocampus: electrophysiological evidence. Eur J Pharmacol 141:479–483
Maura G, Raiteri M (1984) Functional evidence that chronic drugs induce adaptive changes of central autoreceptors regulating serotonin release. Eur J Pharmacol 97:309–313
Middlemiss DN, Bremer ME, Smith SM (1988) A pharmacological analysis of the 5-HT receptor mediating inhibition of 5-HT release in the guinea-pig frontal cortex. Eur J Pharmacol 157:101–107
Moret C, Briley M (1990) Serotonin autoreceptor subsensitivity and antidepressant activity. Eur J Pharmacol 180:351–356
Peroutka SJ (1988) 5-Hydroxytryptamine receptor subtypes. Annu Rev Neurosci 11:45–60
Robinson DS, Roberts DL, Shrotriya RS, Copp JE, Wickramarative P, Alms DR (1989) Clinical effects of the 5-HT-1A partial agonists, buspirone and gepirone, in the treatment of depression. Biol Psychiatry Abstr 25:141A
Schlicker E, Fink K, Göthert M, Hoyer D, Molderings G, Roschke I, Schoeffter P (1989) The pharmacological properties of the presynaptic serotonin autoreceptor in the pig brain cortex conform to the 5-HT_{1D} receptor subtype. Naunyn Schmiedebergs Arch Pharmacol 340:45–51
Schoups AA, De Potter WP (1988) Species dependence of adaptations at the pre- and postsynaptic serotonergic receptors following long-term antidepressant drug treatment. Biochem Pharmacol 37:4451–4460
Sprouse JS, Aghajanian GK (1986) (-)-Propranolol blocks the inhibition of serotoninergic dorsal raphe cell firing by 5-HT_{1A} selective agonists. Eur J Pharmacol 128:295–298
Sprouse JS, Aghajanian GK (1987) Electrophysiological responses of serotoninergic dorsal raphe neurons to 5-HT_{1A} and 5-HT_{1B} agonists. Synapse 1:3–9
Sprouse JS, Aghajanian GK (1988) Responses of hippocampal pyramidal cells to putative serotonin 5-HT_{1A} and 5-HT_{1B} agonists: a comparative study with dorsal raphe neurons. Neuropharmacology 27:707–715
Starke K, Göthert M, Kilbinger H (1989) Modulation of neurotransmitter release by presynaptic autoreceptors. Physiol Rev 69:864–989
Taylor DP (1990) Serotonin agents in anxiety. Ann NY Acad Sci 600:545–557
Traber J, Glaser T (1987) 5-HT_{1A} receptor related anxiolytics. Trends Pharmacol Sci 8:432–437

Traber J, Davies MA, Dompert WU, Glaser T, Schuurman T, Seidel P-R (1984) Brain serotonin receptors as a target for the putative anxiolytic TVX Q 7821. Brain Res Bull 12:741–744
Willner P (1985) Antidepressants and serotonergic neurotransmission: an integrative review. Psychopharmacology (Berl) 85:387–404
Wise CD, Berger BD, Stein L (1972) Benzodiazepines: anxiety-reducing activity by reduction of serotonin turnover in the brain. Science 177:180–183

Brain Serotonin Subsystem Complexity and Receptor Heterogeneity: Therapeutic Potential of Selective Serotonin Agonists and Antagonists

K.P. Lesch, C.S. Aulakh, and D.L. Murphy

1 Introduction

Gaddum and Picarelli (1957) initially suggested the existence of more than one serotonin (5-HT) receptor over 30 years ago. Subsequently, neurophysiological, pharmacological, and other investigative techniques provided evidence that 5-HT could act at presynaptic and postsynaptic sites and could be either excitatory or inhibitory in different systems; however, more definitive evidence of 5-HT receptor heterogeneity did not begin to emerge until the beginning of the last decade (Peroutka and Snyder 1979; Sanders-Bush 1988; Whitaker-Azmitia and Peroutka 1990). There is now molecular and functional evidence for the existence of eight 5-HT receptors, designated 5-HT$_{1A-E}$, 5-HT$_2$, 5-HT$_3$ and 5-HT$_4$; in addition, there is increasingly compelling data indicative of additional 5-HT receptor subtypes or subforms (Sanders-Bush 1988; Schmidt and Peroutka 1989; Frazer et al. 1990). While studies of the multiple 5-HT receptor subtypes and their signal transduction mechanisms have dominated many recent investigations of this neurotransmitter system, there have also been substantial advances in the development of selective receptor subtype agonists and antagonists with therapeutic potentials in a variety of neuropsychiatric disorders.

This review provides a survey of 5-HT receptor pharmacology, physiology and neuroanatomy of relevance to 5-HT subsystems in humans. It specifically emphasizes those receptor subtypes and subsystems which are potential targets for the development of siteselective therapeutic strategies.

2 Multiple Serotonin Receptor Subtypes: Therapeutic Potential of Selective Ligands

2.1 5-HT$_{1A}$ Partial Agonists with Anxiolytic/Antidepressant Properties

Perhaps the strongest association between ligands with highly selective affinity for one 5-HT receptor subtype site and functional activity in a

Laboratory of Clinical Science, National Institute of Mental Health, NIH Clinical 10-3D41, 9000 Rockville Pike, Bethesda, MD 20892, USA

Table 1. Affinities of buspirone, ipsapirone and the prototypical $5\text{-}HT_{1A}$ agonist 8-hydroxy-2(di-n-propylamino) tetralin (8-OH-DPAT) for 5-HT binding sites (p*K*d, -log mol/l). (From Hoyer 1988; Neijt et al. 1988)

	$5\text{-}HT_{1A}$	$5\text{-}HT_{1B}$	$5\text{-}HT_{1C}$	$5\text{-}HT_{1D}$	$5\text{-}HT_2$	$5\text{-}HT_3$
Buspirone	7.58	3.94	5.08	4.48	6.07	–
Ipsapirone	7.73	3.87	4.53	4.88	5.07	–
8-OH-DPAT	8.74	4.22	5.24	5.94	5.04	4.44

neuropsychiatric disorder is that of several $5HT_{1A}$ partial agonists and generalized anxiety disorder. Several of these $5HT_{1A}$ agents – buspirone, gepirone, and ipsapirone – which are now collectively designated the azapirones have markedly higher affinities for the brain $5\text{-}HT_{1A}$ site relative to other 5-HT binding sites (Table 1), and recent reviews suggest that this 5-HT receptor is the primary mediator of their anxiolytic and related actions (Traber and Glaser 1987; Glaser 1988; Marsden 1988; Taylor 1988, 1989; Carli et al. 1989).

These agents have negligible affinity for brain benzodiazepine binding sites and are inactive at the GABA receptor complex (Taylor 1988). $5\text{-}HT_{1A}$ sites are located throughout the brain, although some brain regions such as the brainstem raphe nuclei and the hippocampus have especially high numbers of $5\text{-}HT_{1A}$ sites (Fig. 1). The azapirones have a common effect of acting as agonists at somatodendritic, autoreceptor $5\text{-}HT_{1A}$ sites in the raphe areas, slowing the spontaneous firing rates of serotonergic neurons located in these raphe nuclei (Basse-Tomusk and Rebec 1986; VanderMaelen et al. 1986; Andrade and Nicoll 1987; Sprouse and Aghajanian 1987). All three azapirones can also directly hyperpolarize hippocampal pyramidal cells in vitro, inhibiting their firing (Andrade and Nicoll 1987).

The cumulative reduction in serotonergic impulse flow to septohippocampal and other cortical and limbic areas has been theorized to explain the behavioral effects of the azapirones in some animal models of anxiety (Traber and Glaser 1987; Taylor 1988, 1989). This conclusion is based, in part, on evidence that the effects of buspirone in these behavioral models are prevented when serotonergic system lesions are produced by selective neurotoxins (Eison et al. 1986; Carli et al. 1989). In one animal model, an anxiolytic effect has been attributed, on the basis of lesion studies, to specific serotonergic effects of buspirone on the medial, and not dorsal, raphe nucleus (Carli et al. 1989).

Controlled trials indicate that the most well-studied azapirone, buspirone, is significantly more effective than placebo in the treatment of anxiety (Goa and Ward 1986). In almost all studies, buspirone possessed equal efficacy as diazepam and other benzodiazepines in patients with anxiety; these data have been extensively reviewed (Schuckit 1984; Cohn et al. 1986; Sleight et al. 1991; Glitz and Pohl 1991). More limited studies also suggest likely

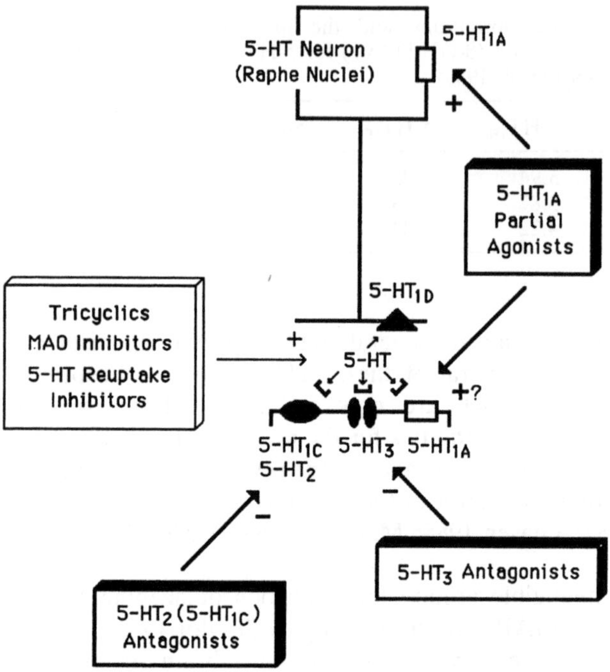

Fig. 1. Mechanism of action of 5-HT agonists and antagonists

equivalent efficacy for gepirone and ipsapirone (Csanalosi et al. 1987; Glaser 1988). Important distinctions between 5-HT_{1A} partial agonists and benzodiazepine-type anxiolytics include the azapirones' lack of the sedative, muscle relaxant, and anticonvulsant effects characteristic of the benzodiazepines. Also, the anxiolytic effects of the azapirones have a slower onset of action, requiring approximately 2 weeks of treatment to gradually develop. Preclinical as well as clinical studies with 5-HT_{1A} partial agonists indicate antidepressant and antiobsessional activity (Glaser 1988; Murphy et al. 1990a; Glitz and Pohl 1991). The spectrum of potential indications and ongoing efficacy evaluation is summarized in Table 2.

Of note, 5-HT_{1A} partial agonists appear to be valid tools in the pharmacological challenge paradigm and have facilitated the assessment of 5-HT_{1A} responsivity in anxiety disorders and depression and its modification by psychotropic drug treatment (Cowen et al. 1990; Lesch et al. 1991; Lesch 1991).

A small amount of evidence suggests that agents acting at 5-HT_2 receptors may possess antianxiety as well as mood stabilizing effects. Ritanserin, a drug with greater affinity for 5-HT_2/5-HT_{1C} sites than other neurotransmitter sites, was reported to be significantly more effective than placebo and equally effective as lorazepam in one controlled study of

Table 2. Clinical application of 5-HT_{1A} partial agonist. (From Glitz and Pohl 1991)

	Entity	Compound	Remarks
Anxiety disorders	Generalized anxiety disorder	Buspirone, gepirone, ipsapirone	Anxiolytic effects (controlled trials; develop gradually over several weeks)
	Panic disorder	Buspirone	Inconclusive (controlled trials)
	Obsessive–compulsive disorder	Buspirone, ipsapirone	Buspirone-clomipramine (cross-over), buspirone Ø (open trial), buspirone augmentation of fluoxetine (open trial)
Depression		Buspirone, gepirone, ipsapirone	Antiderpressant effects (controlled trials: buspirone, gepirone > placebo), ipsapirone effective in dysthymia
Impulse control disorders	Aggressive/self-injurious behavior	Buspirone	Case reports (antidopaminergic effects?)
	Bulimia	Ipsapirone	Reduction of bulemic behavior
	Alcohol abuse	Buspirone	Reduction of craving and consumption

anxious patients and is undergoing clinical trials in dysthymia (Ceulemans et al. 1985a). Although considerably less selective, the 5-HT_2 antagonist mianserin has been shown to possess antidepressant properties (Eklund et al. 1985).

2.2 A 5-HT_{1C} Receptor Agonist with Anxiogenic Effects

One 5-HT agonist, *m*-chlorophenylpiperazine (*m*-CPP), a metabolite of the antidepressant trazodone, was first reported to induce small but statistically significant increases in anxiety ratings when given orally in 0.5 mg/kg doses under double-blind, placebo-controlled conditions to healthy volunteers (Mueller et al. 1985). When *m*-CPP was given orally in smaller doses (0.25 mg/kg) to normal volunteers, no significant anxiogenic effects were observed (Kahn et al. 1988). In contrast, patients with panic disorder in the same study developed panic episodes (Kahn et al. 1988). When patients with obsersive compulsive disorder (OCD) were given *m*-CPP (0.5 mg/kg) orally, they also became significantly more anxious than normal controls, but did not exhibit panic episodes (Zohar et al. 1987). Rather, the OCD patients experienced a transient but marked exacerbation of OC symptoms after *m*-CPP, but not after placebo or after the 5-HT antagonist metergoline. These OC symptoms occurred in 11 of 12 patients, half of whom reported the reemergence of OC symptoms that had not been present for many months or the occurrence of new OC symptoms. A second study also reported that six of eight OCD patients manifested OC symptoms twice the severity of baseline OC symptoms when given *m*-CPP orally (Hollander et al. 1988).

Studies using intravenously administered *m*-CPP revealed somewhat different results from those found in studies using orally administered *m*-CPP. When *m*-CPP was given intravenously to normal volunteers, it produced significantly greater anxiety than when administered orally (Murphy et al. 1989). In another study, intravenous *m*-CPP elicited severe anxiety and panic attacks in both panic disorder patients and normal controls (Charney et al. 1987). Similarly, intravenously administered *m*-CPP markedly increased anxiety and other behavioral changes in OCD patients and normal controls, but produced no concomitant, specific changes in OC symptoms (Charney et al. 1988). These results are in contrast to results of the two studies investigating the effects of oral administration of *m*-CPP in OCD patients. One interpretation of these data suggests that *m*-CPP has dose-dependent anxiogenic properties, which can be modified by method and duration of administration (Kahn et al. 1988; Murphy et al. 1989). Symptoms elicited by *m*-CPP may be specific to a psychobiological substrate characteristic of the patient subgroup, with subsequent differential manifestations of anxiety. This hypothesis is best exemplified by the ability of orally administered *m*-CPP to elicit panic in panic disorder patients (but not in controls) and to increase OC symptoms but not induce panic episodes in OCD patients.

m-CPP possesses an approximately tenfold higher affinity for 5-HT_{1C} versus 5-HT_{1A} and 5-HT_2 sites in vitro (Hoyer 1988). It thus has less selectivity for 5-HT_{1C} sites than the azapirones possess for 5-HT_{1A} sites (Table 1). Nonetheless, a number of studies with different 5-HT antagonists have led to the conclusion that most of *m*-CPP's effects – at least when it is given in low doses – are mediated by its 5-HT_{1C} agonist effects (Fozard and Gray 1989; Kennett and Curzon 1988a,b; Kennett et al. 1989; Whitton and Curzon 1990; Curzon and Kennett 1990; Berendsen et al. 1990). This includes data from studies of rodent models of anxiety such as social interaction and light/dark box explorations (Kennett et al. 1989; Curzon and Kennett 1990).

2.3 5-HT_2 Agonists and Antagonists with Actions Relevant to Psychosis

Several well-studied phenylisopropylamine hallucinogens, including 1-(2,5-dimethoxy-4-bromophenyl)-2-aminopropane (DOB), and 1-(2,5-dimethoxy-4-iodophenyl)-2-aminopropane (DOI), are selective 5-HT_2 agonists (Hoyer 1988; Titeler et al. 1988). It has recently been suggested that phenylisopropylamines such as DOI and DOB may exert their hallucinogenic effects via a subset of 5-HT_2 receptors highly localized in some brain regions, for example, the claustrum (Titeler et al. 1988; McKenna et al. 1989). These agents together with other psychotomimetic indoleamines and phenylethylamines have been suggested to provide a partial model for the schizophrenia syndrome (Bowers 1987).

Some speculation about the mechanism of action of the atypical neuroleptic clozapine, which has been found effective in some otherwise drug treatment-resistant schizophrenic patients and which lacks some typical dopamine antagonist features found with other neuroleptics, has focused on its 5-HT_2 antagonist properties, although other neuroleptics also possess potent 5-HT_2 antagonist actions (Wander et al. 1987; Meltzer 1989). Some 5-HT_2 antagonists, including setoperone and ritanserin, are under study in schizophrenic patients and like clozapine have been reported to be of particular benefit for negative schizophrenic symptoms (Ceulemans et al. 1985b; Gelders et al. 1986). An indirect effect of 5-HT_2 blockade on midbrain dopamine neurons produced by ritanserin, which was blocked by pretreatment with the 5-HT synthesis inhibitor *para*-chlorophenylalanine has been suggested as a possible mechanism whereby 5-HT_2 antagonists might lead to improved mood, drive, and motivation, and thus benefit negative symptoms in schizophrenia, as well as to benefit patients with parkinsonism and anxiety disorders (Ugedo et al. 1989). A selective enhancing action of clozapine on dopamine neurons in the striatum mediated by 5-HT_2 receptors has been suggested to counter the direct dopamine receptor-blocking action of this neuroleptic; this action may be responsible for the low incidence of tardive dyskinesia found with clozapine (Saller et al. 1990).

2.4 5-HT_3 Antagonists – Broad Spectrum Therapeutics?

5-HT_3 receptors are highly concentrated in the entorhinal cortex, amygdala, hippocampus, and nucleus accumbens. In contrast to 5-HT_1, 5-HT_2, and 5-HT_4 receptors, 5-HT_3 receptors are coupled to a ligand-gated cation channel (Hoyer 1990). Growing evidence that 5-HT_3 receptors participate in the control of disturbed behavior in the absence of effort on normal behavior not only has focused research effort on their involvement in the pathophysiology of neuropsychiatric disorders but has also stimulated the development of selective 5-HT_3 antagonists with a potentially broad therapeutic spectrum (Table 3). Several 5-HT_3 receptor antagonists, including MDL 72222, ICS 205-930, granisetron, and ondansetron, have anxiolytic-type effects in rodent and nonhuman primate models (Costall et al. 1987, 1990; Tyers et al. 1987; Jones et al. 1988). 5-HT_3 receptor antagonism in the dorsal raphe nucleus (DRN) and the amygdala appears to be the neuroanatomical site of action. Preliminiary evidence from ongoing controlled clinical trials suggests that ondansetron has, albeit weak, anxiolytic activity with few side effects and no rebound anxiety on discontinuation (Lader 1991).

The property of 5-HT_3 antagonists to inhibit mesolimbic dopaminergic hyperactivity is intriguing in the view that 5-HT_3 antagonists may have an

Table 3. Therapeutic potential of 5-HT_3 antagonists

Neuronal interaction	Therapeutic effects	Potential efficacy
Pre- and/or postsynaptic 5-HT_3 antagonism	Anxiolytic properties (animal models of experimental anxiety)	Anxiety disorders (generalized anxiety, panic, obsessive–compulsive disorder)
Inhibition of mesolimbic dopaminergic hyperactivity	Antipsychotic effects?	Schizophrenia, schizoaffective psychoses
Facilitation of cortical acetylcholine release	Improvement of cognitive deficits and age-related memory impairment	Dementia, Alzheimer's disease
Dopamine and/or serotonin antagonism	Prevention of withdrawal syndromes, rebound phenomena	Benzodiazepine withdrawal, alcoholism, drug addiction

antipsychotic potential and may prevent neuroleptic-induced rebound hyperactivity (Costall et al. 1990). Despite the evidence that 5-HT_3 antagonists are very potent in modulating dopamine function in the animal model, potential efficacy in schizophrenic psychoses, in the prevention of withdrawal syndromes, and in the control of substance abuse has to be substantiated in controlled clinical trials (Meltzer 1991).

Based on in vitro evidence that 5-HT exerts an inhibitory influence on learning and memory, possibly via interaction with the cholinergic system, and that 5-HT_3 antagonists facilitate cortical acetylcholine release, cognitive deficits and age-related memory impairment, most commonly encountered in patients with dementia and Alzheimer's disease, may also be improved by 5-HT_3 antagonists (Barnes et al. 1989).

2.5 Other 5-HT Receptor Subtypes

Only fragmentary data is presently available linking other 5-HT receptors to neuropsychiatric disorders and their treatment. For the most part, this is due to a lack of selective agonists for receptors which can be studied in humans.

In addition, the great majority of studies characterizing brain 5-HT receptor subtypes have been carried out in rodents, with relatively few comparative studies available, especially of human or nonhuman primate brain. Major anatomical differences are well known to exist between primate and rodent brain structures. In addition, a major difference between human brain and rodent brain (and also brains from several other species) is the rodent brain 5-HT_{1B} binding site, which is of considerable functional interest according to the results of drug studies in rodents, but which apparently is not present in human brain (Engel et al. 1983, 1987; Raiteri et al. 1986; Hoyer et al. 1988; Hamik and Peroutka 1989).

Interestingly, however, the 5-HT$_{1D}$ site in human brain possesses a pattern of regional localization and site density highly similar to the 5-HT$_{1B}$ site in rat brain (Waeber et al. 1988; Peroutka et al. 1989). Selective agonists and antagonists for the 5-HT$_{1D}$ site are in early stages of development (Peroutka and McCarthy 1989), and it is not yet clear whether only anatomical but also functional homology may exist across species for these two sites (Hoyer and Middlemiss 1989). A fairly comprehensive autoradiographic survey of 5-HT$_1$, 5-HT$_{1A}$, 5-HT$_{1C}$, 5-HT$_{1D}$, and 5-HT$_2$ binding sites in human brain was completed in the last few years by one research group, permitting some direct comparisons with rodent brain sites (Pazos and Palacios 1985; Pazos et al. 1985, 1987; Hoyer et al. 1986a,b; Waeber et al. 1988).

3 Serotonin Subsystem Complexity: Other Nonreceptor Aspects of Serotonin Pharmacology, Physiology, and Neuroanatomy of Relevance for Strategies in Psychotropic Drug Development

3.1 Brain Serotonin Subsystems

Recent developments in 5-HT neuroanatomy and neurophysiology have clarified earlier data suggesting that cell bodies and projections from different 5-HT neurons in the raphe nuclei have different characteristics. In 5-HT projection areas of the rat brain, two major classes of 5-HT axon terminals are found which differ in axon morphology, cells of origin, regional distribution, and responses to neurotoxic and other drugs. Axons from the DRN as studied, for example, in the frontal cortex are very fine, with small varicosities, and are highly vulnerable to damage by *para*-chloroamphetamine, 3,4-methylene dioxyamphetamine (MDMA), and 3,4-methylene dioxymethamphetamine (MDA). In contrast, axons from the median raphe nucleus (MRN), for example, in the parietal cortex, hippocampus, and lateral hypothalamus, have large varicosities and are resistant to the neurotoxic, substituted amphetamines (Conrad et al. 1974; Moore and Halaris 1975; Kohler and Steinbusch 1982; Kosofsky and Molliver 1987; Molliver 1987; O'Hearn et al. 1988; Mamounas and Molliver 1988; Fritschy et al. 1988). Fine axonal projections from the DRN studied in layer Va of the rat somatosensory cortex are closely associated with a high density of 5-HT$_2$ binding sites in autoradiographic studies, suggesting that 5-HT$_2$ receptors may be selectively linked in this area to one type of 5-HT neuron (Blue et al. 1988).

The evidence from neuroanatomical studies that there are different subclasses of 5-HT neurons in brain is supported by some neurophysiological and neuropharmacological data. For example, the 5-HT$_{1A}$ partial agonists, 8-hydroxy-2-[di-n-propylamino]tetralin (8-OH-DPAT) or ipsapirone, are well known to slow raphe 5-HT neuron firing rates on a dose-dependent basis; however, the 8-OH-DPAT dose (ED_{50}) required to produce the slowing effect in the MRN is 30 times higher than that required for the same effect in the DRN (Sinton and Fallon 1988). Moreover, a range of doses of another serotonergic agent related to *m*-CPP, trifluoromethylphenylpiperazine (TFMPP), yielded no consistent effects on cell firing rates in the DRN, but dose dependently increased firing rates in the MRN (Sinton and Fallon 1988). The 5-HT-selective tricyclic clomipramine affects 5-HT turnover in the MRN more than in the DRN (Meek and Lofstrandh 1976).

In other experiments, direct application of 8-OH-DPAT or 5-HT to the MRN-stimulated rat locomotor activity and exploratory behavior, but similar results were not observed with DRN applications (Hillegaart et al. 1989; Hillegaart and Hjorth 1989). These results may be related to data from earlier studies indicating that electrolytic lesions of the MRN reduced 5-HT concentrations in the hippocampus 82%, while lesions of the DRN produced 5-HT reductions of only 10%, although 5-HT reductions in the cortex and striatum (30%–40%) and hypothalamus (60%) were similar after MRN and DRN lesions (Jacobs et al. 1974). Electrolytic lesions of the MRN, but not the DRN or control lesions in another brain area, produced sustained, 100% increases in locomotor activity in rats; these changes were similar to those which followed lesions placed directly in the dorsal hippocampus, in agreement with the MRN vs DRN lesion effects on 5-HT concentrations in the hippocampus, and a proposed role for modulation of locomotor activity by hippocampal 5-HT (Jacobs et al. 1974, 1975).

The extent to which these examples of DRN vs MRN differences in structure and function have implications for the other B1–B9 grouping of 5-HT cell bodies in the raphe and nonraphe areas of the rodent brain is not yet clear, although there is considerable evidence of different physiological and behavioral functions being mediated by the descending vs ascending projections from these different serotonergic cell body groups, and other evidence of functional differences among different ascending 5-HT projections (Consolazione and Cuello 1982; Azmitia 1987).

While evidence for multiple 5-HT neuronal subsystems is accumulating from studies in rodents, less is known about primate, including human, brain 5-HT subsystems. Some general similarities exist between rat and primate 5-HT neuroanatomy, but recent reviews (Azmitia 1987; Takeuchi 1988) have noted some substantial differences. In rats, the majority of serotonergic cell body groups are indeed in the raphe nuclei, with cells clustered tightly in the midline; in primates, relatively few cells lie directly in the midline, but are more scattered, with a paramedian organization. While the DRN is the most prominent nuclear group in the rat, the MRN equivalent (the nucleus centralis superior, with its dorsalis portion) is larger and comprises the major group of ascending 5-HT neurons in primates. Also in primates, the dorsal raphe cortical tract contains more ascending fibers than does the median forebrain bundle, the reverse of the situation in the rat. Also, more myelinated 5-HT fibers (approximately 25%) are found in primates than in the rat (<1%) (Azmitia 1987; Takeuchi 1988).

3.2 Multiple Synaptic and Nonsynaptic Serotonergic Terminals

Direct synaptic contacts appear to be the exception rather than the rule of 5-HT neurons; that is, only 5%–40% of 5-HT varicosities in different rodent brain regions make synaptic junctions (Descarries et al. 1990). This data has been interpreted as indicating a more common neuromodulatory role for 5-HT. When 5-HT acts as a direct synaptic neurotransmitter in brain, some unexpectedly complex actions have been observed. In a study using intracellular recording of rat single cortical pyramidal cells, evidence was found for two distinct, functional 5-HT receptors on the same cell (Davies et al. 1987). Activation of these two receptors by 5-HT produced opposing effects on membrane potentials and conductance. A depolarizing effect of 5-HT (probably produced by decreasing a resting K^+ conductance) was blocked by the 5-HT antagonists ritanserin and cinanserin. A hyperpolarizing effect of 5-HT associated with a state of increased conductance was insensitive to these 5-HT_2 antagonists, but could be mimicked by 8-OH-DPAT (Davies et al. 1987).

3.3 Serotonin Transport and the Tricyclic Binding Site

In regard to 5-HT reuptake, much still remains unknown about many aspects of the sequence of steps involved in this major mechanism for inactivating released 5-HT, and likewise for the release process itself. One issue was recently clarified, however. It now appears that the tricyclic antidepressant binding site that was once thought to be a closely associated modulatory site separate from the 5-HT uptake site is, rather, one and the same, i.e., [^{3}H]paroxetine and other highly selective ligands for what was originally described as the [^{3}H]imipramine binding site actually bind directly and solely to the 5-HT uptake site itself (Marcusson et al. 1988, 1989; Graham et al. 1989).

Significant progress has been made towards the purification of the 5-HT uptake site (Graham and Langer 1988), but molecular biological studies have not yet been reported. Autoradiographic studies using [^{3}H]paroxetine and other ligands have revealed considerable diversity in numbers of binding sites in different brain areas (Fuxe et al. 1983; Kovachich et al. 1988). Similar results have been obtained in studies in human brain (Cortes et al. 1988; Plenge et al. 1990). Cortical areas contain relatively few 5-HT uptake sites, while the substantia nigra, among different projection areas, contains a relatively high number of sites. The raphe nuclei possess the highest density of sites, a finding interpreted as reflecting the possibility that the entire 5-HT neuron – not only terminals but the cell body dendrites and axons – possess 5-HT uptake capacity (Fuxe et al. 1983). This would seem to open the door to speculation about effects of uptake inhibiting drugs directly on the 5-HT cell body as well as at terminals.

3.4 Synthetic and Degradatory Enzymes for Serotonin

Tryptophan hydroxylase, the principal enzyme in 5-HT synthesis, has been cloned and sequenced from preparations of rat and rabbit pineal bodies. The enzyme shows considerable homology with phenylalanine hydroxylase (58% identity) and tyrosine hydroxylase (46% identity) and has been mapped to the human chromosome 11 (Darmon et al. 1986, 1988; Grenett et al. 1987; Ledley et al. 1987).

Aromatic L-amino acid decarboxylase (AADC), which converts 5-HTP to 5-HT, appears to be a single enzyme serving general decarboxylase functions in neuronal (brain, adrenal) and nonneuronal (liver, kidney) tissues; this conclusion is based on an aggregate of studies of immunological cross-reactivity, molecular size, biochemical properties, and hybridization analysis using a cDNA probe complementary to bovine adrenal AADC mRNA which indicated the presence of a single mRNA in these different tissues (Albert et al. 1987; Shirota and Fujisawa 1988). Southern blot analysis of bovine genomic DNA suggests that a single gene codes for AADC (Albert et al. 1987).

Monoamine oxidase (MAO), the principal degradatory enzyme for 5-HT, exists in two forms, MAO-A and MAO-B. While 5-HT is a better substrate for MAO-A than MAO-B, 5-HT cell bodies in brain and in human platelets (which selectively take up and store 5-HT) contain MAO-B either exclusively or predominantly (Thorpe et al. 1987; Donnelly and Murphy 1977). Nonetheless, there is functional evidence that serotonergic synaptosomes preferentially deaminate 5-HT by MAO-A (Ross 1987). Recently, both MAO-A and MAO-B have been sequenced and cloned, and it is now clear that separate genes located closely together on the short arm of the X chromosome encode MAO-A and MAO-B (Hsu et al. 1989). Humans with an X chromosome deletion and lacking both forms of MAO have markedly reduced urinary concentrations of the deaminated norepinephrine metabolite MHPG but, surprisingly, near normal urinary concentrations of the 5-HT metabolite 5-HIAA (Sims et al. 1989a,b; Murphy et al. 1990b).

4 Overview

In conclusion, there is now considerable, detailed information indicating that there are not only multiple 5-HT receptor subtypes, but also multiple anatomical and functional brain 5-HT subsystems. Considerable progress in the clinical applications of selective agents has resulted from the preclinical development of potent and selective 5-HT receptor ligands, each of which allows modification of specific 5-HT receptor subtypes and/or 5-HT subsystems. Activation/inhibition of a given 5-HT cell body by selective agonists/antagonists may lead to very different consequences, depending upon the cell subtypes of origin, their projection networks, and, of course, the multiple pre- and postsynaptic receptors that various transmitter/cotransmitter systems may activate. From the observations to date, it is likely that the clinical indications for selective 5-HT receptor subtype drugs will increase substantially in the years ahead.

The complexity of serotonergic subsystems has also obvious implications for cautious interpretation of the meaning of any changes in global measures such as 5-HIAA or 5-HT in brain tissue, cerebrospinal fluid, or other body fluids; changes in 5-HT receptor densities; or responses to 5-HT precursors such as L-tryptophan and to 5-HT semiselective as well as 5-HT receptor subtype selective agents that may reflect the interactive consequences of many changes in the multiple 5-HT subsystems. Nevertheless, the development of new, even more selective agents will facilitate the assessment of 5-HT receptor subtype responsivity and its involvement in the mechanisms of action of 5-HT receptor subtype selective drugs.

References

Albert VR, Allen JM, Joh TH (1987) A single gene codes for aromatic L-amino acid decarboxylase in both neuronal and non-neuronal tissues. J Biol Chem 262:9404–9411

Andrade R, Nicoll RA (1987) Novel anxiolytics discriminate between postsynaptic serotonin receptors mediating different physiological responses on single neurons of the rat hippocampus. Naunyn Schmiedebergs Arch Pharmacol 336:5–10

Azmitia EC (1987) The CNS serotonergic system: progression toward a collaborative organization. In: Meltzer HY (ed) Psychopharmacology: the third generation of progress. Raven, New York, pp 61–74

Barnes JM, Barnes NM, Costall B, Naylor RJ, Tyers MB (1989) 5-HT3 receptors mediate inhibition of acetylcholine release in cortical tissue. Nature 338:762–763

Basse-Tomusk A, Rebec GV (1986) Ipsapirone depresses neuronal activity in the dorsal raphe nucleus and the hippocampal formation. Eur J Pharmacol 130:141–143

Berendsen HHG, Jenck F, Broekkamp CLE (1990) Involvement of 5-HT_{1C}-receptors in drug-induced penile erections in rats. Psychopharmacology (Berl) 101:57–61

Blue ME, Yagaloff KA, Mamounas LA, Hartig PR, Molliver ME (1988) Correspondence between 5-HT_2 receptors and serotonergic axons in rat neocortex. Brain Res 453:315–328

Bowers MB (1987) The role of drugs in the production of schizophreniform psychoses and related disorders. In: Meltzer HY (ed) Psychopharmacology: the third generation of progress. Raven, New York, pp 819–823

Carli M, Prontera C, Samanin R (1989) Evidence that central 5-hydroxytryptaminergic neurones are involved in the anxiolytic activity of buspirone. Br J Pharmacol 96:829–836

Ceulemans DLS, Hoppenbrouwers M-LJA, Gelders YG, Reyntjens AJM (1985a) The influence of ritanserin, a serotonin antagonist, in anxiety disorders: a double-blind placebo-controlled study versus lorazepam. Pharmacopsychiatry 18:303–305

Ceulemans DLS, Gelders Y, Hoppenbrouwers M-L, Reyntjens A, Janssen P (1985b) Effect of serotonin antagonism in schizophrenia: a pilot study with setoperone. Psychopharmacology (Berl) 85:329–332
Charney DS, Woods SW, Goodman WK, Heninger GR (1987) Serotonin function in anxiety. II. Effects of the serotonin agonist m-CPP in panic disorder patients and healthy subjects. Psychopharmacology (Berl) 92:14–24
Charney DS, Goodman WK, Price LH, Woods SW, Rasmussen SA, Heninger GR (1988) Serotonin function in obsessive-compulsive disorder: a comparison of the effects of tryptophan and m-chlorophenylpiperazine in patients and healthy subjects. Arch Gen Psychiatry 45:177–185
Cohn JB, Bowden CL, Fisher JG, Rodos JJ (1986) Double-blind comparison of buspirone and clorazepate in anxious outpatients. Am J Med 80 Suppl 3B:10–16
Conrad LC, Leonard CM, Pfaff DW (1974) Connections of the median and dorsal raphe nuclei in the rat: an autoradiographic and degeneration study. J Comp Neurol 156:179–205
Consolazione A, Cuello AC (1982) CNS serotonin pathways. In: Osborne NN (ed) Biology of serotonergic transmission. Wiley, Chichester, pp 29–61
Cortes R, Soriano E, Pazos A, Probst A, Palacios JM (1988) Autoradiography of antidepressant binding sites in the human brain: localization using [^{3}H]imipramine and [^{3}H]paroxetine. Neuroscience 27:473–496
Costall B, Domeney AM, Naylor RJ, Tyers MB (1987) Effects of the 5-HT3 receptor antagonist, GR38032F, on raised dopaminergic activity in the mesolimbic system of the rat and marmoset brain. Br J Pharmacol 92:881–894
Costall B, Naylor RJ, Tyers MB (1990) The pharmacology of 5-HT_3 receptors. Pharmacol Ther 47:181–202
Cowen PJ, Anderson IM, Grahame-Smith DG (1990) Neuroendocrine effects of azapirones. J Clin Psychopharmacol 10:21S–25S
Csanalosi I, Schweizer E, Case WG, Rickels K (1987) Gepirone in anxiety: a pilot study. J Clin Psychopharmacol 7:31–33
Curzon G, Kennett GA (1990) m-CPP: a tool for studying behavioral responses associated with 5-HT_{1C} receptors. Trends Pharmacol Sci 11:181–182
Darmon MC, Grima B, Cash CD, Maitre M, Mallet J (1986) Isolation of a rat pineal gland cDNA clone homologous to tyrosine and phenylalanine hydroxylases. FEBS Lett 206:43–46
Darmon MC, Guibert B, Leviel V, Ehret M, Maitre M, Mallet J (1988) Sequence of two mRNAs encoding active rat tryptophan hydroxylase. J Neurochem 51:312–316
Davies MF, Deisz RA, Prince DA, Peroutka SJ (1987) Two distinct effects of 5-hydroxytryptamine on single cortical neurons. Brain Res 423:347–352
Descarries L, Audet MA, Doucet G, Garcia S, Oleskevich S, Seguela P, Soghomonian JJ, Watkins KC (1990) Morphology of central serotonin neurons: brief review of quantified aspects of their distribution and ultrastructural relationships. Ann NY Acad Sci 600:81–92
Donnelly CH, Murphy DL (1977) Substrate- and inhibitor-related characteristics of human platelet monoamine oxidase. Biochem Pharmacol 26:853–858
Eison AS, Eison MS, Stanley M, Riblet LA (1986) Serotonergic mechanisms in the behavioral effects of buspirone and gepirone. Pharmacol Biochem Behav 24:701–707
Eklund K, Dunhar GC, Pinder RM, Steffensen K (1985) Minaserin and imipramine in the treatment of elderly depressed patients. Acta Psychiatr Scand 72:54–59
Engel G, Gothert M, Muller-Schweinitzer E, Schlicker E, Sistonen L, Stadler PA (1983) Evidence for common pharmacological properties of [^{3}H]5-hydroxytryptamine binding sites, presynaptic 5-hydroxytryptamine autoreceptors in CNS and inhibitory presynaptic 5-hydroxytryptamine receptors on sympathetic nerves. Naunyn Schmiedebergs Arch Pharmacol 324:116–124
Engel G, Gothert M, Hoyer D, Schlicker E, Hillenbrand K (1987) Identity of inhibitory presynaptic 5-hydroxytryptamine (5-HT) autoreceptors in the rat brain cortex with 5-HT_{1B} binding sites. Naunyn Schmiedebergs Arch Pharmacol 332:1–7

Fozard JR, Gray JA (1989) $5\text{-}HT_{1C}$ receptor activation: a key step in the initiation of migraine? Trends Pharmacol Sci 10(8):307–309
Frazer A, Maayani S, Wolfe BB (1990) Subtypes of receptors for serotonin. Annu Rev Pharmacol Toxicol 30:307–348
Fritschy JM, Lyons WE, Molliver ME, Grzanna R (1988) Neurotoxic effects of p-chloroamphetamine on the serotoninergic innervation of the trigeminal motor nucleus: a retrograde transport study. Brain Res 473:261–270
Fuxe K, Calza L, Benfenati F, Zini I, Agnati LF (1983) Quantitative autoradiographic localization of [^{3}H]imipramine binding sites in the brain of the rat: relationship to ascending 5-hydroxytryptamine neuron systems. Proc Natl Acad Sci USA 80:3836–3840
Gaddum JH, Picarelli ZP (1957) Two kinds of tryptamine receptor. Br J Pharmacol 12:323–328
Gelders Y, Vanden Bussche G, Reyntjens A, Janssen P (1986) Serotonin-S2 receptor blockers in the treatment of chronic schizophrenia. Clin Neuropharmacol 9 Suppl 4:325–327
Glaser T (1988) Ipsapirone, a potent and selective $5\text{-}HT_{1A}$-receptor ligand with anxiolytic and antidepressant properties. Drugs Future 13:429–439
Glitz DA, Pohl R (1991) $5\text{-}HT_{1A}$ partial agonists: what is their future? Drugs 41:11–18
Goa KL, Ward A (1986) Buspirone: a preliminary review of its pharmacological properties and therapeutic efficacy as an anxiolytic. Drugs 32:114–129
Graham D, Langer SZ (1988) The neuronal sodium-dependent serotonin transporter: studies with [3H]imipramine and [3H]paroxetine. In: Osborne NN, Hamon M (eds) Neuronal serotonin. Wiley, Chichester, pp 367–391
Graham D, Esnaud H, Habert E, Langer SZ (1989) A common binding site for tricyclic and nontricyclic 5-hydroxytryptamine uptake inhibitors at the substrate recognition site of the neuronal sodium-dependent 5-hydroxytryptamine transporter. Biochem Pharmacol 38:3819–3826
Grenett HE, Ledley FD, Reed LL, Woo SL (1987) Full-length cDNA for rabbit tryptophan hydroxylase: functional domains and evolution of aromatic amino acid hydroxylases. Proc Natl Acad Sci USA 84:5530–5534
Hamik A, Peroutka SJ (1989) 1-(m-Chlorophenyl)piperazine (mCPP) interactions with neurotransmitter receptors in the human brain. Biol Psychiatry 25:569–575
Hillegaart V, Hjorth S (1989) Median raphe, but not dorsal raphe, application of the $5\text{-}HT_{1A}$ agonist 8-OH-DPAT stimulates rat motor activity. Eur J Pharmacol 160:303–307
Hillegaart V, Ahlenius S, Larsson K (1989) Effects of local application of 5-HT into the median and dorsal raphe nuclei on male rat sexual and motor behavior. Behav Brain Res 33:279–286
Hollander E, Fay M, Cohen B, Campeas R, Gorman JM, Liebowitz MR (1988) Serotonergic and noradrenergic sensitivity in obsessive-compulsive disorder: behavioral findings. Am J Psychiatry 145:1015–1017
Hoyer D (1988) Functional correlates of serotonin $5\text{-}HT_1$ recognition sites. J Recept Res 8:59–81
Hoyer D (1990) Serotonin $5\text{-}HT_3$, $5\text{-}HT_4$, and 5-HT-M receptors. Neuropsychopharmacology 3:371–383
Hoyer D, Middlemiss DN (1989) Species differences in the pharmacology of terminal 5-HT autoreceptors in mammalian brain. Trends Pharmacol Sci 10:130–132
Hoyer D, Pazos A, Probst A, Palacios JM (1986a) Serotonin receptors in the human brain. I. Characterization and autoradiographic localization of $5\text{-}HT_{1A}$ recognition sites: apparent absence of $5\text{-}HT_{1B}$ recognition sites. Brain Res 376:85–96
Hoyer D, Pazos A, Probst A, Palacios JM (1986b) Serotonin receptors in the human brain. II. Characterization and autoradiographic localization of $5\text{-}HT_{1C}$ and $5\text{-}HT_2$ recognition sites. Brain Res 376:97–107
Hoyer D, Waeber C, Pazos A, Probst A, Palacios JM (1988) Identification of a $5\text{-}HT_1$ recognition site in human brain membranes different from $5\text{-}HT_{1A}$, $5\text{-}HT_{1B}$ and $5\text{-}HT_{1C}$ sites. Neurosci Lett 85:357–362

Hsu YP, Powell JF, Sims KB, Breakefield XO (1989) Molecular genetics of the monoamine oxidases. J Neurochem 53:12–18

Jocobs BL, Wise WD, Taylor KM (1974) Differential behavioral and neurochemical effects following lesions of the dorsal or median raphe nuclei in rats. Brain Res 79:353–361

Jacobs BL, Trimbach C, Eubanks EE, Trulson M (1975) Hippocampal mediation of raphe lesion- and PCPA-induced hyperactivity in the rat. Brain Res 94:253–261

Jones BJ, Costall B, Domeney AM, Kelly ME, Naylor RJ, Oakley NR, Tyers MB (1988) The potential anxiolytic activity of GR38032F, a 5-HT3-receptor antagonist. Br J Pharmacol 93:985–993

Kahn RS, Wetzler S, Van Praag HM, Asnis GM, Strauman T (1988) Behavioral indiactions for serotonin receptor hypersensitivity in panic disorder. Psychiatry Res 25:101–104

Kennett GA, Curzon G (1988a) Evidence that hypophagia induced by m-CPP and TFMPP requires 5-HT_{1C} and 5-HT_{1B} receptors; hypophagia induced by RU24969 only requires 5-HT_{1B} receptors. Psychopharmacology (Berl) 96:93–100

Kennett GA, Curzon G (1988b) Evidence that m-CPP may have behavioral effects mediated by central 5-HT_{1C} receptors. Br J Pharmacol 94:137–147

Kennett GA, Whitton P, Shah K, Curzon G (1989) Anxiogenic-like effects of mCPP and TFMPP in animal models are opposed by 5-HT_{1C} receptor antagonists. Eur J Pharmacol 164(3):445–454

Kohler C, Steinbusch H (1982) Identification of serotonin and non-serotonin-containing neurons of the mid-brain raphe projecting to the entorhinal area and the hippocampal formation. A combined immunohistochemical and fluorescent retrograde tracing study in the rat brain. Neuroscience 7:951–975

Kosofsky BE, Molliver ME (1987) The serotoninergic innervation of cerebral cortex: different classes of axon terminals arise from dorsal and median raphe nuclei. Synapse 1:153–168

Kovachich GB, Aronson CE, Brunswick DJ, Frazer A (1988) Quantitative autoradiography of serotonin uptake sites in rat brain using [^{3}H]cyanoimipramine. Brain Res 454:78–88

Lader MH (1991) Ondansetron in the treatment of anxiety. In: The role of ondansetron, a novel 5-HT_3 antagonist, in the treatment of psychiatric disorders. 5th World Congress of Biological Psychiatry, Satellite Symposium, abstract book, pp 17–19

Ledley FD, Grenett HE, Bartos DP, van Tuinen P, Ledbetter DH, Woo SL (1987) Assignment of human tryptophan hydroxylase locus to chromosome 11: gene duplication and translocation in evolution of aromatic amino acid hydroxylases. Somat Cell Mol Genet 13:575–580

Lesch KP (1991) The ipsapirone/5-HT_{1A} receptor challenge in anxiety disorders and depression. In: Stahl SM, Gastpar M, Keppel Hesselink J, Traber J (eds) Serotonin 1A receptors in depression and anxiety. New York, Raven, pp 135–162

Lesch KP, Hoh A, Disselkamp-Tietze J, Wiesmann M, Osterheider M, Schulte HM (1991) 5-Hydroxytryptamine$_{1A}$ receptor responsivity in obsessive-compulsive disorder: comparison of patients and controls. Arch Gen Psychiatry 48:540–547

Mamounas LA, Molliver ME (1988) Evidence for dual serotonergic projections to neocortex: Axons from the dorsal and median raphe nuclei are differentially vulnerable to the neurotoxin p-chloroamphetamine (PCA). Exp Neurol 102:23–36

Marcusson JO, Bergstrom M, Eriksson K, Ross SB (1988) Characterization of [^{3}H]paroxetine binding in rat brain. J Neurochem 50:1783–1790

Marcusson JO, Andersson A, Backstrom I (1989) Drug inhibition indicates a single-site model of the 5-HT uptake site/antidepressant binding site in rat and human brain. Psychopharmacology (Berl) 99:17–21

Marsden CA (1988) 5-Hydroxytryptamine receptor subtypes and new anxiolytic drugs: an appraisal. In: Tyrer P (ed) Psychopharmacology of anxiety. Oxford University Press, Oxford, pp 3–27

McKenna DJ, Nazarali AJ, Hoffman AJ, Nichols DE, Mathis CA, Saavedra JM (1989) Common receptors for hallucinogens in rat brain: a comparative autoradiographic study using [^{125}I]LSD and [^{125}I]DOI, a new psychotomimetic radioligand. Brain Res 476:45–56

Meek JL, Lofstrandh S (1976) Tryptophan hydroxylase in discrete brain nuclei: comparison activity in vitro and in vivo. Eur J Pharmacol 37:377–380

Meltzer HY (1989) Clozapine: clinical advantages and biologic mechanisms. In: Schulz SC, Tamminga CA (eds) Schizophrenia: scientific progress. Oxford University Press, New York, pp 302–309

Meltzer HY (1991) Studies of ondansetron in schizophrenia. In: The role of ondansetron, a novel 5-HT$_3$ antagonist, in the treatment of psychiatric disorders. 5th World Congress of Biological Psychiatry, Satellite Symposium, abstract book, pp 25–27

Molliver ME (1987) Serotonergic neuronal systems: what their anatomic organization tells us about function. J Clin Psychopharmacol 7 Suppl 6:3S–23S

Moore RY, Halaris AE (1975) Hippocampal innervation by serotonin neurons of the midbrain raphe in the rat. J Comp Neurol 164:171–183

Mueller EA, Murphy DL, Sunderland T (1985) Neuroendocrine effects of m-chlorophenylpiperazine, a serotonin agonist, in humans. J Clin Endocrinol Metab 61:1179–1184

Murphy DL, Mueller EA, Hill JL, Tolliver TJ, Jacobsen FM (1989) Comparative anxiogenic, neuroendocrine, and other physiologic effects of m-chlorophenylpiperazine given intravenously or orally to healthy volunteers. Psychopharmacology (Berl) 98:275–282

Murphy DL, Pigott TA, Insel TR (1990a) Obsessive-compulsive disorder and anxiety. In: Burrows GD, Noyes R, Roth M (eds) Handbook of anxiety, vol 3. Elsevier, Amsterdam

Murphy DL, Sims KB, Karoum F, de la Chapelle A, Norio R, Sankila E-M, Breakefield XO (1990b) Marked amine and amine metabolite changes in Norrie disease patients with an X-chromosomal deletion affecting monoamine oxidase. J Neurochem 54:242–247

Neijt HC, Karpf A, Schoeffter P, Engel G, Hoyer D (1988) Characterization of 5-HT$_3$ recognition sites in membranes of NG 108-15 neuroblastoma-glioma cells with [^{3}H]ICS 205-930. Naunyn Schmiedebergs Arch Pharmacol 337:493–499

O'Hearn E, Battaglia G, DeSouza EB, Kuhar MJ, Molliver ME (1988) Methylenedioxyamphetamine (MDA) and methylenedioxymethamphetamine (MDMA) cause selective ablation of serotonergic axon terminals in forebrain: immunocytochemical evidence for neurotoxicity. J Neurosci 8:2788–2803

Pazos A, Palacios JM (1985) Quantitative autoradiographic mapping of serotonin receptors in the rat brain. I. Serotonin-1 receptors. Brain Res 346:205–230

Pazos A, Cortes R, Palacios JM (1985) Quantitative autoradiographic mapping of serotonin receptors in the rat brain. II. Serotonin-2 receptors. Brain Res 346:231–249

Pazos A, Probst A, Palacios JM (1987) Serotonin receptors in the human brain. III. Autoradiographic mapping of serotonin-1 receptors. Neuroscience 21:97–122

Peroutka SH, McCarthy BG (1989) Sumatriptan (GR 43175) interacts selectively with 5-HT$_{1B}$ and 5-HT$_{1D}$ binding sites. Eur J Pharmacol 163:133–136

Peroutka SJ, Snyder SH (1979) Multiple serotonin receptors: differential binding of ^{3}H-serotonin, ^{3}H-lysergic acid diethylamide and ^{3}H-spiroperidol. Mol Pharmacol 16:687–699

Peroutka SJ, Switzer JA, Hamik A (1989) Identification of 5-hydroxytryptamine$_{1D}$ binding sites in human brain membranes. Synapse 3:61–66

Plenge P, Mellerup ET, Laursen H (1990) Regional distribution of the serotonin transport complex in human brain, identified with ^{3}H-paroxetine, ^{3}H-citalopram and ^{3}H-imipramine. Prog Neuropsychopharmacol Biol Psychiatry 14:61–72

Raiteri M, Maura G, Bonanno G, Pittaluga A (1986) Differential pharmacology and function of two 5-HT$_1$ receptors modulating transmitter release in rat cerebellum. J Pharmacol Exp Ther 237:644–648

Ross SB (1987) Distribution of the two forms of monoamine oxidase within monoaminergic neurons of the guinea pig brain. J Neurochem 48:609–614

Shaller CF, Czupryna J, Salama AI (1990) 5-HT_2 receptor blockade by ICI 169,369 and other 5-HT_2 antagonists modulates the effects of D-2 dopamine receptor blockade. J Pharmacol Exp Ther 253:1162–1170
Sanders-Bush E (1988) The serotonin receptors. Humana, Clifton
Schmidt AW, Peroutka SJ (1989) 5-Hydroxytryptamine receptor "families". FASEB J 3:2242–2249
Schuckit MA (1984) Clinical studies of buspirone. Psychopathology 17 Suppl 3:61–68
Shirota K, Fujisawa H (1988) Purification and characterization of aromatic L-amino acid decarboxylase from rat kidney and monoclonal antibody to the enzyme. J Neurochem 51:426–434
Sims KB, de la Chapelle A, Norio R, Sankila E-M, Hsu Y-PP, Rinehart WB, Corey TJ, Ozelius L, Powell JF, Bruns G, Gusella JF, Murphy DL, Breakefield XO (1989a) Monoamine oxidase deficiency in males with an X chromosome deletion. Neuron 2:1069–1076
Sims KB, Ozelius L, Corey T, Rinehart WB, Liberfarb R, Haines J, Chen WJ, Norio R, Sankila E, de la Chapelle A, Murphy DL, Gusella J, Breakefield XO (1989b) Norrie disease gene is distinct from the monoamine oxidase genes. Am J Hum Genet 45:424–434
Sinton CM, Fallon SL (1988) Electrophysiological evidence for a functional differentiation between subtypes of the 5-HT1 receptor. Eur J Pharmacol 157:173–181
Sleight AJ, Pierce PA, Schmidt AW, Hekmatpanah CR, Peroutka SJ (1991) The clinical utility of serotonin receptor active agents in neuropsychiatric disease. In: Peroutka SJ (ed) Serotonin receptor subtypes: basic and clinical aspects. New York, Wiley, pp 211–227
Sprouse JS, Aghajanian GK (1987) Electrophysiological responses of serotonergic dorsal raphe neurons to 5-HT_{1A} and 5-HT_{1B} agonists. Synapse 1:3–9
Takeuchi Y (1988) Distribution of serotonin neurons in the mammalian brain. In: Osborne NN, Hamon M (eds) Neuronal serotonin. Wiley, New York, pp 25–56
Taylor DP (1988) Buspirone, a new approach to the treatment of anxiety. FASEB J 2:2445–2452
Taylor DP (1989) Serotonin agents in anxiety. Ann NY Acad Sci 600:545–557
Thorpe LW, Westlund KN, Kochersperger LM, Abell CW, Denney RM (1987) Immunocytochemical localization of monoamine oxidases A and B in human peripheral tissues and brain. J Histochem Cytochem 35:23–32
Titeler M, Lyon RA, Glennon RA (1988) Radioligand binding evidence implicates the brain 5-HT_2 receptor as a site of action for LSD and phenylisopropylamine hallucinogens. Psychopharmacology (Berl) 94:213–216
Traber J, Glaser T (1987) 5-HT_{1A} receptor-related anxiolytics. Trends Pharmacol Sci 8:432–437
Tyers MB, Costall B, Domeney A, Jones BJ, Kelly ME, Naylor RJ, Oakley NR (1987) The anxiolytic activities of 5-HT_3 antagonists in laboratory animals. Neurosci Lett 29 Suppl:S68
Ugedo L, Grenhoff J, Svensson TH (1989) Ritanserin, a 5-HT_2 receptor antagonist, activates midbrain dopamine neurons by blocking serotonergic inhibition. Psychopharmacology (Berl) 98:45–50
Vandermaelen CP, Matheson GK, Wilderman RC, Patterson LA (1986) Inhibition of serotonergic dorsal raphe neurons by systemic and iontophoretic administration of buspirone, a non-benzodiazepine anxiolytic drug. Eur J Pharmacol 129:123–130
Waeber C, Dietl MM, Hoyer D, Probst A, Palacios JM (1988) Visualization of a novel serotonin recognition site (5-HT_{1D}) in the human brain by autoradiography. Neurosci Lett 88:11–16
Wander TJ, Nelson A, Okazaki H, Richelson E (1987) Antagonism by neuroleptics of serotonin 5-HT_{1A} and 5-HT_2 receptors of normal human brain in vitro. Eur J Pharmacol 143:279–282
Whitaker-Azmitia PM, Peroutka SJ (1990) The neuropharmacology of serotonin. Ann NY Acad Sci 600:1–718

Whitton P, Curzon G (1990) Anxiogenic-like effect of infusing 1-(3-chlorophenyl) piperazine (mCPP) into the hippocampus. Psychopharmacology (Berl) 100(1):138–140

Zohar J, Mueller EA, Insel TR, Zohar-Kadouch RC, Murphy DL (1987) Serotonergic responsivity in obsessive-compulsive disorder: comparison of patients and healthy controls. Arch Gen Psychiatry 44:946–951

Serotonin Receptors and Antipsychotic Drug Action

H.Y. Meltzer

1 Introduction

The effect of serotonin (5-HT) to modulate dopaminergic activity in the nigrostriatal system has been known for some time (Dray et al. 1976). Generally, 5-HT has an inhibitory effect on dopaminergic output (see Meltzer and Nash 1991, for review). However, there is also evidence that 5-HT can enhance some aspects of dopaminergic function; thus, an over-simplistic one-way model should not be considered (Meltzer and Nash 1991). The effect of 5-HT in modulating dopaminergic activity is mediated via specific 5-HT receptors, the nature of which will be discussed subsequently. Due to the central role that antagonism of dopamine (DA) receptors has in the ability of antipsychotic drugs to reduce psychotic symptoms and in producing side effects such as extrapyramidal symptoms, tardive dyskinesia, and stimulation of prolactin secretion (Meltzer and Stahl 1976), it is necessary to consider whether serotonergic influences modulate the action of at least some antipsychotic drugs. As will be discussed, it has been suggested that serotonergic effects are particularly relevant to the action of clozapine and some other so-called atypical antipsychotic drugs (see Meltzer 1989; Deutch et al. 1991, for reviews). This article will consider the evidence for the action of antipsychotic drugs on specific 5-HT receptors as a contributing factor to their antipsychotic action or unique side effect profile.

2 Serotonin Receptors

Four "families" of 5-HT receptors have been identified by receptor binding methods and, in some instances, the genes which direct the synthesis of the receptor have been cloned. These families are the 5-HT_1, 5-HT_2, 5-HT_3, and 5-HT_4 receptors (Schmidt and Peroutka 1989). The molecular biology of these receptors is discussed in detail in other chapters in this book (see

Departments of Psychiatry and Pharmacology, Case Western Reserve University School of Medicine, Cleveland, OH 44106, USA

Ciaranello et al.; Hartig et al.). The receptors most clearly linked to the actions of antipsychotic drugs are the 5-HT_2, 5-HT_{1C}, and 5-HT_3 receptors and the effect of antipsychotic drugs on these receptors will be the major focus of this chapter. The 5-HT_2 and 5-HT_{1C} receptors, though nominally related to different families, share more common features with regard to molecular biology, pharmacology, and biochemistry than do the 5-HT_{1C} and other members of the 5-HT_1 family (5-$HT_{1A,B,C,D}$). Thus, the 5-HT_2 family and 5-HT_{1C} receptors are generally considered to be members of the 5-HT_2 family (Pazos et al. 1984; Yagaloff and Hartig 1985; Schmidt and Peroutka 1989; Julius et al. 1988, 1989).

The 5-HT_2 receptor is present in moderately high concentrations in the terminal regions of the A9 and A10 neurons, including the striatum, nucleus accumbens, and frontal cortex, but is present in low concentrations in the substantia nigra and ventral tegmentum (Pazos et al. 1985; McKenna et al. 1989). Thus, effects on 5-HT_2 receptors of direct-acting 5-HT_2 agonists, selective 5-HT_2 antagonists, or antipsychotics with 5-HT_2 antagonist properties which are produced at clinically relevant doses have the potential to modulate mesostriatal, mesolimbic, and mesocortical dopaminergic activity.

5-HT_{1C} receptor mRNA is present in many brain areas but is expressed in high concentrations only in the choroid plexus (Molineaux et al. 1989). It has been reported that mRNA levels of the 5-HT_{1C} receptor are high in the substantia nigra but not in the striatum and in the nucleus accumbens but not in the ventral tegmentum (Molineaux et al. 1989). Thus, if the mRNA is expressed under the right conditions, it is possible that 5-HT_{1C} agonists or antagonists could modulate mesostriatal and mesolimbic dopaminergic activity.

5-HT_3 receptors are present in the striatum, limbic region, and various regions of the cortex, although higher levels are present in hind brain areas (Palacios et al. 1990). They have been reported to have a direct effect in inhibiting DA release (Blandina et al. 1989; Imperato and Angelucci 1989). Thus, antipsychotic drugs with potent 5-HT_3 blocking properties at clinically effective doses may directly influence mesostriatal, mesolimbic, and mesocortical dopaminergic function by inhibiting 5-HT_3-mediated release of DA.

3 Classification of Typical and Atypical Antipsychotic Drugs

It has become commonplace to classify antipsychotic drugs as typical or atypical. The designation of a drug as antipsychotic is usually unambiguous. In humans, it should be able to alleviate positive symptoms (delusions, hallucinations, formal thought disorder) in schizophrenic patients in a double-blind, placebo-controlled trial or prevent the reemergence of such symptoms in a drug substitution trial, with a standard drug and preferably a placebo for comparison. The designation of an antipsychotic as typical is based upon its ability to produce extrapyramidal syndromes (EPS) and stimulate prolactin secretion at clinically effective doses. The rodent equivalent of EPS is catalepsy. Antipsychotic drugs are classified as atypical if they produce little or no EPS and in humans no or slight transient increases in prolactin secretion (Meltzer et al. 1989c). However, these drugs usually produce marked but brief increases in prolactin secretion in rodents (Meltzer et al. 1975; Gudelsky and Meltzer 1989). There are, however, some drugs which are sometimes labeled as atypical, e.g., the substituted benzamides and thioridazine, because of evidence that they produce low EPS. However, substituted benzamides and thioridazine produce marked increases in plasma prolactin levels in humans. Moreover, while some substituted benzamides, e.g., remoxipride (Lewander et al. 1990), may produce fewer EPS, this is not the case for sulpiride (Harnryd et al. 1984; Gerlach et al. 1985). There is some question whether amisulpride, a recently introduced benzamide, produces fewer EPS (Mann et al. 1984). The few EPS induced by thioridazine are most likely the result of thioridazine's potent anticholinergic properties (Miller and Hiley 1974), whereas the reason why the benzamides produce fewer EPS has not been entirely established. It may be due to selective action on D_2 receptors within the limbic system or a subgroup of striatal D_2 receptors. Relatively poor penetration into the brain has also been suggested as an explanation but seems unlikely (Köhler et al. 1990). It may be useful to designate those atypical antipsychotic drugs which do not produce EPS or elevate plasma prolactin in humans as type A (e.g., clozapine, fluperlapine) and those which do as type B (e.g., remoxipride, amisulpride). This review of the effects of antipsychotic drugs on 5-HT receptors will focus on the type A atypical antipsychotic drugs, since the type B atypicals are selective D_2 antagonists. Thioridazine seems to be best classified as a typical antipsychotic drug (Meltzer et al. 1989c).

4 Atypical Antipsychotic Drugs and DA Receptors

This section will consider the interaction of antipsychotic drugs in relation to their affinity for DA D_1, D_2, D_3, D_4, and D_5 receptors. D_2 receptor antagonism has been thought to be the major basis for the action of neuroleptic drugs, based on the high correlation between the log of antipsychotic dose and the log of the affinity for the striatal D_2 receptor (Creese et al. 1976; Seeman et al. 1975). It is now clear that interaction of antipsychotic drugs with other types of DA receptors is also of importance. It is beyond the scope of this review to discuss these issues in detail, except in so far as they affect the hypothesis concerning the mechanism of action of type A atypical antipsychotic drugs such as clozapine. Clozapine's affinity for the D_1 receptor is approximately the same as for the D_2 receptor. Both are relatively weak (Meltzer et al. 1989c). We have reviewed elsewhere the earlier evidence which suggested that clozapine has a unique effect compared to typical antipsychotic drugs on some subtypes of the D_1 receptor (Meltzer 1990a). Recently, the D_3 and D_5 receptors have been cloned (Sokoloff et al. 1990; Sunahara et al. 1991). The D_3 is a member of the D_2 family while the D_5 is a member of the D_1 family. The affinity of clozapine for the D_3 receptor was reported to be 180 ± 17 n*M* vs 56 ± 2 n*M* for the D_2 receptor. Although Sokoloff et al. (1990) suggested that the ability of both type A and type B atypical antipsychotic drugs to antagonize D_3 receptors might be related to their atypical properties, examination of the relative affinities for D_2 and D_3 receptors of the typical and atypical antipsychotic drugs does not suggest that a differential relationship exists. For example, chlorpromazine and pimozide, two typical drugs, have higher K_i D_2/K_i D_3 ratios (0.52 and 0.65, respectively) than do clozapine (0.31) and amisulpride (0.45). The other atypical drugs have much lower ratios than clozapine. Nevertheless, further study of the relevance of D_3 receptors to antipsychotic drug action is warranted on the basis of their localization, especially in the limbic area.

The D_4 receptor is an isoform of the D_2 receptor (Van Tol et al. 1991). It has been called the clozapine receptor because the affinity of clozapine for this receptor is nearly eight times greater than for the D_2 receptor. D_4 receptor mRNA is present in the mesolimbic and mesocortical system so it is a candidate for some of the important properties of clozapine in producing greater effects on positive and negative symptoms than typical neuroleptic drugs (Kane et al. 1988). It will be necessary to characterize the functional role of the D_4 receptor before it can be assigned the role of the clozapine receptor. It will be of particular interest to determine whether other atypical antipsychotic drugs of the type A variety, e.g., fluperlapine, melperone, sertindole, Org 5222 (see Meltzer 1991; Meltzer et al. 1989c; Meltzer and Nash 1991, for references), are also relatively more potent antagonists of the D_4 than the D_2 receptor.

5 Effect of Clozapine and Type A Atypical Antipsychotic Drugs on the Serotonergic System

There have been numerous studies of the effect of clozapine on 5-HT in rat brain. Clozapine has been reported to increase brain 5-HT concentrations (Maj et al. 1974; Burki et al. 1975; Ruch et al. 1976). However, in vivo studies of the effect of clozapine on 5-HT synthesis and release suggest only a small influence, if any (Ruch et al. 1976). Drescher and Hetey (1988) reported that clozapine enhanced 5-HT release in vitro from prelabeled rat nucleus accumbens synaptosomes by blocking 5-HT autoreceptors and DA heteroreceptors which inhibit 5-HT release. In vivo microdialysis studies found no effect of acute or chronic clozapine in enhancing the release of 5-

Table 1. pK_d or pK_i values of antipsychotic drugs

	5-HT_{1A}	5-HT_2	5-HT_{1C}	5-HT_3	References
Typical					
Chlorpromazine	5.5	8.7	7.9	5.1	3–6
Clothiapine	–	9.2	6.5	–	4, 6
Fluphenazine	4.4	8.6	7.0	<5.0	1, 4, 5, 7
Haloperidol	5.3	7.7	5.2	5.5	2, 4, 6
Loxapine	5.5	8.7	–	6.9	3–5
Spiperone	6.3	9.4	6.0	–	2, 4
Thioridazine	6.5	8.4	7.2	–	4, 5
Atypical					
Amperozide	7.10	8.0	<6.0	–	4, 8, 9
Clozapine	5.7	8.3	8.1	7.0	4–6, 10
Fluperlapine	–	8.1	–	–	4
Melperone	–	7.5	–	–	4
Sulpiride	–	<5	<5	–	6

References: 1, Barnes et al. (1989); 2, Hoyer (1988); 3, Hoyer et al. (1989); 4, Meltzer et al. (1989c); 5, Wander et al. (1987); 6, Canton et al. (1990); 7, Palacios and Hoyer (1989, personal communication); 8, Roth (1991, personal communication); 9, Svartengren and Simonsson (1990); 10, Watling et al. (1990).

hydroxyindoleacetic acid (5-HIAA) in the striatum of nucleus accumbens of awake freely moving rats (Ichikawa and Meltzer 1990, 1991).

6 In Vitro Receptor Binding of Antipsychotic Drugs to 5-HT Receptors

The pK_d or pK_i values for representative typical and type A atypical antipsychotic drugs are given in Table 1. The affinities of those antipsychotic drugs for the 5-HT_{1A} binding site which have been studied are quite low (Wander et al. 1987). The affinities of typical and atypical antipsychotic drugs for the 5-HT_2 binding site are more variable. We have presented evidence elsewhere, based upon the 20 typical and 17 type A atypical antipsychotic drugs, that there is no significant difference between the pK_i values of the 5-HT_2 binding site for these two groups of drugs (Meltzer et al. 1989c). The pK_i 5-HT_2/pK_i D_2 ratio and, to a lesser extent, the pK_i 5-HT_2/pK_i D_1 ratio did distinguish these two classes of drugs (Meltzer et al. 1989c). However, discriminant function analysis showed that only the pK_i values for the D_2 and the 5-HT_2 binding sites were needed to distinguish these two classes of drug. All but three of the type A atypical drugs had a weaker 5-HT_2 than D_2 profile whereas the reverse was true of the typical drugs. A stepwise discriminant function revealed that the D_1 affinity did not contribute to the classification of the drugs studied as typical or atypical. The 5-HT_2/D_2 ratio may not be the optimal way to express the difference between these classes of drugs. Rather, the differences between the pK_i values may be a more appropriate measure since log units are involved. The type A atypical antipsychotic drugs have a greater affinity for the $5\text{-}HT_2$ than the D_2 site by 1.30 log units, whereas the typical drugs are more potent antagonists at the D_2 than the $5\text{-}HT_2$ site by 0.26 log units. Thus, there is a 1.56 log unit (36.3-fold) difference between the two classes of antipsychotic drugs on average, suggesting that in vivo there should be marked differences in occupancy of $5\text{-}HT_2$ and D_2 receptors between the two groups. Specifically, $5\text{-}HT_2$ occupancy should be greater than D_2 occupancy in the cortex and limbic system and striatum at atypical drug doses which result in only partial occupation of D_2 sites (Meltzer et al. 1990; Meltzer and Nash 1991; Meltzer and Stockmeier 1992). To the extent that $5\text{-}HT_2$ receptors mediate the serotonergic influence on dopaminergic neurotransmission, this may be highly relevant.

There is very little data on $5\text{-}HT_{1C}$ and $5\text{-}HT_3$ binding of antipsychotic drugs. It has been reported that clozapine has a greater affinity for the $5\text{-}HT_{1C}$ than the $5\text{-}HT_2$ site (Canton et al. 1990); however, this needs to be confirmed. The affinity of other atypical antipsychotic drugs for the $5\text{-}HT_{1C}$ site, with the exception of fluperlapine, is relatively weak. Chlorpromazine has a high affinity for the $5\text{-}HT_{1C}$ site relative to clozapine when adjustment is made for clinical dose. Available data suggest that the $5\text{-}HT_{1C}/D_2$ ratio does not differentiate between typical and atypical antipsychotic drugs as well as the $5\text{-}HT_2/D_2$ ratio does (Meltzer and Nash 1992). Further study of the affinity of other typical and atypical antipsychotic drugs for the $5\text{-}HT_{1C}$ is needed.

As previously indicated, $5\text{-}HT_3$ receptor agonists may stimulate DA release while $5\text{-}HT_3$ antagonists may have the opposite effect and would therefore be of interest as antipsychotic drugs (Costall et al. 1990). Clozapine has a moderate affinity for the $5\text{-}HT_3$ receptor (Watling et al. 1990) and has been found to antagonize the inhibitory effect of the $5\text{-}HT_3$ agonist 2-methylserotonin on cortical neurons (Ashby et al. 1989). The affinity of clozapine for the $5\text{-}HT_3$ receptor ($pK_i = 7.0$; Watling et al. 1990) is the same as that for the D_2 receptor (Meltzer et al. 1989c) suggesting that $5\text{-}HT_3$ receptor blockade might be contributing to its mechanism of action.

7 In Vivo Receptor Occupancy

In vivo binding studies are of significant value in determining whether the in vitro affinities reflect what is happening in specific brain regions following systemic drug administration. There may be significant differences between in vitro affinities and in vivo effects because of differences in absorption, metabolism, binding to plasma proteins, whole body and regional brain differences in distribution, and intracerebral metabolism. We have studied

Table 2. ED_{50} values for blockade of cortical 5-HT_2 and striatal and olfactory tubercle D_2 binding of [^{3}H]N-methylspiperone

Drug	ED_{50}		
	Cortex	Striatum	Olfactory tubercle
Ritanserin	>20	>20	1.0
Raclopride	3.4	3.2	>30
Haloperidol	0.13	0.17	1.5
Clozapine	16.9	5.5	0.73
Amperozide	≫40	≫40	1.07

the in vivo binding of a group of typical and atypical antipsychotic drugs to frontal cortical 5-HT_2 and striatal and olfactory tubercle (OT) D_2 binding sites using [^{3}H]N-methylspiperone (NMSP) as a ligand (Meltzer et al. 1990). A more extensive group of typical and atypical drugs has been studied (Stockmeier and Meltzer, in preparation). The dose which produced 50% occupancy of cortical 5-HT_2 and striatal and OT D_2 binding sites was determined by pretreating groups of male Sprague-Dawley rodents with five to six doses of a given antipsychotic drug. The ED_{50} values for a group of typical and atypical antipsychotic drugs to block cortical 5-HT_2 and striatal and OT D_2 sites are given in Table 2. Ritanserin had no effect on [^{3}H]NMSP binding in the striatal and OT, despite a pK_i of 7.9 for the striatal D_2 receptor in vitro (Meltzer et al. 1989c). This indicates that in vivo ritanserin has no significant effect on the D_2 binding site, at least acutely, and illustrates how the in vitro binding data may be misleading. There was no effect on cortical 5-HT_2 sites, indicating that ritanserin is a selective D_2 antagonist in vivo. Haloperidol was 10 times more potent at D_2 than 5-HT_2 sites and had an equivalent action at the limbic and striatal D_2 sites. By contrast, clozapine had a threefold greater effect at the limbic (OT) D_2 binding site than on the striatal D_2 site but was 23 and 7.5 times more potent at cortical 5-HT_2 than striatal and OT D_2 sites in vivo, consistent with the in vitro data. Amperozide, a novel atypical antipsychotic drug (Mertens et al. 1989), had no effect on striatal or OT D_2 occupancy. At the low doses used clinically, it should not occupy any D_2 sites if this rodent data can be extrapolated to humans. This will be discussed subsequently.

8 Clozapine and Other Atypical Antipsychotic Drugs as 5-HT_2 Antagonists In Vivo

There is extensive evidence that clozapine, fluperlapine, melperone, and amperozide can antagonize the effect of 5-HT itself and of 5-HT_2 agonists in particular (see Meltzer 1990b, for references). For example, clozapine can block the effect of MK-212, a $5\text{-HT}_2/5\text{-HT}_{1C}$ agonist, on rat corticosterone secretion and MK-212-induced hyperthermia (Nash et al. 1988). Melperone, fluperlapine, and amperozide also block the effects of $5\text{-HT}_2/5\text{-HT}_{1C}$ stimulation in rodents (Nash et al. 1988; Christensson and Björk 1990). We have found that clozapine can block the effect of 5-HTP and MK-212 on cortisol secretion in humans (Meltzer 1988), an indication of 5-HT_2 antagonism. Thus, it is quite possible that 5-HT_2 antagonism may be a component of the action of clozapine and other atypical antipsychotic drugs.

Clozapine has been found to down-regulate the number of cortical 5-HT_2 receptors even following a single administration (Helmeste and Tang 1983; Matsubara and Meltzer 1989). This effect is, however, shared by typical neuroleptics such as ioxapine and is not common to the action of all type A atypical drugs, e.g., melperone (Matsubara and Meltzer 1989; Andree et al. 1986). Therefore, it is unlikely to be important to the action of atypical antipsychotic drugs.

9 Role of 5-HT_2 Antagonism in the Action of Clozapine and Type A Atypical Antipsychotic Drugs

If any of the effects of clozapine and other type A atypical antipsychotic drugs on 5-HT receptors is important, it seems most likely to be a potent 5-HT_2 receptor antagonism compared to weak D_2 antagonism. The critical issue appears to be how much D_2 antagonism is present along with 5-HT_2 antagonism. Farde et al. (1989), using C-raclopride, have demonstrated that clozapine produces 40%–50% occupancy of *striatal* D_2 receptors during clinical treatment compared to 80%–90% occupancy, even with low, perhaps subtherapeutic, doses of typical antipsychotics. The rodent in vivo binding data we have obtained (Table 2) are consistent with the low level occupancy of striatal D_2 receptors by clozapine, although greater limbic occupancy may occur in humans. Addition of a selective 5-HT_2 antagonist to a potent D_2 blocker such as haloperidol may not produce the equivalent of clozapine in terms of weak D_2 and strong 5-HT_2 receptor antagonism. Clinical trials of ritanserin alone or ritanserin plus haloperidol suggest that 5-HT_2 antagonism may improve positive and negative symptoms as well as diminish EPS (Bersani et al. 1986; Reyntjens et al. 1986), but these studies need to be replicated with better controls and determination of 5-HT_2 and D_2 occupancy with positron emission tomography if possible.

10 Conclusions

There is extensive preclinical evidence to support the biological basis for a 5-HT_2-mediated influence of dopaminergic activity (Meltzer 1988, 1989;

Meltzer and Nash 1991; Deutch et al. 1991). Through receptor-mediated interaction at the level of the cell bodies and terminal regions, 5-HT_2 antagonism may lead to a normalization of dopaminergic activity that is not possible with D_2 receptor blockade alone. For example, chronic clozapine was reported not to diminish DA release in the nucleus accumbens or the striatum compared to chronic haloperidol (Ichikawa and Meltzer 1990).

To argue for the importance of 5-HT_2 antagonism relative to D_2 antagonism for clozapine does not imply that other effects of clozapine, such as antagonism of D_1 or D_4 receptors or effects on neurotensin, α_1-adrenergic receptors, or muscarinic receptors (see Meltzer 1991), are not also of importance. It may be, as we have suggested, that stronger 5-HT_2 antagonism relative to D_2 antagonism in an antipsychotic only serves to identify the drug as a candidate atypical antipsychotic drug (Meltzer et al. 1989c; Meltzer and Nash 1991). There are, in fact, a number of such atypical antipsychotic candidates which have now been identified, e.g., amperozide, sertindole, ICI 204-636, and Org 5222 (see Meltzer 1991; Meltzer and Nash 1991, for references). Clinical results of current studies with these agents will provide meaningful tests of this hypothesis.

Acknowledgements. The research reported was supported in part by USPHS MH 41684, GCRC MO1RR00080, the Department of Veterans Affairs, and a grant from the Cleveland Foundation. H.Y.M. is the recipient of a USPHS Research Career Scientist Award MH 47808. The secretarial assistance of Ms. Lee Mason is greatly appreciated.

References

Andree TH, Mikuni M, Tong CY, Koenig JI, Meltzer HY (1986) Differential effect of subchronic treatment with various neuroleptic agents on serotonin$_2$ receptors in rat cerebral cortex. J Neurochem 46:191–197

Ashby CR Jr, Edwards E, Harkius KL, Wang RY (1989) Differential effect of typical and atypical antipsychotic drugs on the suppressant action of 2-methylserotonin on medial prefrontal cortical cells: a micioiontophoretic study. Eur J Pharmacol 166: 583–584

Barnes JM, Barnes NM, Costall B, Ironside JW, Naylor RJ (1989) Identification and characterizations of 5-hydroxytryptamine$_3$ recognition sites in human brain tissue. J Neurochem 53:1787–1793

Bersani G, Grispini A, Marini S, Pasini A, Valducci M, Ciani N (1986) Neuroleptic-induced extrapyramidal side effects: clinical perspectives with ritanserin (R35667), a new selective 5-HT_2 receptor blocking agent. Curr Ther Res 40:492–499

Blandina P, Goldfarb J, Craddock-Royal B, Green JP (1989) Release of endogenous dopamine by stimulation of 5-hydroxytryptamine receptors in rat striatum. J Pharmacol Exp Ther 251:803–809

Burki HR, Ruch W, Asper H (1975) Effects of clozapine, thioridazine, perlapine and haloperidol on the metabolism of the biogenic amines in the brain of the rat. Psychopharmacologia (Berl) 41:27–33

Canton H, Verrièle L, Colpaert FC (1990) Binding of typical and atypical antipsychotics to 5-HT_{1C} and 5-HT_2 sites: clozapine potently interacts with 5-HT_{1C} sites. Eur J Pharmacol 191:93–96

Christensson E, Björk A (1990) Amperozide: a new pharmacological approach in the treatment of schizophrenia. Pharmacol Toxicol Suppl 1:5–7
Costall B, Naylor R, Tyers M (1990) The psychopharmacology of 5-HT receptors. Pharmacol Ther 47:181–202
Creese I, Burt DR, Snyder SH (1976) Dopamine receptor binding predicts clinical and pharmacological potencies of antischizophrenic drugs. Science 192:481–483
Deutch AY, Moghaddam B, Innis RB, Krystal JH, Aghajanian GK, Bunney BS, Charney DS (1991) Mechanisms of action of atypical antipsychotic drugs. Implications for novel therapeutic strategies for schizophrenia. Schizophr Res 4:121–156
Dray A, Gonye TJ, Oakley NR, Tanner T (1976) Evidence for the existance of a raphe projection to the substantia nigra in rat. Brain Res 113:45–57
Drescher K, Hetey L (1988) Influence of antipsychotics and serotonin antagonists on presynaptic receptors modulating the release of serotonin in synaptosomes of the nucleus accumbens of rats. Neuropharmacology 27(1):31–36
Farde L, Wiesel FA, Nordstrom A-L, Sedvall G (1989) D1- and D2-dopamine receptor occupancy during treatment with conventional and atypical neuroleptics. Psychopharmacology (Berl) 99 Suppl:S-28–S-31
Gerlach J, Behuke K, Heltberg J, Munk-Anderson E, Nielsen H (1985) Sulpiride and haloperidol in schizophrenia: a double-blind cross over study of therapeutic efficacy, side effects and plasma concentrations. Br J Psychiatry 147:283–288
Gudelsky GA, Meltzer HY (1989) Activation of tuberoinfundibular dopamine neurons following the acute administration of atypical antipsychotics. Neuropsychopharmacology 2:45–51
Harnryd C, Bjerkenstedt L, Bjork K, Gullberg B, Oxenstierna G, Sedvall G, Weisel F-A, Wik G, Aberg-Wistedt A (1984) Clinical evaluation of sulpiride in schizophrenic patients–a double-blind comparison with chlorpromazine. Acta Psychiatr Scand 69 Suppl 311:7–20
Helmeste DM, Tang SW (1983) Unusual acute effects of antidepressants and neuroleptics on S_2-serotonergic receptors. Life Sci 33:2527–2533
Hoyer D (1988) Functional correlates of serotonin 5-HT_1 recognition sites. J Recept Res 8:59–81
Hoyer D, Gozlan H, Bolanos F, Schechter LE, Hamon M (1989) Interaction of psychotropic drugs with central 5-HT_3 recognition sites: fact or artifact. Eur J Pharmacol 171:137–139
Ichikawa J, Meltzer HY (1990) The effect of chronic clozapine and haloperidol on basal dopamine release and metabolism in rat striatum and nucleus accumbens studied by in vivo microdialysis. Eur J Pharmacol 176:371–374
Ichikawa J, Meltzer HY (1991) Differential effects of repeated treatment with haloperidol and clozapine on dopamine release and metabolism in the striatum and nucleus accumbens. J Pharmacol Exp Ther 256:348–357
Imperato A, Angelucci L (1989) 5-HT_3 receptors control dopamine release in the nucleus accumbens of freely moving rats. Neurosci Lett 101:214–217
Julius D, Macdermott AB, Axe R, Jessell TM (1988) Molecular characterization of a functional cDNA encoding the $serotonin_{1C}$ receptor. Science 241:558–564
Julius D, Livelli TJ, Jessell TM, Axel R (1989) Ectopic expression of the $serotonin_{1C}$ receptor and the triggering of malignant transformation. Science 244:1057–1062
Kane J, Honigfeld G, Singer J, Meltzer HY (1988) Clozapine for the treatment-resistant schizophrenic. Arch Gen Psychiatry 45:789–796
Köhler C, Hall H, Magnusson O, Lewander T, Gustafsson K (1990) Biochemical pharmacology of the atypical neuroleptic remoxipride. Acta Psychiatr Scand 82 Suppl 358:27–36
Lewander T, Westerberg S-E, Morrison D (1990) Clinical profile of remoxipride – a combined analysis of a comparative double-blind multicenter trial programme. Acta Psychiatr Scand 82 Suppl 358:92–98
Maj J, Sowinska H, Baran L, Palider W (1974) The central action of clozapine. Pol J Pharmacol Pharm 26:425–435

Mann JJ, Bartles M, Bauer H, Gaertner HJ (1984) Amisulpride–an open clinical study of a new benzamide in schizophrenic patients. Pharmacopsychiatry 17:111–115

Matsubara S, Meltzer HY (1989) Effect of typical and atypical antipsychotic drugs on 5-HT_2 receptor density in rat cerebral cortex. Life Sci 45:1397–1406

McKenna DJ, Nazarali AJ, Hoffman AJ, Nichols DE, Mathis CA, Saavedra JM (1989) Common receptors for hallucinogens in rat brain: a comparative autoradiographic study using [^{125}I]LSD and [^{125}I]DOI, a new psychotomimetic radioligand. Brain Res 476:45–56

Meltzer HY (1988) Clozapine: clinical advantages and biological mechanisms. In: Schulz C, Tamminga C (eds) Schizophrenia: a scientific focus. International conference on schizophrenia. Oxford University Press, New York, pp 302–309

Meltzer HY (1989) Clinical studies on the mechanism of action of clozapine: the dopamine-serotonin hypothesis of schizophrenia. Psychopharmacology (Berl) 99: S18–S27

Meltzer HY (1990a) Clozapine: mechanism of action in relation to its clinical advantages. In: Kales A, Stefanos GN, Talbott JA (eds) Recent advances in schizophrenia. Springer, Berlin Heidelber New York, pp 237–246

Meltzer HY (1990b) The role of serotonin in the action of atypical antipsychotic drugs. Psychiatr Ann 20(10):571–579

Meltzer HY (1991) The mechanism of action of novel antipsychotic drugs. Schizophr Bull 17:263–287

Meltzer HY, Nash JF (1991) The effects of antipsychotic drugs on serotonin receptors. Pharmacol Rev 43:587–604

Meltzer HY, Stahl SM (1976) The dopamine hypothesis of schizophrenia: a review. Schizophr Bull 2(1):19–76

Meltzer HY, Stockmeier CA (1992) The influence of 5-HT_2/5-HT_{1C} receptor blockade on the action of clozapine and other Type A atypical antipsychotic drugs. Br J Psychiatry (in press)

Meltzer HY, Daniels S, Fang VS (1975) Clozapine increases rat serum prolactin levels. Life Sci 17:339–342

Meltzer HY, Young M, Metz J, Fang VS, Schyve PM, Arora RC (1985) Extrapyramidal side effects and increased serum prolactin following fluoxetine, a new antidepressant. J Neural Transm 45:165–175

Meltzer HY, Sommers AA, Luchins DJ (1986) The effect of neuroleptics and other psychotropic drugs on negative symptoms in schizophrenia. J Clin Psychopharmacol 6:329–338

Meltzer HY, Alphs LD, Bastani B, Ramirez L (1989a) Effect of melperone in treatment resistant schizophrenia (Abstr). Excerpta Med Int Congr Ser 889:502

Meltzer HY, Bastani B, Kwon KY, Ramirez L, Burnett S, Sharpe J (1989b) A prospective study of clozapine in treatment resistant schizophrenic patients. I. Preliminary report. Psychopharmacology (Berl) 99 Suppl:S68–S72

Meltzer HY, Matsubara S, Lee J-C (1989c) Classification of typical and atypical antipsychotic drugs on the basis of dopamine D_1, D_2 and serotonin$_2$ pKi values. J Pharmacol Exp Ther 251:238–246

Meltzer HY, Zhang Y, Stockmeier CA (1990) Effect of typical and atypical antipsychotic drugs (APD) on frontal cortical (FC), serotonin$_2$ (5-HT_2) and striatal (STR) dopamine$_2$ (DA_2) binding in vivo. Neurosci Abstr 16:586

Mertens C, Dewilds J, Dierick M, Bergman I, Gustavsson G (1989) Clinical trials of amperozide in schizophrenia (Abstr). Excerpta Med Int Congr Ser 889:502

Miller RJ, Hiley CR (1974) Anti-muscarinic properties of neuroleptics and drug-induced parkinsonism. Nature 248:596–597

Molineaux SM, Jessell TM, Axel R, Julius D (1989) 5-HT_{1C} receptor is a prominent serotonin receptor subtype in the central nervous system. Proc Natl Acad Sci USA 86:6793–6797

Nash JF, Meltzer HY, Gudelsky GA (1988) Antagonism of serotonin receptor mediated neuroendocrine and temperature responses by atypical neuroleptics in the rat. Eur J Pharmacol 151:463–469

Palacios JM, Waeber C, Hoyer D, Mengod G (1990) Distribution of serotonin receptors. The neuropharmacology of serotonin. Ann NY Acad Sci 600:36–52

Pazos A, Hoyer D, Palacios J (1984) The binding of serotonergic ligands to the porcine choroid plexus: characterization of an new type of serotonin recognition site. Eur J Pharmacol 106:539–546

Pazos A, Cortes R, Palacios JM (1985) Quantitative autoradiographic mapping of serotonin receptors in the rat brain. II. Serotonin-2 receptors. Brain Res 346: 231–249

Reyntjens A, Gelders YG, Hoppenbrouwers M-L, Vanden Bussche G (1986) Thymosthenic effects of ritanserin (R 55667), a centrally acting serotonin-S_2 blocker. Drug Dev Res 8:205–211

Ruch W, Asper H, Burki HR (1976) Effect of clozapine on the metabolism of serotonin in rat brain. Psychopharmacologia (Berl) 46:103–109

Schmidt AW, Peroutka SJ (1989) 5-Hydroxytryptamine receptor "families". FASEB J 3:2242–2249

Seeman P, Chau-Wong M, Tedesco J, Wong K (1975) Brain receptors for antipsychotic drugs and dopamine: direct binding assays. Proc Natl Acad Sci USA 72:4376–4380

Sokoloff P, Giros B, Martres M-P, Bouthenet M-L, Schwartz J-C (1990) Molecular cloning and characterization of a novel dopamine receptor (D_3) as a target for neuroleptics. Nature 347:146–151

Sunahara RK, Guan H-C, O'Dowd BF, Seeman P, Laurier LG, Ng G, George SR, Torchia J, Van Tol HHM, Niznik HB (1991) Cloning of the gene for a human dopamine 5 receptor with higher affinity for dopamine than D_1. Nature 350:614–619

Svartengren J, Simonsson P (1990) Receptor binding properties of amperozide. Pharmacol Toxicol Suppl 1:8–11

Van Tol HHM, Bunzow JR, Guan H-C, Sunahara RK, Seeman P, Niznik HB, Civelli O (1991) Cloning of the gene for a human dopamine D_4 receptor with high affinity for the antipsychotic clozapine. Nature 350:610–614

Wander TJ, Nelson A, Okazaki H, Richelson E (1987) Antagonism by neuroleptics of serotonin 5-HT_{1A} and 5-HT_2 receptors of normal human brain in vitro. Eur J Pharmacol 143:279–282

Watling KJ, Beer MS, Stanton JA, Newberry NR (1990) Interaction of the atypical neuroleptic clozapine with 5-HT_3 receptors in the cerebral cortex and superior ganglion of the rat. Eur J Pharmacol 182:465–472

Yagaloff KA, Hartig GR (1985) ^{125}I-lysergic acid diethylamide binds to a novel serotonergic site on rat choroid plexus epithelial alls. J Neurosci 5:3718–3183

The Third Dopamine Receptor (D_3): New Perspectives in Therapeutics

B. GIROS, P. SOKOLOFF, M.P. MARTRES, L. LANNFELT, M. ANDRIEUX, R. BESANÇON, C. PILON, M.L. BOUTHENET, E. SOUIL, and J.C. SCHWARTZ

1 Introduction

Until recently it was widely accepted that dopamine affects its target cells in brain and endocrine tissues via interaction with only two receptor subtypes, termed D_1 and D_2, differing from each other by their pharmacological specificity and their opposite effect on adenylate cyclase (Kebabian and Calne 1979). It was also generally admitted that the therapeutic efficacy of antipsychotics derived from their high affinity binding to D_2 receptors.

However, we have repeatedly raised the idea that antipsychotic agents interact to a variable extent with more than a single dopamine receptor subtype, i.e., that the dual categorization of dopamine receptors was incomplete. Our conviction was mainly based upon the observation that a series of "atypical antipsychotics" that we termed the "discriminant benzamide derivatives," whereas inactive at D_1 receptors, were able to distinguish subclasses of D_2 receptors in both binding studies in brain (but not pituitary) and in behavioral studies (Schwartz et al. 1984). However, the discriminant factor of these compounds was rather limited in both series of studies, i.e., no highly selective agent could be identified. In addition, the idea that dopamine autoreceptors, although well recognized by antipsychotics, might differ pharmacologically from postsynaptic D_2 receptors was put forward but did not gain general acceptance (Starke et al. 1989).

Hence the idea that more than a single molecular entity, the D_2 receptor, was responsible for the various actions of antipsychotics remained controversial, in spite of its substantial clinical relevance. Dopaminergic agents are currently used in the treatment of neurological and psychiatric diseases. Their varying therapeutic properties as well as their adverse side effects justify the search for more effective and safer drugs.

The situation has started to change with the advent of molecular biology in this field, which has confirmed the existence of additional dopamine receptors. Besides the cloning of D_1 and D_2 receptor genes (Bunzow et al. 1988; Zhou et al. 1990; Dearry et al. 1990; Sunahara et al. 1990), two

Unité de Neurobiologie et Pharmacologie (U. 109) de l'INSERM, Centre Paul Broca, 2ter rue d'Alésia, 75014 Paris, France receptor isoforms generated from a single D_2 receptor gene by alternative splicing were identified (Giros et al. 1989; Dal Toso et al. 1989). However, there is no evidence yet that these isoforms differ pharmacologically (Giros et al. 1989) or functionally (Dal Toso et al. 1989; Einhorn et al. 1990).

More recently, we have cloned and characterized in rat (Sokoloff et al. 1990) and human (Giros et al. 1990) a novel dopamine receptor which differs from the D_1 and D_2 receptors by its gene, chromosome localization, sequence, pharmacology, signaling system, and tissue localization, hence its designation as the D_3 receptor. Two main features of the D_3 receptor, i.e., its unique localization to limbic brain areas and its differential recognition of various antipsychotics, suggest that the D_3 receptor may play a major role in schizophrenia and the treatment of this affection.

2 Molecular Structure of the Rat and Human D_3 Receptors

Like that of the other catecholamine receptor subtypes, the D_3 receptor sequence contains seven putative transmembrane domains which have come to be recognized as hallmarks of all members of the superfamily of G protein-coupled receptors.

The open reading frame of the D_3 receptor corresponds to a sequence of 446 amino acid residues in the rat (Fig. 1) but only 400 residues in humans. The main difference in homology resides at the level of the third putative intracytoplasmic loop, where these receptors are thought to interact with G proteins. There is relatively little sequence homology at the level of this loop between D_2 and D_3 receptors, contrasting with the high amino acid sequence homology at the level of the transmembrane domains where the dopaminergic ligands are thought to bind (for instance homology is as high as 78% between the human D_2 and D_3 receptors).

Like the rhodopsin gene, the D_2 and D_3 dopamine receptor genes have their coding sequence interrupted by six and five introns, respectively, among which four are located at strictly similar positions. These features suggest that the D_2 and D_3 receptor genes diverged from a common ancestral gene in recent evolutionary history.

The human D_3 receptor gene was assigned to chromosome 3 on band 13.3 (Giros et al. 1990; Leconiat et al. 1991), whereas D_1 and D_2 receptor genes are on chromosomes 5 (Zhou et al. 1990) and 11 (Grandy et al. 1989), respectively.

3 Splice Variants of D_3 Receptor mRNA

Polymerase chain reaction (PCR) amplification, using primers flanking the entire coding sequence, and mRNAs of various rat brain areas in which the

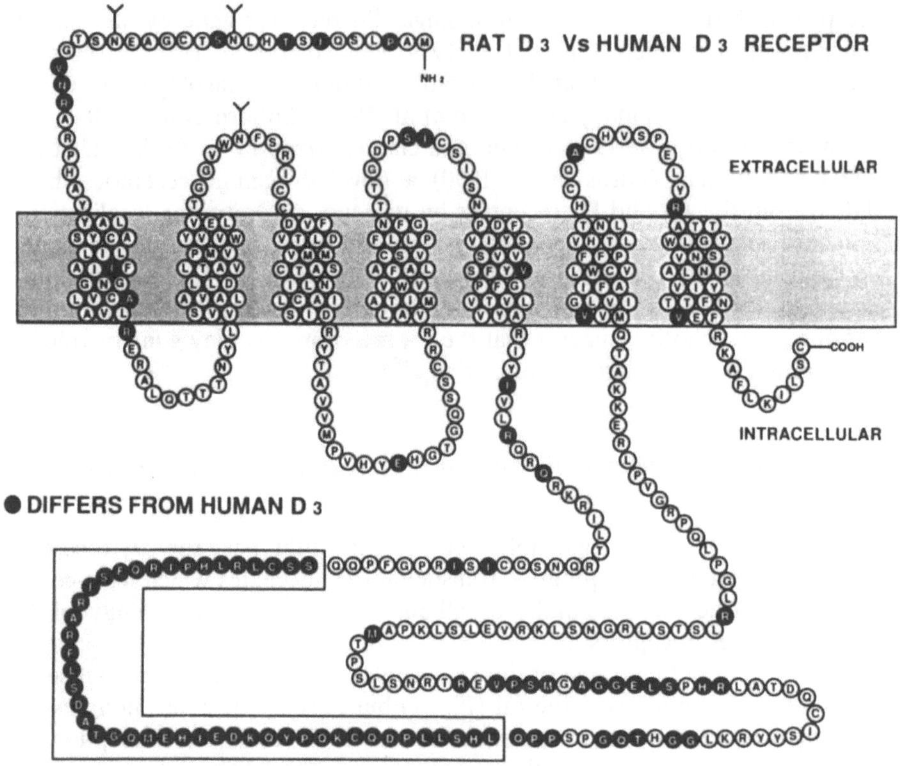

Fig. 1. Proposed membrane topography of the rat D_3 dopamine receptor. *Darkened circles* represent residues which differ between rat and human D_3 receptors. The *boxed portions* of the third intracytoplasmic loop represent the stretch of 46 residues absent in the human D_3 receptor

D_3 receptor is expressed (Sokoloff et al. 1990) gave rise, in addition to the D_3 receptor cDNA, to two other products with sizeable deletions of 113 bp in TM3 and 54 bp in 02, respectively. Thus, the proteins potentially encoded by these two transcripts are designated D_3(TM3-del) and D_3(02-del), respectively (Giros et al. 1991).

Two distinct alternative splicing mechanisms underlie the production of mRNAs corresponding to D_3(TM3-del) and D_3(02-del). In the first case, the process involves combinatorial exons, the "cassette" exon being the second exon which does not comprise n × 3 nucleotides. Therefore, this introduces a frameshift in the sequence and the splice product encodes a 109 amino acid protein. By contrast, in D_3(02-del) mRNA, the in-frame 54 bp deletion does not correspond to a full exon: alternative splicing occurs within the fourth exon where an internal acceptor site can be used by the splicing machinery, giving rise to mRNA encoding a 428 amino acid protein (Fig. 2).

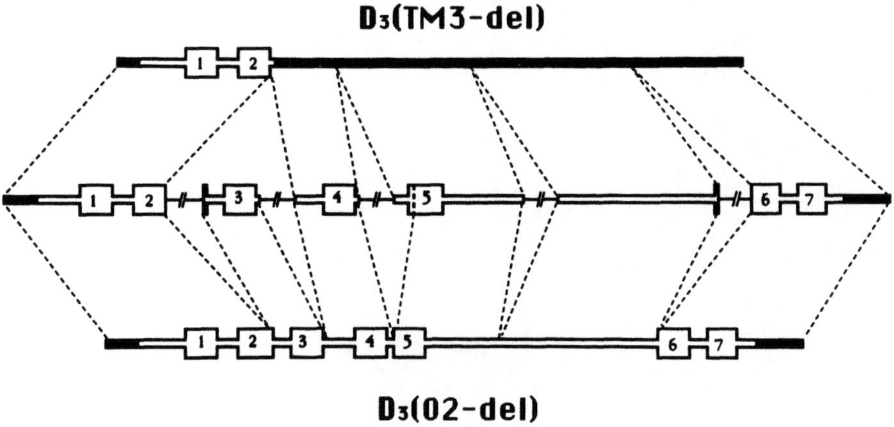

Fig. 2. The D_3 receptor gene and the production of D_3 (TM3-del) and D_3 (02-del). The D_3 receptor gene is represented in the *middle*. *Open boxes* represent the open reading frame and transmembrane segments are enlarged and numbered *1–7*. *Dark open boxes* represent the untranslated reading frame. *Thin lines* represent introns *1–5*. The *dotted line* within TM5 represents the internal acceptor splicing site

Whereas the structure of D_3(TM3-del) makes it unlikely that the protein may function as a receptor, this is not so clear in the case of D_3(02-del), whose structure may still be compatible with the occurrence of seven transmembrane domains, as revealed by the hydropathy profile. However, CHO clones stably expressing D_3(02-del) mRNA failed to show any dopaminergic binding activity as assessed with various radioactive ligands. This could be expected since the deletion affects one of the two serine residues implicated in the binding of catecholamines (Strader et al. 1989).

What could be the function, if any, of these truncated products of the D_3 receptor gene? Indeed, both the D_3(TM3-del) and the D_3(02-del) encode potential integral membrane proteins, possibly involved in cell signaling. Nevertheless the idea that these truncated forms lack any direct biological activity in signal transduction cannot be discarded. They could be formed at random during biosynthesis of the functionally active D_3 receptor. Alternatively, if the process of alternative splicing is physiologically regulated in some manner and variously occurs in different cells or under various circumstances, this may represent a mechanism controlling the abundance of the active D_3 receptor. Finally, since multiple D_3 receptor gene transcripts are also found in human brain (Giros et al. 1990) it cannot be excluded that defects in the alternative splicing mechanisms, leading to the formation of either modified or inactive receptors, might occur during psychiatric diseases in which several features of the D_3 receptor, such as its pharmacology and limbic localization, suggest its involvement.

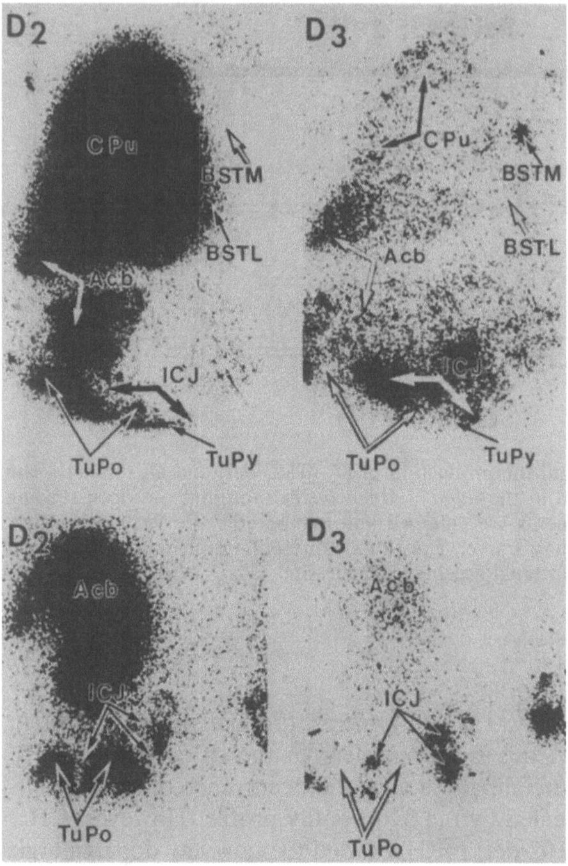

Fig. 3. Compared distributions of D_2 and D_3 receptor mRNAs established by in situ hybridization in sagittal (*top*) and frontal (*bottom*) sections performed in rat telencephalon. *Acb*, accumbens nucleus; *BSTL* and *BSTM*, bed nucleus of the stria terminalis, lateral or medial part; *ICj*, islands of Calleja; *CPu*, caudate putamen; *TuPo* and *TuPy*, polymorph and pyramidal layers of the olfactory tubercle

4 Anatomical Distribution of D_3 Receptor mRNA in Rat Brain

The distribution of D_3 receptor gene transcripts in rat brain areas, as established using northern or PCR analysis or visualized by in situ hybridization histochemistry, markedly differs from that of the D_2 receptor gene transcripts. For instance, only a weak D_3 receptor hybridization signal was detected in restricted parts of the striatum, while the whole striatum contains the highest densities of dopamine axons and D_2 receptor mRNA (Fig. 3). By contrast, the D_3 receptor mRNA is highly expressed in the olfactory tubercle – island of Calleja complex, the bed nucleus of stria terminalis and nucleus accumbens. These areas constitute, with the ventral and ventromedial parts of the caudate putamen, the "ventral striatum," a territory receiving afferents from the prefrontal or allocortex and amygdala and its major dopamine inputs from the A10 cell group in the ventral tegmental area. It projects to ventral pallidum and the latter to the mediodorsal thalamic nucleus which selectively innervates the prefrontal cortex (Björklund and Lindvall 1984). This connectivity has led to the designation of this territory as the "limbic" part of the striatal complex, in which D_3 receptors may therefore mediate a large part of dopamine signals. The remainder of the striatal complex, which is mainly innervated by dopamine projections from the substantia nigra, receives its cortical inputs from the somatic neocortex and is highly enriched in D_2 receptors. D_3 receptor signals were also detected in other "limbic" areas such as the hippocampus, septum, or mammillary nuclei in the hypothalamus. This suggests a major participation of D_3 receptors in dopaminergic transmissions in limbic areas known to be associated with cognitive, emotional, and endocrine functions.

D_2 receptor mRNA is also highly expressed in these areas but there is *no strict overlap* with D_3 receptor mRNA: for instance, the highest levels of D_3 receptor mRNA in brain are detected in the islands of Calleja, in which the D_2 receptor signal is weak, whereas a reverse situation is found in the olfactory tubercles (Fig. 3). In the bed nucleus of the stria terminalis, only cells of the medial division strongly and selectively express D_3 receptor mRNAs, whereas those of the lateral and ventral divisions selectively express D_2 receptor mRNAs; in the posterior hypothalamus, D_2 and D_3 receptor mRNAs are selectively expressed in the lateral and medial mammillary nuclei, respectively. The functional significance of these selective expressions is not entirely clear at the present stage but it is already known that the two receptor subtypes differ by the much higher affinity of dopamine for the D_3 receptor (see below) and, possibly, by their intracellular signaling systems. Hence, it seems likely that different kinds of signal might be generated by dopamine in neighboring but topographically distinct cerebral structures. Nonetheless, several structures contain both D_2 and D_3 receptor mRNAs (e.g., several layers of the olfactory bulb or the cerebral cortex).

5 The D_3 Receptor as a Second Autoreceptor

In situ hybridization reveals a weak but clearly detectable D_3 receptor signal at the level of the substantia nigra. The hypothesis that D_3 receptors are expressed by dopamine neurons themselves was verified after lesioning these areas by 6-hydroxydopamine, a toxin selectively ablating catecholaminergic neurons. After degeneration of these neurons, we found a marked ipsilateral reduction of the PCR-generated signal for the D_3 receptor in both the substantia nigra (−65% ± 10%) and the ventral tegmental area (−69% ± 14%). In the same tissue extracts, the D_2 receptor mRNA levels were similarly affected, i.e., by −88% and −65%, respectively (Sokoloff et al. 1990).

This establishes that both D_2 and D_3 receptors are expressed by dopamine neurons belonging to the A_9 and A_{10} cell groups and suggests that both play the role of autoreceptors. Such a role for the D_3 receptor is consistent with its high apparent affinity for dopamine since this amine, in very low concentrations, reduces, for instance, the electrical activity of dopaminergic neurons (Starke et al. 1989); but even more convincing is the pharmacological profile of the D_3 receptor (see below).

Many distinct functions were previously attributed to dopamine autoreceptors, i.e., inhibitions of impulse flow, dopamine synthesis and release at either nerve terminals or dendrites, and cotransmitter release. D_2 and D_3 autoreceptors might variously participate in all these actions and in various brain areas. Finally, the question as to whether a single cell expresses both D_2 and D_3 receptors remains to be answered, namely, by in situ hybridization studies at the cellular level.

6 Pharmacology of the D_3 Receptor

In order to compare signal transduction pathways and pharmacological properties of D_2 and D_3 receptors, two cell lines expressing each type of receptor were created by transfecting the corresponding cDNAs into Chinese hamster ovary cells (CHO). These cell lines express high levels of binding site (1–5 pmol mg protein^{-1}) which can be labeled with high affinity by the D_2 receptor selective radioligand [^{125}I]iodosulpride (Martres et al. 1985).

In view of the possible therapeutical implications of the interaction of drugs with the D_3 receptor, we have used the clonal cell lines expressing the human D_2 or D_3 receptors to compare the affinities of various dopamine receptor agonists and antagonists, namely, those currently used in the treatment of neurological and psychiatric disorders.

Like dopamine itself, several agonists (TL99, pergolide, quinpirole, and quinerolane) display higher affinities at the D_3 receptor than at the D_2 receptor (Table 1). These agonists presumably act preferentially at presynaptic autoreceptors, an assumption supported by their high potencies in animal autoreceptor models, such as reversion of the γ-butyrolactone-induced increase of in vivo dopamine synthesis (Martin et al. 1982). This suggests that some functions attributed to autoreceptor stimulation actually involve the D_3 receptor, which is consistent with the expression of this receptor mRNA by dopaminergic neurons (Sokoloff et al. 1990). In agreement, AJ76 and UH232, which are the only antagonists exhibiting a partial

Table 1. Dissociation constants of dopaminergic drugs for D_2 and D_3 human dopamine receptors on CHO transfected cell membranes

Agents	K_i values (nM)		K_iD_2/K_iD_3
	D_2 receptor	D_3 receptor	
Agonists			
Apomorphine	63 ± 14	73 ± 20	0.87
Pergolide	19 ± 5	2.3 ± 0.6	8.4
Dopamine	544 ± 70	23 ± 2	24
Dopamine + Gpp(NH)p	2059 ± 183	34 ± 2	61
TL99	66 ± 14	2.3 ± 0.4	29
Quinpirole	1402 ± 204	39 ± 2	36
Quinerolane	341 ± 27	3.6 ± 0.9	95
Antagonists			
Remoxipride	198 ± 46	2300 ± 248	0.086
Clozapine	69 ± 18	479 ± 68	0.14
Domperidone	1.3 ± 0.1	7.5 ± 0.9	0.18
Haloperidol	0.6 ± 0.1	2.9 ± 0.5	0.21
Prochlorperazine	0.4 ± 0.07	1.8 ± 0.15	0.22
Iodosulpride	0.5 ± 0.06	1.3 ± 0.05	0.38
Chlorpromazine	2.3 ± 0.4	5.9 ± 1.2	0.39
Thioproperazine	0.45 ± 0.07	1.2 ± 0.1	0.44
(−)Sulpiride	10 ± 2	20 ± 3	0.50
Amisulpride	1.3 ± 0.1	2.4 ± 0.1	0.53
Carpipramine	8.7 ± 2	15 ± 3	0.58
Pipotiazine	0.20 ± 0.01	0.28 ± 0.03	0.72
Pimozide	9.8 ± 0.6	11 ± 1	0.88
AJ 76	311 ± 14	139 ± 14	2.2
UH 232	36 ± 5	11 ± 1	3.2

The terms agonist and antagonist refer to the known action of drugs at the D_2 receptor. Drugs were ranked according to their K_iD_2/K_iD_3 ratios in human.

selectivity towards the D_3 receptor, have behavioral stimulating properties in animals attributed to autoreceptor blockade (Svensson et al. 1986). These pharmacological data suggest that the D_3 receptor plays a major role in the feedback inhibition of dopamine function.

Most antipsychotics tested displayed high affinities at the D_3 receptor, indicating that it is probably blocked during the treatment of schizophrenia and other psychiatric disorders. The degree of this blockade would, however, depend on the antipsychotics used, since their recognition by the D_3 receptor relative to that of the D_2 receptor is variable. The compounds for which the ratios between K_i values for D_2 and D_3 receptors (K_iD_2/K_iD_3 ratios) are the highest would exert a more complete blockade of dopamine receptors in the limbic areas, where the D_3 receptor is selectively expressed. Conversely, those for which the ratios are the lowest would preferentially block the D_2 receptor present in other dopaminergic areas, including the extrapyramidal system implicated in the control of motor function. This could be one of the molecular bases of the distinction of "atypical" neuroleptics. Consistent with this hypothesis is the present observation of a high K_iD_2/K_iD_3 ratio measured with atypical neuroleptics such as sulpiride and amisulpride. Nevertheless, there is no strict overlap, since other atypical neuroleptics (clozapine and remoxipride) share low K_iD_2/K_iD_3 ratios. An efficient blockade of either D_2 or D_3 receptors by these latter compounds is almost questionable in view of their low affinities at both sites, suggesting that they might primarily act through metabolites or at other receptor sites.

Interestingly, among antipsychotics having the highest K_iD_2/K_iD_3 ratios are amisulpride, carpipramine, pipothiazine, and pimozide, which all exhibit definite disinhibitory actions sought in the treatment of negative symptoms in schizophrenia. Conceivably, the more efficient blockade of D_3 autoreceptors by these compounds could lead to accelerated dopaminergic functions in some brain areas, which might be beneficial in the treatment of those symptoms for which a hypoactivity rather than a hyperactivity of dopamine has been advocated. To address these questions, further studies will be necessary using more selective compounds, the design of which should be facilitated by the use of clonal cell lines expressing D_2 and D_3 receptors.

7 Polymorphism of the Human D_3 Gene

Despite decades of biologically oriented research, little is known about the most fundamental biological basis of the major psychiatric disorders. For schizophrenia, if it seems clear that the dopamine neurotransmission system is deeply involved in the etiology of the disease, as revealed by the antipsychotic effects of dopamine antagonists, attempts to explain this disease as a simple molecular dysfunction have not been successful.

Since vulnerability to schizophrenia has been shown to be inherited and since D_3 receptor mRNA is enriched in limbic areas, we began to search for gene polymorphisms in order to test the hypothesis that the D_3 receptor gene could be a candidate for the inheritance of schizophrenia.

By sequencing several human genomic clones, we first found point mutations in the coding sequence, among which was one that created a novel *Bal*I (TGGCCA) restriction site. This polymorphism is located in the ninth amino acid, a serine residue (AGC; Giros et al. 1990), which is changed to a glycine residue (*G*GC).

We then synthesized two oligonucleotides flanking this polymorphism, which delineated a 462 bp fragment containing, in addition, two invariant *Bal*I restriction sites, and used them for PCR amplification of human genomic DNA. The amplified DNA was thereafter cut with the enzyme *Bal*I. We obtained three fragments in the case of allele 1 (304, 111, and 47 bp), four fragments in the case of allele 2 (206, 111, 98, and 47 bp), and a combination of fragments from alleles 1 and 2 when the individuals were

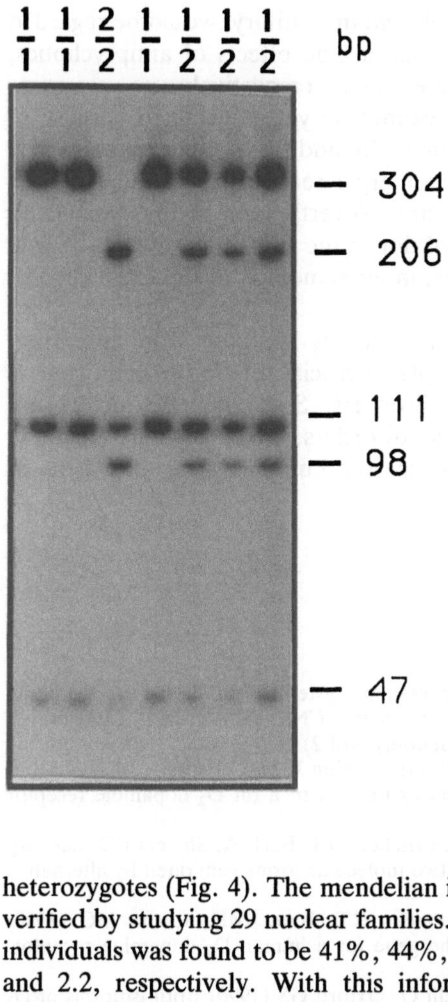

Fig. 4. *Bal*I polymorphism of the D_3 receptor gene. DNA from seven unrelated individuals was amplified by PCR in the presence of a trace amount of radiolabeled nucleotides and digested with *Bal*I. An aliquot of the reaction was resolved by polyacrylamide gel electrophoresis and exposed to X-ray sensitive film. The haplotype is indicated at the *top* and the restriction fragment size (bp) on the *right*

heterozygotes (Fig. 4). The mendelian inheritance of this polymorphism was verified by studying 29 nuclear families. The allele frequency in 41 unrelated individuals was found to be 41%, 44%, and 15% for the haplotypes 1.1, 1.2, and 2.2, respectively. With this information, it will be now possible to perform linkage and association studies with the dopamine D_3 receptor gene.

8 Conclusion: D_3 Receptor Function and Implication in Mental Diseases

The high affinity of most antipsychotics for the D_3 receptor and the selective expression of this receptor in limbic areas known to control cognitive and emotional functions possibly affected in psychotic patients are consistent with the idea that blockade of the D_3 receptor has a predominant role in the therapeutic activity of antipsychotics. According to this hypothesis, interaction of antipsychotics with the D_2 receptor, mainly expressed in cerebral areas involved in motor controls and in pituitary, would be regarded as being at the origin of some of the major side effects of antipsychotics, i.e., extrapyramidal and neuroendocrine effects, respectively.

The precise D_3 receptor function cannot be yet ascertained because of the lack of highly selective antagonists. In addition, other factors such as interactions of drugs with other aminergic receptors and in vivo drug metabolism should be taken into account. Nevertheless, its involvement as autoreceptor in the feedback control of dopamine function seems to be well established on a pharmacological basis, in agreement with the expression of this receptor by dopaminergic neurons.

These various features suggest that the D_3 receptor is an important target for antipsychotic drugs and may play a crucial role in the pathogenesis of schizophrenia and other mental disorders. Since genetic factors are implicated in the susceptibility to these disorders, which tend to cluster in families, it will be of great interest to use the human D_3 receptor gene in linkage studies.

References

Björklund A, Lindvall O (1984) dopamine-containing systems in the CNS. In: Björklund P, Hökfelt T (eds) Classical transmitters in the CNS. Amsterdam, Elsevier, pp 55–122 (Handbook of chemical neuroanatomy, vol 2)

Bunzow JR, Van Tol HHM, Grandy DK, Albert P, Salon J, McChristie D, Machida CA, Neve KA, Civelli O (1988) Cloning and expression of a rat D_2 dopamine receptor cDNA. Nature 336:783–787

Dal Toso R, Sommer B, Ewert M, Herb A, Pritchett DB, Bach A, Shivers BD, Seeburg PH (1989) The dopamine D_2 receptor: two molecular forms generated by alternative splicing. EMBO J 8:4025–4034

Dearry A, Gingrich JA, Falardeau P, Fremeau RT, Bates MD, Caron MG (1990) Molecular cloning and expression of the gene for a human D_1 dopamine receptor. Nature 347:72–76

Einhorn LC, Falardeau P, Caron MG, Civelli O, Oxford GS (1990) Both isoforms of D_2 dopamine receptor couple to a G protein activated K^+ channel when expressed in GH_4 cells. Soc Neurosci Abstr 16:382

Giros B, Sokoloff P, Martres MP, Riou JF, Emorine LJ, Schwartz JC (1989) Alternative splicing directs the expression of two D_2 dopamine receptor isoforms. Nature 342:923–926

Giros B, Martres MP, Sokoloff P, Schwartz JC (1990) cDNA cloning of the human dopaminergic D_3 receptor and chromosome identification. C R Acad Sci [III] 311:501–508

Giros B, Martres MP, Pilon C, Sokoloff P, Schwartz JC (1991) Shorter variants of the D_3 dopamine receptor produced through various patterns of alternative splicing. Biochem Biophys Res Commun (in press)

Grandy DK, Litt M, Allen L, Bunzow JR, Marchionni M, Makam H, Reed L, Magenis RE, Civelli O (1989) The human dopamine D_2 receptor gene is located on chromosome 11 at q22-q23 and identifies a TaqI RFLP. Am J Hum Genet 45:778–785

Kebabian JW, Calne DB (1979) Multiple receptors for dopamine. Nature 277:93–96

Leconiat M, Sokoloff P, Hillion J, Martres MP, Giros B, Pilon C, Schwartz JC, Berger R (1991) Chromosomal localization of the human D_3 dopamine receptor gene. Hum Genet 87:618–620

Martin GE, Williams M, Haubrich DR (1982) A pharmacological comparison of 6,7 dihydroxy-2 dimethyl-aminotetralin (TL 99) and N-n-propyl-3(3-hydroxyphenyl) piperidine (3-PPP) with selected dopamine agonists. J Pharmacol Exp Ther 223:298–304

Martres MP, Bouthenet ML, Salès N, Sokoloff P, Schwartz JC (1985) Widespread distribution of brain dopamine receptors evidenced with ^{125}I-iodosulpride, a highly selective ligand. Science 228:752–755

Schwartz JC, Delandre M, Martres MP, Sokoloff P, Protais P, Vasse M, Costentin J, Laibe P, Wermuth CG, Gulat C, Lafitte A (1984) Biochemical and behavioral identification of discriminant benzamide derivatives: new tools to differentiate subclasses of dopamine receptors. In: Usdin E, Carlsson A, Dahlstrom A, Engel J (eds) Catecholamines: neuropharmacology and central nervous system – theoretical aspects. Liss, New York, pp 59–72

Sokoloff P, Giros B, Martres MP, Bouthenet ML, Schwartz JC (1990) Molecular cloning and characterization of a novel dopamine receptor (D_3) as a target for neuroleptics. Nature 347:146–151

Starke K, Göthert M, Kilbinger H (1989) Modulation of neurotransmitter release by presynaptic autoreceptors. Physiol Rev 69:864–989

Strader DC, Sigal SI, Dixon AFR (1989) Mapping of functional domains of the β-adrenergic receptor. Am J Respir Cell Mol Biol 1:81–86

Sunahara RK, Niznik DB, Weiner DM, Stormann TM, Brann MR, Kennedy JL, Gelernter JE, Rozmahel R, Yang Y, Israel Y, Seeman P, O'Dowd BF (1990) Human dopamine D_1 receptor encoded by an intronless gene on chromosome 5. Nature 347:80–83

Svensson K, Johansson AM, Magnusson T, Carlsson A (1986) (+)-AJ 76 and (+)-UH 232: central stimulants acting as preferential dopamine autoreceptor antagonists. Naunyn Schmiedebergs Arch Pharmacol 334:234–245

Zhou QZ, Grandy DK, Thambi L, Kushner JA, Van Tol HHM, Cone R, Pribnow D, Salon J, Bunzow JR, Civelli O (1990) Cloning and expression of human and rat D_1 dopamine receptors. Nature 347:76–80

PET Examination of Central D_2 Dopamine Receptor Occupancy in Relation to Extrapyramidal Syndromes in Patients Being Treated with Neuroleptic Drugs

L. FARDE and A.-L. NORDSTRÖM

1 Introduction

Positron emission tomography (PET) and suitable radioligands have been used to determine D_2 dopamine receptor occupancy in the basal ganglia of patients undergoing neuroleptic drug treatment. The dopamine hypothesis of antipsychotic drug action has been supported by consistent PET findings of a high D_2 dopamine receptor occupancy in patients treated with conventional clinical doses of chemically distinct classes of antipsychotic drugs (Farde et al. 1988; Smith et al. 1988; Baron et al. 1989).

Extrapyramidal syndromes (EPS) are frequently recorded during neuroleptic drug treatment. Long before the advent of neuroleptic drugs EPS were described in assocation with degenerative disorders of the basal ganglia (Bing 1923; Wilson and Kinnier 1940). It is generally assumed that neuroleptic-induced EPS are mediated by drug interference with dopamine transmission in the basal ganglia.

Dopamine receptor binding can be quantitatively determined in the human basal ganglia (Farde et al. 1986; Wong et al. 1986), the proposed site of action for drug-induced EPS. A potential with PET is to relate central receptor binding *quantitatively* to pharmacological effects induced in the same human subject. It is accordingly of interest to examine the degree of central D_2 dopamine receptor occupancy and its relationship to EPS in patients treated with neuroleptics (Farde et al. 1992).

2 Subjects and Methods

The study was approved by the Ethics and Radiation Safety Committees of the Karolinska Hospital. The subjects participated after having given informed consent.

For the calculation of D_2 dopamine receptor occupancy a control group of 18 neuroleptic-naive schizophrenic patients was used, average age 24

Department of Psychiatry and Psychology, Karolinska Institutet and Hospital, 104 01 Stockholm, Sweden years (range 18–29). This patient group is described in detail in Farde et al. (1990). They were healthy according to history, physical examination, and blood and urine biochemistry. Exclusion criteria were: present or previous neuroleptic drug treatment, organic mental disorder (DSM-III), alcohol or substance abuse, somatic disorder, history of head injury, and pregnancy.

Patients with a schizophreniform or schizophrenic disorder according to DSM-III and on monotherapy with a conventional dosage of an antipsychotic drug were selected. Patients should have been on neuroleptic drug treatment with a fixed dosage for at least 4 weeks. The exclusion criteria were those listed above for the control patients.

Twenty-two patients, average age 30 years (range 20–51), were recruited at the Department of Psychiatry and Psychology, the Karolinska Hospital. Seventeen patients were treated with oral doses and five patients with a depot formulation of a classical neuroleptic (Table 1).

Concomitant medication for sedation was allowed with occasional doses of oxazepam (T. Sobril 15 or 25 mg, Kabi, Sweden) or diazepam (T. Valium 2 or 5 mg, Roche, Sweden). To treat EPS biperiden (Akineton, 2 mg, Meda, Sweden) was allowed but not during the 72 h preceding the PET examination.

All 22 patients had responded to neuroleptic drug treatment. In relation to the PET examination all the patients were rated "much improved" or "very much improved" on the Clinical Global Impression Scale (ECDEU 1976).

EPS were recorded immediately before the PET examination on the basis of a neurological examination and according to "The Rating Scale For Extrapyramidal Side Effects" (Simpson and Angus 1970) and "The Rating Scale for Drug Induced Akathisia" (Barnes 1989). The rater knew the drug and dosage used for the treatment but not the dopamine receptor occupancy.

In all 22 drug-treated patients a PET examination was performed to determine D_2 dopamine receptor occupancy. In the patients treated with oral formulations the PET examination was performed at 2 p.m., i.e., 6 h after the morning dose was given. In patients treated with depot formulations the PET examinations were performed at 2 p.m., 1 week after the last injection.

2.1 PET Determination of Dopamine Receptor Occupancy

The radioligand for PET determination of D_2 receptor occupancy was $[^{11}C]$raclopride (Farde et al. 1985; Halldin et al. 1991). At time of injection the specific activity was 100–1200 Ci/mmol.

The PET system (Scanditronix, PC-384-7B) at the Department of Neuroradiology, Karolinska Hospital, Stockholm, Sweden, was used to follow radioactivity in seven sections of the brain (Litton et al. 1984). Each

Table 1. D_2 dopamine receptor occupancy in 22 schizophrenic patients treated with neuroleptic drugs

Drug	Dosage (mg)	Serum concentration (nmol/l)	D_2 Occupancy (%)	EPS
Phenothiazines				
Chlorpromazine	100 × 2	100	78	–
Thioridazine	150 × 2	620	74	–
Thioridazine	200 × 2	900	81	
Trifluoperazine	5 × 2	N.A.	75	–
Perphenazine enantate (7 days)	100	5	76	Parkinsonism
Butyrophenones				
Haloperidol	6 × 2	19	84	Akathisia
Haloperidol	3 × 2	13	89	Parkinsonism
Haloperidol	3 × 2	9	84	Parkinsonism
Haloperidol	2 × 2	6	75	Akathisia
Haloperidol	2 × 2	11	84	Akathisia, parkinsonism
Haloperidol	3 × 2	9	86	Akathisia
Haloperidol decanoate (28 days)	50	9	85	Parkinsonism
Haloperidol decanoate (28 days)	70	4	74	–
Melperone	125 × 2	240	71	–
Melperone	100 × 3	270	70	–
Thioxanthenes				
Flupentixol	3 × 2	2	71	–
Flupentixol	3 × 2	5	70	–
Flupentixol decanoate (7 days)	40	19	81	Parkinsonism
Zuclopentixol decanoate (14 days)	200	50	81	Dystonia
Diphenylbutyls				
Pimozide	4 × 2	4	79	Akathisia
Substituted benzamides				
Remoxipride	200 × 2	325	71	–
Sulpiride	400 × 2	490	78	–

N.A., not assessed.

study comprised 11–12 sequential scans during a period of 45–51 min. A fiberglass helmet was made for each individual and used with a head fixation system both during computed tomography (CT) and PET (Bergström et al. 1981). The head fixation system made transfer of the positioning from CT to PET feasible. To optimize and standardize the position of the caudate nucleus and the putamen within a PET section, foramen of Monroe was identified by CT. A level 3 mm above the foramen of Monroe was chosen as the transaxial midpoint of the PET and the CT section 4.

Regions of interest were drawn for the cerebellum and the putamen. Regional radioactivity was measured for each sequential scan, corrected for ^{11}C decay and plotted versus time. Total radioactivity in the cerebellum, a region with negligible densities of D_2 dopamine receptors (Cortés et al. 1989), was used as an estimate of C_f, the free radioligand concentration in brain. Specific binding (C_b) in the putamen, a region with a high density of D_2 dopamine receptors, was defined as the difference between total radioactivity (C_t) in the putamen and the free radioligand concentration (C_f).

The theory underlying calculation of dopamine receptor occupancy by PET has been presented earlier (Farde et al. 1988). In summary, the ratio of C_b to C_f was calculated for each experiment at time of equilibrium. If a neuroleptic drug binds to the receptor population of interest and thereby occupies a certain proportion of the receptors, this will be reflected in a reduced number of receptors available for radioligand binding. The reduction in number of available receptors is proportional to a reduction in the ratio C_b/C_f. Dopamine receptor occupancy (R) was expressed in percent and calculated according to the equation

$$R = \frac{C_b/C_f\ (\text{ref}) - C_b/C_f\ (\text{drug})}{C_b/C_f\ (\text{ref})} \times 100$$

where the reference value C_b/C_f (ref) is the average ratio obtained in control subjects and C_b/C_f (drug) is the individual ratio in a drug-treated patient.

2.1.1 Statistics

D_2 dopamine receptor occupancy was determined in patients treated with classical neuroleptics ($n = 22$) with EPS ($n = 11$) and without EPS ($n = 11$). The groups were normally distributed according to Shapiro-Wilk test indicating normality on the $p < 0.01$ level (Shapiro and Wilk 1972). Groups were compared by Students *t*-test for independent samples, taking the different standard deviations into account using the program MINITAB (Ryan et al. 1985) implemented in a VAX computer.

3 Results

After i.v. injection of [^{11}C]raclopride into the 18 neuroleptic-naive schizophrenic patients there was a high accumulation of radioactivity in the basal ganglia. The average ratio, C_b/C_f, for [^{11}C]raclopride binding in the 18 patients was 3.04 (SEM = 0.11; range 2.3–4.3).

After i.v. injection of [^{11}C]raclopride in the 22 antipsychotic drug-treated patients there was a markedly reduced accumulation of radioactivity in the basal ganglia when compared to the control patients. The ratio of specific [^{11}C]raclopride binding to free radioligand concentration, C_b/C_f,

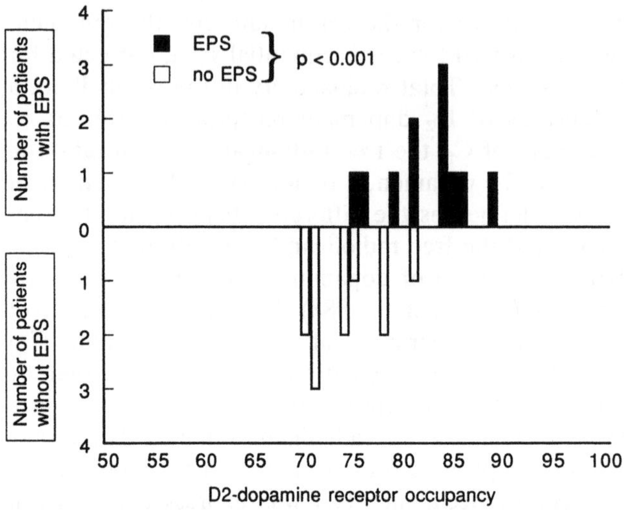

Fig. 1. D_2 dopamine receptor occupancy in relation to extrapyramidal syndromes (*EPS*) in 22 schizophrenic patients treated with classical neuroleptics

ranged between 0.33 and 0.90 and the D_2 dopamine receptor occupancy between 70% and 89% (78% ± 6%, average ± SD; Table 1).

EPS were recorded in 11 of the 22 patients. (Table 1; Fig. 1). The 11 patients who had EPS had an average D_2 dopamine receptor occupancy of 82% (SD = 4%). The 11 patients who did not have EPS had an average occupancy of 74% (SD = 4%) which is significantly lower ($p < 0.001$) than in the patients with EPS.

3.1 D_2 Dopamine Receptor Occupancy and Extrapyramidal Syndromes

We have previously reported a high D_2 dopamine receptor occupancy in schizophrenic patients treated with conventional doses of all the chemically distinct classes of classical neuroleptics (Farde et al. 1988). Other PET centers have mainly examined patients treated with butyrophenons and have also reported high occupancy (Smith et al. 1988; Baron et al. 1989). A D_2 dopamine receptor occupancy ranging between 70% and 89% was also found in the presently reported extended series of patients treated with classical neuroleptics.

Since EPS appeared in some of these patients it was possible to compare the D_2 occupancy found in these patients to that found in patients who did not show any side effects. The patients who had EPS had a significantly higher D_2 dopamine receptor occupancy than those who did not ($p <$ 0.001). This finding was the first direct demonstration that EPS are quantitatively related to central D_2 dopamine receptor occupancy (Farde et al. 1992).

3.2 Hypothesis of Distinct Thresholds

Both for EPS and for the antipsychotic effect there may be thresholds in terms of the D_2 dopamine receptor occupancy required to induce the effect. The patients who did not have EPS were clinical responders to neuroleptic drug treatment. The results of the present study indicate that there may be a threshold for EPS at about 80% (Fig. 1). This threshold seems to be higher than the D_2 occupancy required for the antipsychotic effect. Further confirmation of such hypothesis has implications for optimal dose finding in clinical neuroleptic drug treatment. The hypothesis has to be tested in controlled clinical studies designed for indentification of sigmoid-shaped occupancy–response relationships.

Recently, several new dopamine receptor subtypes have been cloned (Sokoloff et al. 1990; Van Tol et al. 1991). A D_3 dopamine receptor seems to be found predominantly in the nucleus accumbens, a limbic brain region of particular interest for the antipsychotic effect (Andén and Stock 1970; Sokoloff et al. 1990). With the new PET systems with improved resolution and with new selective radioligands it will be possible to determine binding to dopamine receptor subtypes both in the basal ganglia and in other brain regions suggested as site of action for the antipsychotic effect.

Acknowledgement. This study was supported by grants from the National Institute of Mental Health (MH 41205-05), the Swedish Medical Research Council B91-21X-09114-02A, The Karolinska Pharmacy, and the Ulf Lundahl Memorial Foundation.

References

Andén NE, Stock G (1973) Effect of clozapine on the turnover of dopamine in the corpus striatum and the limbic system. J Pharm Pharmacol 25:346

Baron JC, Martinot JL, Cambon H, Boulenger JP, Poirier MF, Caillard V, Blin J, Huret JD, Loc'h C, Maziére B (1989) Striatal dopamine receptor occupancy during and following withdrawal from neuroleptic treatment: correlative evaluation by positron emission tomography and plasma prolactine levels. Psychopharmacology (Berl) 99:463–472

Barnes TRE (1989) A rating scale for drug-induced akathisia. Br J Psychiatry 154: 672–676

Bergström M, Boethius J, Eriksson L, Greitz T, Ribbe T, Widen L (1981) Head fixation device for reproducible positron alignment in transmission CT and positron emission tomography. J Comput Assist Tomogr 8:74–87

Bing R (1923) Über einige bemerkenswerte Begleiterscheinigungen der extrapyramidalen Rigidität (Akathesie – Mocrographie – Kinesia paradoxica). Schweiz Med Wochenschr 53:167–171

Cortés R, Camps M, Gueye B, et al. (1989) Dopamine receptors in human brain: autoradiographic distribution of D1 and D2 sites in Parkinson syndrome of different etiology. Brain Res 483:30–38

ECDEU (1976) Assessment manual for psychopharmacology. US Department of Health, Education and Welfare, Washington

Farde L, Ehrin E, Eriksson L, Greitz T, Hall H, Hedström C-G, Litton J-E, Sedvall G (1985) Substituted benzamides as ligands for visualization of dopamine-D2 receptor binding in the living human brain by poistron emission tomography. Proc Natl Acad Sci USA 82:3863–3867

Farde L, Hall H, Ehrin E, Sedvall G (1986) Quantitative analysis of dopamine-D2 receptor binding in the living human brain by positron emission tomography. Science 231:258–261

Farde L, Wiesel F-A, Halldin C, Sedvall G (1988) Central D_2-dopamine receptor occupancy in schizophrenic patients treated with antipsychotic drugs. Arch Gen Psychiatry 45:71–78

Farde L, Wiesel F-A, Halldin C, Stone-Elander S, Nordström A-L, Hall H, Sedvall G (1990) D2-dopamine receptor characteristics in neuroleptic-naive patients with schizophrenia – a PET-study with [11C]raclopride. Arch Gen Psychiatry 47:213–219

Farde L, Nordström A-L, Wiesel F-A, Pauli S, Halldin C, Sedvall G (1992) PET-analysis of central D1- and D2-dopamine receptor occupancy in patients treated with classical neuroleptics and clozapine – relation to extrapyramidal side effects. Arch Gen Psychiatry 49:538–544

Halldin C, Farde L, Högberg T, Hall H, Stöm P, Ohlberger A, Solin O (1991) A comparative PET-study of five carbon-11 or fluorine-18 labelled salicylamides: preparation and in vitro dopamine D_2 receptor binding. Nucl Med Biol 8:871–881

Litton J, Bergström L, Eriksson L, Bohm C, Blomqvist G, Kesselberg M (1984) Performance study of the PC-384 positron camera system for emission tomography of the brain. J Comput Assist Tomogr 8:74–87

Ryan F, Joiner L, Ryan A Jr (1985) The minitab handbook, 2nd edn. Duxbury Boston, pp 185–190

Shapiro SS, Wilk MB (1972) An analysis of variance test for normality (complete samples). Biometrika 52:591

Simpson GM, Angus JWS (1970) A rating scale for extrapyramidal side effects. Acta Psychiatr Scand 45 Suppl 212:11–19

Smith M, Wolf AP, Brodie JD, Arnett CD, Barouche F, Shiue CY, Fowler JS, Russell JAG, MacGregor RR, Wolkin A, Angrist B, Rotrosen J, Peselow E (1988) Serial [18F]N-methylspiperone PET studies to measure changes in antipsychotic drug D-2 receptor occupancy in schizophrenic patients. Biol Psychiatry 23:653–663

Sokoloff P, Giros B, Martres MP, Bouthenet ML, Schwartz JC (1990) Molecular cloning and characterization of a novel dopamine receptor (D3) as a target for neuroleptics. Nature 347:146–151

Van Tol H, Bunzow J, Guan H, Sunahara R, Seeman P, Niznik H, Civelli O (1991) Cloning of the gene for a human dopamine D4 receptor with high affinity for the antipsychotic clozapine. Nature 350:610–614

Wilson SA, Kinnier JW (1940) Encephalitis. In: Bruce AN (ed) Neurology, vols 1 and 2. A William Wood book. Williams and Wilkins, Baltimore, pp 118, (vol 1), 793 (vol 2)

Wong DF, Gjedde A, Wagner HN Jr (1986) Quantification of neuroreceptors in the living human brain. I. Irreversible binding of ligands. J Cereb Blood Flow Metab 6: 137–146

Dopaminergic and Serotonergic Aspects of Acute Extrapyramidal Syndromes

D.E. Casey

1 Introduction

Neuroleptic (antipsychotic) drugs have become the primary pharmacological method for controlling both acute and chronic psychotic symptoms. Since these drugs were introduced in the 1950s, acute extrapyramidal syndromes have been associated with these neuroleptic agents. Indeed, the word "neuroleptic," meaning "to take the neuron," was intentionally created to encompass the concept that both antipsychotic benefits and motor side effects occurred at or near the same dose (Deniker 1984). Thus, these two clinical effects were considered to be inextricably linked. It is now widely recognized that this concept is incorrect and that the antipsychotic benefits and extrapyramidal side effects are potentially separable. Some patients obtain benefit without developing any motor side effects, whereas other patients develop incapacitating motor syndromes before any antipsychotic benefit is derived. However, the majority of patients who experience extrapyramidal side effects have these symptoms develop at doses that are close to those that also produce antipsychotic benefit. Thus, most of the commercially available neuroleptics have a narrow therapeutic index separating desirable from undesirable effects.

Any treatment approach that reduces or prevents these extrapyramidal symptoms while maintaining the antipsychotic benefits would be a clear advancement in managing psychoses. With a much broader therapeutic index it would be possible to treat patients across a wider dose range in an attempt to find the lowest effective dose, but spare patients the morbidity of extrapyramidal side effects, which may occur in up to 75% of patients receiving neuroleptics (Casey and Keepers 1988).

The biochemical basis of acute extrapyramidal syndromes is thought to be related to the blockade of dopamine D2 receptors in the basal ganglia. This property is common to all the commercially available neuroleptics used to treat schizophrenia and other psychoses. The one possible exception to this principle is clozapine, a compound with weak dopamine D2 antagonist

Psychiatry Service (116A), V.A. Medical Center, 3710 S.W. U.S. Veterans Hospital Road, Portland, OR 97207, USA properties that also antagonizes many other neurotransmitter receptors but produces minimal extrapyramidal symptoms (Casey 1989a).

As part of the support for the D2 receptor blockade hypotheses of acute extrapyramidal syndromes, there is a relatively strong correlation between a drug's ability to block dopamine D2 receptors, its milligram potency, and clinical dose. Also correlating with these observations are the inversely related anticholinergic properties intrinsic to many of these drugs. Thus, compounds with less potent D2 antagonism and high anticholinergic antagonism are considered as high milligram, low potency compounds producing fewer extrapyramidal syndromes, such as thioridazine. Conversely, drugs with high D2 antagonism and low anticholinergic activity are considered low milligram, high potency drugs with higher rates of extrapyramidal syndromes. However, the D2/anticholinergic recepor antagonism ratio is not the whole explanation of relative rates of extrapyramidal symptoms. For example, combining haloperidol, a low milligram, high potency compound, with an anticholinergic does not equal the effects of clozapine, a drug with low D2 antagonism and high anticholinergic activity (Bürki et al. 1975).

Alternatively, it has been proposed that some neuroleptics might have regional selectivity with a preference for limbic rather than basal ganglia dopamine receptors (Bischoff et al. 1986). However, this concept is not well-established and no neuroleptics have been unequivocally proven to have regional central nervous system selectivity (Wetzel et al. 1991).

The hypothesis explaining acute extrapyramidal syndromes on the basis of D2 antagonism is somewhat challenged by observations with the antipsychotic substituted benzamides. These compounds are highly specific D2 antagonists and span the range of milligram potency from low to high, yet have relatively low rates of extrapyramidal symptoms (Tamminga and Gerlach 1987). With this class of drugs, akathisia appears to be more common than acute dystonia or drug-induced parkinsonism. This is in the context of well-documented antipsychotic efficacy. Sulpiride produces little or no catalepsy in rodents and is a high milligram, low potency compound that has been effectively used for many years to treat psychosis. Remoxipride is a moderate potency compound that also produces low extrapyramidal syndrome rates (Lewander et al. 1990). It is characterized in animal models by a very wide separation between the catalepsy (model of extrapyramidal syndromes) and antistereotypic stimulant-induced behavior (model of antipsychotic effects) dose-response curves (Ögren et al. 1986; Hall et al. 1986; Gerlach and Casey 1990; Casey 1991a). Raclopride is a low milligram, high potency substituted benzamide with antipsychotic efficacy that also produces lower than expected extrapyramidal syndrome rates (Farde et al. 1988; Casey 1991b).

The role of dopamine D1 receptors has been controversial in the area of extrapyramidal syndromes. SCH 23390, a compound with high D1 and low to moderate 5-HT2 antagonism (McQuade et al. 1988), produces catalepsy in rodents and acute dystonia in both neuroleptic-sensitized and neuroleptic-naive *cebus* monkeys when the compound is given intramuscularly (Gerlach et al. 1986; Casey 1988, 1992). However, when this drug is given orally to drug-naive monkeys it does not produce extrapyramidal symptoms (Coffin et al. 1989). To further complicate matters, SCH 23390 can desensitize previously haloperidol-sensitized monkeys so that SCH 23390 produces far fewer dystonic symptoms after multiple treatments compared to the initial SCH 23390 exposure (Casey 1989b).

Recent studies have suggested that ratios between serotonin 5-HT2 and dopamine D2 receptor antagonism may greatly decrease or prevent the development of extrapyramidal symptoms. This hypothesis derives from earlier rodent studies demonstrating that 5-HT2 antagonism significantly decreased D2 antagonist-induced catalepsy in rodents (Balsara et al. 1979; Waldmeier and Delini-Stula 1979), though this has not always been observed (Arnt 1986). More recently this hypothesis has been explicitly formulated to suggest that pK_i values with a ratio of 5-HT2/D2 greater than 1.1 identify neuroleptics which will have an antipsychotic effect but be relatively or completely free of extrapyramidal syndromes (Meltzer et al. 1989). Thus, compounds meeting this criterion, such as clozapine, will be considered atypical. Other compounds with 5-HT2/D2 ratios that approximate this criterion are melperone and risperidone, and one compound, ritanserine, clearly exceeds the proposed minimum 5-HT2/D2 pK_i ratio.

Studies in nonhuman primates have also produced somewhat conflicting results for and against the 5-HT2/D2 ratio hypothesis. One study noted statistically significant but clinically modest decreases in neuroleptic-induced acute dystonia in *cebus* monkeys with serotonin antagonists and an increase in symptoms with serotonin agonists (Korsgaard et al. 1985). In contrast, another study did not find such changes (Povlsen et al. 1986). This study may have had negative results because of the narrow drug dose range tested. However, additional support for this latter study comes from another report that noted compounds with varying ranges of 5-HT2/D2 antagonist ratios produced similar extrapyramidal syndrome rates in nonhuman primates (Casey 1989c).

The aim of these studies was to evaluate the acute dystonia extrapyramidal syndrome liability of currently available and potentially new antipsychotic agents in *cebus* monkeys. Drugs with varying antagonist properties for D1, D2, and 5-HT2 receptors were evaluated. Much of the extrapyramidal syndrome data focused on the role of variable 5-HT2/D2 antagonist ratios in drugs since agents with preferential 5-HT2/D2 ratios have been hypothesized to be atypical neuroleptics that will be free of extrapyramidal symptoms.

2 Subjects and Methods

Cebus albifrons monkeys (22–28 years old) were tested across wide dose ranges for each drug. Group size varied from $n = 20$ to $n = 6$; the smaller

Table 1. The dystonia-inducing threshold in monkeys receiving dopamine and serotonin antagonists

Drug (dose range, mg/kg)	Serotonin and dopamine receptor antagonism (reference)	Dystonia-inducing threshold dose (mg/kg)
SCH 23390 (0.01–0.25)	Low-moderate 5-HT2/high D1 (McQuade et al. 1988)	0.025
Remoxipride (2.5–25.0)	No 5-HT2/high D2 (Hall et al. 1986)	5.0
Haloperidol (0.01–0.25)	Low 5-HT2/high D2 (Leysen 1981)	0.025
Clopenthixol (0.01–0.50)	Low-moderate 5-HT2/moderate D2 (Hyttel et al. 1985)	0.05
Melperone (0.05–5.0)	Moderate 5-HT2/moderate D2 (Meltzer et al. 1989)	1.0
Tefludazine (0.01–0.25)	Moderate 5-HT2/moderate D2 (Svendsen et al. 1986)	0.025
Setoperone (0.01–1.0)	High 5-HT2/moderate D2 (Niemegeers et al. 1984)	0.05
Risperidone (0.01–0.25)	High 5-HT2/high D2 (Leysen et al. 1988)	0.025
Clozapine (0.5–25.0)	Moderate-high 5-HT2/low D2, D1 (Meltzer et al. 1989)	>25.0
Ritanserine (0.1–5.0)	High 5-HT2/moderate D2 (Leysen et al. 1988)	>5.0

groups were subsets of the larger $n = 20$ cohort. These monkeys had previously received haloperidol and other neuroleptics and thus were considered "sensitized" with stable extrapyramidal syndrome response rates.

The agents tested, their dose range, and biochemical profile regarding D1, D2, and 5-HT2 are detailed in Table 1. Saline (0.25 ml) was used as a control with each drug tested.

All drugs were prepared fresh each day and administered intramuscularly. The full dose range was tested for each drug prior to starting evaluations with the next compound. Single doses were randomly sequenced and given at 7-day intervals. Behaviors were scored by an experienced rater who was blind to dose. In a combination haloperidol-ritanserine test, ritanserine doses were given 1 h after haloperidol, which was the time required for a stable dystonia syndrome to be established.

Animal behavior was scored before and at 30 min intervals for 3 h, then hourly for the next 3 h, and once again at 24 h after drug administration. Acute dystonia was scored in four different body regions (head and neck, trunk, upper limbs, lower limbs) on a scale of 0 to +3 (0 = normal, 1 = mild, 2 = moderate, 3 = severe). The threshold dose for inducing dystonia was defined for each drug as that dose which produced dystonic symptoms for at least two consecutive observation periods and gave a mean group score of 20 or more.

3 Results

All drugs produced acute dystonia, with the exception of clozapine, ritanserine, and saline. Threshold dystonia-inducing doses are shown in Table 1. Dystonia syndromes were clinically indistinguishable. Dose-response curves had similar slopes. The factor that mainly discriminated between these drugs was their duration of action.

Ritanserine, when given 1 h after haloperidol-induced dystonia was stabilized, did not affect the haloperidol syndrome. Also, there were no other new abnormal behaviors observed when ritanserine and haloperidol were combined.

4 Discussion

The drugs tested span a wide range of specific aminergic actions and ratios of serotonin and dopamine interactions. The results support a primary role of dopamine D2 antagonism in producing acute dystonia. Yet, this is unlikely to be the sole explanation. Dopamine D1 antagonism also caused dystonia in *cebus* monkeys that had previously received neuroleptics and thus had a stable sensitized prior response to intramuscular neuroleptic treatment. The role of D1 antagonism in dystonia is controversial, however, as others have not found drug-induced dystonia when D1 antagonists were administered orally to drug-naive monkeys (Coffin et al. 1989). In contrast, parenteral (intramuscular) administration of the D1 antagonist SCH 23390 to drug-naive monkeys did produce dystonia (Casey 1992). Since SCH 23390 has low to moderate 5-HT2 antagonism in addition to high D1 blockade (McQuade et al. 1988), this may have led to lower extrapyramidal syndromes than a pure D1 antagonist would produce if the 5-HT2/D2 antagonism ratio hypothesis of low extrapyramidal syndromes is correct. Thus there are several questions that remain unanswered. Is there any dose of the D1 antagonist given orally to neuroleptic-naive monkeys that produces dystonia? Where is the dose response curve in relation to both oral and parenteral administration? Are these conflicting findings due primarily to bioavailability and route of drug delivery? Further evidence supporting the role of D1 antagonists having the liability to produce dystonia comes from the reports of SCH 23390-induced catalepsy in rodents. Evidence supporting the low likelihood of D1 antagonists producing acute extrapyramidal syndromes comes from the observation that repeated treatment with SCH 23390 desensitized previously haloperidol-sensitized monkeys that showed much greater SCH 23390-induced dystonia prior to receiving the desensitizing doses of this drug (Casey 1989b).

Remoxipride, a D2 specific antagonist, had a much higher than expected threshold dose for inducing dystonia. Since remoxipride and other substituted benzamides are D2-specific antagonists, it would be anticipated that these compounds would produce rates of dystonia and other extrapyramidal syndromes that were similar to haloperidol, another highly specific D2 antagonist. When antipsychotic equipotency ratios are calculated from the clinic, haloperidol and remoxipride are approximately 1:30 as represented by commonly used antipsychotic doses of 5–20 mg per day for haloperidol and 150–600 mg per day for remoxipride. Yet remoxipride has a significantly lower extrapyramidal syndrome profile in the clinic (Lewander et al. 1990). Also, in the nonhuman primate model, there is a much wider difference (of approximately 200-fold) in the threshold for dystonia-inducing doses of these two compounds (Casey 1991a). This is consistent with the rodent studies of a very wide separation between catalepsy and blockade of stimulant-induced stereotypic behavior (Ögren et al. 1986).

What could account for this low extrapyramidal syndrome liability with remoxipride and other substituted benzamides? There are no readily available answers. These effects could not be explained by high anticholinergic antagonistic activity, as the substituted benzamides are devoid of this function (Hall et al. 1986). Perhaps there is a subtype of dopamine receptors that is selectively or preferentially bound by substituted benzamides, as has been proposed for clozapine (VanTol et al. 1991). Or perhaps there are other binding sites, such as sigma sites, that are affected by remoxipride and similar substituted benzamides which may have a mitigating effect on extrapyramidal syndromes. If so, identifying these mechanisms may open many new avenues to neuroleptic drug development.

These data are not supportive of the preferential 5-HT2/D2 antagonism ratio hypothesis from several perspectives. Agents that are very similar to clozapine in 5-HT2/D2 pK_i ratios of 1.1, such as melperone and risperidone, clearly produce extrapyramidal syndromes at doses given to monkeys that are clinically equipotent. For example, risperidone shows antipsychotic efficacy at doses similar to haloperidol, and both these drugs have similar dystonia-inducing capacity in monkeys. Similarly, melperone is used in the clinic for controlling psychoses at doses that are approximately 30 times higher than haloperidol (haloperidol = 5–20 mg/day vs melperone = 150–600 mg/day) (Bjerkenstedt et al. 1978), and the dystonia-inducing threshold dose for melperone is approximately 40 times higher than that for haloperidol in these monkeys.

Other drugs across a range of 5-HT2/D2 ratios seem not to identify a critically specific ratio for predicting low extrapyramidal syndromes. Compounds like clopenthixol with low-moderate 5-HT2/moderate D2 ratios also produce extrapyramidal syndromes in both monkeys and humans. Compounds such as tefludazine with a moderate 5-HT2/moderate D2 ratio and setoperone with a high 5-HT2/moderate D2 antagonist ratio also produced dystonia in monkeys (Casey 1989c). Setoperone has been evaluated only once in the clinic at low doses and was found to have modest antipsychotic effects with a low extrapyramidal syndrome profile (Ceulemans et al. 1985);

however, this compound has not been studied further. Tefludazine has yet to be evaluated in psychotic patients (Svendsen et al. 1986).

Though one could argue that ritanserine's inability to produce extrapyramidal syndromes, up to 5.0 mg/kg, supports the high 5-HT2/D2 antagonist ratio hypothesis for no extrapyramidal syndromes, this must be tempered by the lack of compelling data that ritanserine is antipsychotic in doses used in the clinic. Since clozapine and ritanserine have closely similar 5-HT2/D2 pK_i ratios, it may be necessary to give far higher doses of ritanserine to achieve an antipsychotic effect. However, this is unlikely as clinical doses are limited to below 20 mg per day because of side effect toxicity.

The study evaluating ritanserine's effect on existing haloperidol-induced dystonia also does not support a specific 5-HT2/D2 antagonist ratio for limiting extrapyramidal syndromes. The complete inability of ritanserine, at dose ranges from 0.10–5.0 mg/kg, to alter D2 antagonist haloperidol-induced dystonia suggests that, at least in these dose ratios, it was not possible to exploit a beneficial anti-extrapyramidal syndrome effect of high 5-HT2 antagonism. The inability to reverse haloperidol-induced dystonia is not due to a ceiling effect of severe symptoms that are not treatable because apomorphine and anticholinergics can reverse these symptoms (Casey et al. 1980). This is consistent with prior observations that 5-HT2 antagonists have little or no beneficial effect on neuroleptic-induced dystonia in rodents (Arnt et al. 1986) and nonhuman primates (Povlsen et al. 1986; Casey 1989c). Others have found a strong anti-extrapyramidal syndrome effect with 5-HT2 antagonists in rodent catalepsy (Balsara et al. 1979) and a weak but statistically significant decrease in haloperidol-induced dystonia in monkeys (Korsgaard et al. 1985).

Finally, the relatively low extrapyramidal syndrome rate in monkeys and humans from remoxipride and other substituted benzamides conflicts with this 5-HT2/D2 hypothesis. Remoxipride and the other clinically used drugs in this class are virtually devoid of 5-HT2 antagonistic properties, yet have lower than expected extrapyramidal syndrome liability. While it is possible that a uniquely specific 5-HT2/D2 antagonist ratio is necessary for a neuroleptic to have antipsychotic benefits without substantial extrapyramidal syndrome liability, such as clozapine, it seems unlikely. Even if such a compound were to have these highly desirable effects, it would be very difficult to exploit in the clinic since patients have widely ranging pharmacokinetic profiles with psychoactive drugs.

In conclusion, the data indicate that dopamine D2 (and possibly dopamine D1) receptor antagonism plays a primary role in neuroleptic-induced acute dystonia and, by inference, other extrapyramidal syndromes. However, this is not suitable as a full explanation because remoxipride and other substituted benzamides, which are highly specific D2 antagonists, have a low extrapyramidal syndrome profile that is much less than that predicted by a one-factor model of dopamine receptor antagonism. Similarly, preferential

5-HT2/D2 antagonist ratios do not indicate this is an explanation for the low extrapyramidal syndrome profile of clozapine, nor is there an indication that this strategy can be exploited to develop new antipsychotic compounds that are free of acute extrapyramidal syndromes. While both dopamine and serotonin antagonism undoubtedly play important roles in both the antipsychotic and extrapyramidal syndrome liability, a recurring question remains: "How much is enough?" How much dopamine receptor antagonism is enough for an antipsychotic effect since either highly potent receptor antagonists, such as haloperidol, or weakly potent antagonists, such as clozapine, both have antipsychotic efficacy? Similarly, how much 5-HT2 antagonism is enough to influence extrapyramidal syndromes? Low to moderate 5-HT2/D2 antagonist ratios appear not to produce much anti-extrapyramidal syndrome activity, whereas highly potent 5-HT2 antagonists, such as ritanserine, appear not to be antipsychotic and also do not produce acute extrapyramidal syndromes.

The ultimate value of these hypotheses explaining the pharmacological basis of acute extrapyramidal syndromes is that they increase our understanding of the basic mechanisms of action of drugs as well as the pharmacology and physiology of motor systems. They also foster hypotheses and stimulate leads to pursue that will undoubtedly lead to advances in the drug therapy of psychoses.

Acknowledgements. This work was supported in part by funds from the Veterans Administration Research Program and by NIMH grant MH36657. Kristina Wells prepared the typescript.

References

Arnt J, Hyttel J, Bach-Lauritsen T (1986) Further studies of the mechanism behind scopolamine-induced reversal of antistereotypic and cataleptogenic effects of neuroleptics in rats. Acta Pharmacol Toxicol (Lopenh) 59:319–324

Balsara JJ, Jadhav JH, Chandorkar AG (1979) Effect of drugs influencing central serotonergic mechanisms on haloperidol-induced catalepsy. Psychopharmacology (Berl) 62:67–69

Bischoff S, Vassout A, Delini-Stula A, Waldmeier P (1986) Interactions of cipazoxapine, citatepine, eresepine, and maroxepine with central dopamine (DA) receptors: effects of in vivo [^{3}H]spiperone binding, DA metabolism, and behavioral parameters. Pharmacopsychiatry 19:306–307

Bjerkenstedt L, Härnryd C, Grimm V, Gullberg B (1978) A double-blind comparison of melperone and thiothixene in psychotic women using a new rating scale, the CPRS. Arch Psychiatr Nervenkr 226:157–172

Bürki HR, Ruch W, Asper H (1975) Effects of clozapine, thioridazine, perlapine and haloperidol on the metabolism of the biogenic amines in the brain of the rat. Psychopharmacologia (Berl) 41:27–33

Casey DE (1988) Tardive dyskinesia and dopamine receptor hypersensitivity: pros and cons. In: Belmaker RH, Sandler M, Dahlström (eds) Progress in catecholamine

research. Part C: Clinical aspects. New York, pp 9–12 (Neurology and neurobiology, vol 42C)
Casey DE (1989a) Clozapine: neuroleptic-induced EPS and tardive dyskinesia. Psychopharmacology (Berl) 99:S47–S53
Casey DE (1989b) Desensitization to dopamine D1 and D2 antagonist-induced dystonia. Abstracts of the proceedings of the VIIIth World Congress of Psychiatry 1989
Casey DE (1989c) Serotonergic aspects of acute extrapyramidal syndromes in nonhuman primates. Psychopharmacol Bull 25(3):457–459
Casey DE (1992) Dopamine D1 (SCH 23390) and D2 (haloperidol) antagonists in drug-naive monkeys. Psychopharmacology 107:18–22
Casey DE (1991a) Extrapyramidal syndromes in nonhuman primates: typical and atypical neuroleptics. Psychopharmacol Bull 27(1):47–50
Casey DE (1991b) Raclopride versus haloperidol: comparative efficacy in a double-blind multicenter investigation. Proc Soc Biol Psychiatry 144a:110A
Casey DE, Keepers GA (1988) Neuroleptic side effects: acute extrapyramidal syndromes and tardive dyskinesia. In: Casey DE, Christensen AV (eds) Psychopharmacology: current trends. Springer, Berlin Heidelberg New York, pp 74–93
Casey DE, Gerlach J, Christensson E (1980) Dopamine, acetylcholine, and GABA effects in acute dystonia in primates. Psychopharmacology (Berl) 70:83–87
Ceulemans DLS, Gelders YG, Hoppenbrouwers M-LJA, Reyntjens AJM, Janssen PAJ (1985) Effect of serotonin antagonism in schizophrenia: a pilot study with setoperone. Psychopharmacology (Berl) 85:329–332
Coffin VL, Latranyi MB, Chipkin RE (1989) Acute extrapyramidal syndrome in cebus monkeys: development mediated by dopamine D2 but not D1 receptors. J Pharmacol Exp Ther 249(3):769–774
Deniker P (1984) Introduction of neuroleptic chemotherapy into psychiatry. In: Ayd FJ, Blackwell B (eds) Discoveries in biological psychiatry. Ayd Medical Communications, Baltimore, pp 155–164
Farde L, Wiesel F-A, Jansson P, Uppfeldt G, Wahlen A, Sedvall G (1988) An open label trial of raclopride in acute schizophrenia. Confirmation of D2-dopamine receptor occupancy by PET. Psychopharmacology (Berl) 94:1–7
Gerlach J, Casey DE (1990) Remoxipride, a new selective D2 antagonist, and haloperidol in cebus monkeys. Prog Neuropsychopharmacol Biol Psychiatry 14:103–112
Gerlach J, Casey DE, Kistrup K (1986) D1 and D2 receptor manipulation in cebus monkeys: implication for extrapyramidal syndromes in humans. Clin Neuropharmacol 9 Suppl 4:131–133
Hall H, Sällemark M, Jerning E (1986) Effects of remoxipride and some related new substituted salicylamides on rat brain receptors. Acta Pharmacol Toxicol (Lopenh) 58:61–70
Hyttel J, Larsen J-J, Christensen AV, Arnt J (1985) Receptor binding profiles of neuroleptics. In: Casey DE, Chase TN, Christensen AV, Gerlach J (eds) Dyskinesia: research and treatment. Springer, Berlin Heidelberg New York, pp 9–18
Korsgaard S, Gerlach J, Christensson E (1985) Behavioral aspects of serotonin-dopamine interaction in the monkey. Eur J Pharmacol 118:245–252
Lewander T, Westerbergh S-E, Morrison D (1990) Clinical profile of remoxipride – a combined analysis of a comparative double-blind multicentre trial programme. Acta Psychiatr Scand Suppl 358(82):92–98
Leysen JE (1981) Review on neuroleptic receptors: specificity and multiplicity of in vitro binding related to pharmacological activity. In: Usdin E, Dahl SG, Gram LF, Lingjaerde O (eds) Clinical pharmacology in psychiatry: neuroleptic and antidepressant research. Macmillan, London, pp 35–62
Leysen JE, Gommeren W, Eens A, deChaffoy deCourcelles D, Stoof JC, Janssen PAJ (1988) Biochemical profile of risperidone, a new antipsychotic. J Pharmacol Exp Ther 247(2):661–670
McQuade RD, Ford D, Duffy RA, Chipkin RE, Iorio LC, Barnett A (1988) Serotonergic component of SCH 23390: in vitro and in vivo binding analyses. Life Sci 43: 1861–1869

Meltzer HY, Matsubara S, Lee JC (1989) Classification of typical and atypical antipsychotic drugs on the basis of dopamine D1, D2 and serotonin pKi values. J Pharmacol Exp Ther 251(1):238–246

Niemegeers CJE, Leysen JE, Laduron PM, Janssen PAJ (1984) Differential pharmacological and biochemical profiles of serotonin-S2 antagonists. Collegium Internationale Neuropsychopharmacologicum, 14th CINP Congress, Abstract 667

Ögren SO, Hall H, Köhler CH, Magnusson O, Sjöstrand SE (1986) The selective dopamine D2 receptor antagonist raclopride discriminates between dopamine mediated motor functions. Psychopharmacology (Berl) 90:287–294

Povlsen UJ, Noring J, Laursen AL, Korsgaard S, Gerlach J (1986) Effects of serotonergic and anticholinergic drugs in haloperidol-induced dystonia in cebus monkeys. Clin Neuropharmacol 9:84–90

Svendsen O, Arnt J, Boeck J, Bøgesø KP, Christensen AV, Hyttel J, Larsen J-J (1986) The neuropharmacological profile of tefludazine, a potential antipsychotic drug with dopamine and serotonin receptor antagonistic effects. Drug Dev Res 7:35–47

Tamminga CA, Gerlach J (1987) New neuroleptics and experimental antipsychotics in schizophrenia. In: Meltzer HY (ed) Psychopharmacology: the third generation of progress. Raven, New York, pp 1129–1140

VanTol HHM, Bunzow JR, Guan H-C, Sunahara RK, Seeman P, Niznik HB, Civelli O (1991) Cloning of the gene for a human dopamine D4 receptor with high affinity for the antipsychotic clozapine. Nature 350:610–614

Waldmeier PC, Delini-Stula AA (1979) Serotonin-dopamine interactions in the nigrostriatal system. Eur J Pharmacol 55:363–373

Wetzel H, Wiedemann K, Holsboer F, Benkert O (1991) Savoxepine: invalidation of an "atypical" neuroleptic response pattern predicted by animal models in an open clinical trial with schizophrenic patients. Psychopharmacology (Berl) 103:280–283

Methods to Facilitate Early Exploratory Testing of Novel Psychopharmacologic Agents in Humans

W.Z. POTTER[1] and R.P. IRWIN[2]

The starting point for this chapter follows from three assumptions: (1) substantial numbers of patients seriously ill with psychiatric illnesses such as schizophrenia and depression show inadequate therapeutic responses to all available classes of drugs; (2) decisions to take new potential psychotropic compounds into humans are more and more based on judgments as to the likelihood of there being a reasonable market for that specific compound; and (3) pharmacologic guidance can greatly enhance the efficiency of the clinical development process both in terms of reducing wasted effort in Phase I testing and of deriving maximum information concerning the appropriate dose to test the therapeutic potential of a novel compound. With regard to this latter point, it is well known that even marketed psychotropic drugs have had very misleading dose recommendations because what is required for marketing is to establish safe doses which *on average* have a positive effect rather than doses which produce the maximum possible benefit.

In the first two decades of the development of psychotropic medications, following the discovery that certain phenothiazines were antipsychotic compounds in humans, many exploratory clinical studies of various chemical relatives were carried out (DeLini-Stula 1990) in order to see if they had any interesting properties. Moreover, investigators were able to obtain and administer a variety of novel compounds to small numbers of subjects to test theories of drug action. For instance, parachlorophenylalinine (PCPA) was administered to block tryptophan hydroxylase and perhaps reverse antidepressants' effects and to reduce 5-hydroxyindoleacetic acid (5HIAA) in CSF (Sjoerdsma et al. 1970; Shopsin et al. 1976); fusaric acid was given to block dopamine β-hydroxylase in attempts to identify new antimanic agents (Goodwin and Sack 1974). The preclinical toxicity requirements for these very brief investigations in small numbers of subjects were not that onerous nor expensive. The sense derived today from both academic investigators and individuals representing different companies' neuropharmacologic

[1] Section on Clinical Pharmacology, Experimental Therapeutics Branch, National Institute of Mental Health, Bethesda, MD 20892, USA
[2] National Institute of General Medical Sciences and Clinical Neuroscience Branch, National Institute of Mental Health, Bethesda, MD 20892, USA

groups is that even "exploratory testing" represents major funding and corporate decision-making (Dreyfus et al. 1989; Delini-Stula 1990). At least in the United States, for industry to take a compound into humans now seems to entail extensive enough preclinical toxicity testing with the compound synthesized under the "good manufacturing practices" (GMP) to support ultimate Phase II trials with the desired route of administration (mostly oral for psychotropics). This, in turn, requires a commitment to GMP bulk synthesis of sufficient amounts of compound in order to move forward to long-term Phase II studies in humans. Having recently compared costs to us as academic investigators working under an investigational new drug (IND) protocol, *with no consideration* of undertaking the development of an new drug application (NDA) to support marketing, to costs for industry, one discovers that the latter are conservatively five times as expensive. Given limited resources, one obviously is not going to make a commitment to an expensive process without reasonable hope of some success.

Reasonable hope of success is usually based on the availability of a predictive model. In the field of psychopharmacology we have used behavioral and physiological animal models that reflect the actions of drugs already known to be neuroleptics, antidepressants, anxiolytics, etc. This has proven to be an excellent method of finding compounds with a similar therapeutic profile to the original serendipitously discovered psychotherapeutic compounds. It is not clear, however, that the field has yet developed a widely accepted drug whose therapeutic biochemical principle was not present or inherent in drugs discovered in the 1950s. For instance, norepinephrine and serotonin uptake inhibitors dominate the field of antidepressants with monoamine oxidase and perhaps dopamine uptake inhibitors held in reserve for more difficult to treat depressions (Osman and Potter 1991). Compare this to the evolution of antihypertensive compounds which have included but are not limited to amine depletors (reserpine), ganglionic blockers, various types of vasodilators, α- and β-adrenergic blockers, various classes of calcium channel blockers, angiotensin converting enzyme inhibitors and, in the past, even monoamine oxidase inhibitors. This variety has depended on studying blood pressure regulation in animal models which are not simply based on the observed clinical efficacy of other drugs in hypertension. This admittedly oversimplified comparison captures the dilemma that, in psychopharmacology, when we "discover" a biochemically distinct compound with therapeutic properties (e.g., valproic acid in mania), it is usually because of clinical observation and not because of efficacy in some animal model.

As with most generalizations there are exceptions, and one could argue that the development of, for instance, selective serotonin receptor subtype antagonists and agonists has been based, at least in part, on findings in animal models, particularly with regard to anxiety (Taylor et al. 1984). One might add that these have yet to prove as truly efficacious as the existing standards for any major indication, although many of the modulators of serotonin receptors are remarkably free of troubling side effects.

There remain, however, substantial proportions of patients with the highly prevalent serious psychiatric illnesses schizophrenia and affective disorders who do not respond satisfactorily to existing treatments (Kane et al. 1988; Prien and Potter 1990). Neuroscience, now employing the tools of molecular biology, identifies growing numbers of highly specific processes in the brain that, if manipulated, must produce some functional biochemical change which in humans may or may not be detectable with available methods. For instance, the field has or is in the process of developing compounds selective not only for monoamine neurotransmitter receptor subtypes but also for those reacting with a growing array of peptide receptors such as cholecystokinin (CCK) (Gariano and Groves 1989). There are multiple sites distal to receptors involved in coupling, second messenger function, control of regulatory phosphorylation, etc., which could be and perhaps are the primary sites of psychotropic drug action (e.g., lithium). Should the field depend on our existing animal models to discriminate the therapeutic potential of manipulating such sites in the brain?

If not, it will be necessary either to wait for animal (or in vitro) models comparable to those enjoyed in the fields of, for instance, hypertension and oncology, or to be willing to test compounds in psychiatric patients to see if a particular novel biochemical property (e.g., blockade of receptor "x" or altered regulation of proteins involved in control of signal transduction) has a therapeutic effect. Some possible applications of pharmacologic principles and knowledge will be explored below to facilitate the process of going as quickly as possible into humans within the limits of safety and of ensuring that a compound is producing its maximum pharmacologic effect in the central nervous system.

To this end, the considerations of the Pharmacokinetics and Neurochemical Group of the European Organization for Research and Treatment of Cancer (EORTC 1985, 1987) and the Blood Level Group of the U.S. National Cancer Institute (Collins et al. 1986; Davis et al. 1988) will first be briefly discussed with an eye to their generic recommendations which may be applicable to psychopharmacology. Both groups have struggled with the basically empirical approach to establishing doses in humans and questioned whether current practice in antitumor drug development is necessary, whereby ten or more escalations of acute single doses may be required to reach a dose that produces side effects judged to be dose-limiting. Oncology provides the extreme example of viewing risk of serious toxicity as an almost certain corollary of therapeutic efficacy. With this consideration in mind, Collins et al. (1986) have proposed an approach that may get one to the maximal tolerated dose (MTD) using significantly fewer escalations from the starting dose. This is based on aiming for a dose that produces the same area under the drug concentration vs time curve (AUC) observed in mice at the

Table 1. Proposal for pharmacokinetically guided Phase 1 dose escalation

Preclinical
1. Determine metabolites and effect of host metabolism on drug activity and toxicity.
2. Develop assay for parent drug and any active metabolites with adequate sensitivity for 1/10th LD_{10} dose.
3. Randomize mice and, using the proposed clinical route, vehicle and schedule, determine:
   a. LD_{10}
   b. AUC at the LD_{10} for the parent drug and active metabolites
   c. AUC at $0.5 \times LD_{10}$ and $0.1 \times LD_{10}$ to assess if non-linear kinetics
   d. If possible, correlate AUCs and toxicity
4. Determine protein binding in mouse and human plasma at observed concentrations.

Clinical
1. Initiate the clinical study at 1/10th mouse LD_{10} and treat 3–5 patients to determine AUC with acceptable accuracy.
2. Use appropriate escalation scheme to attain projected MTD AUC monitoring drug and active metabolite concentrations at every dose level modifying for nonlinearity.

Modified from EORTC (1987).
AUC, area under the drug vs time curve; MTD, maximum tolerated dose.

LD_{10} (expressed on a mg/m^2 basis). The process of establishing a MTD, which is taken to be the principal goal of Phase I trials of antitumor drugs, is inherently conflictual. A standard scheme in oncology which attempts to combine efficiency and safety is known as the "modified Fibonacci" (Goldsmith et al. 1975) involving an initial "rapid" escalation of 100% from 1/10th of the murine LD_{10} dose falling to 30%–35% increases over the previous dose by the fifth escalation. Simply by making the first escalation step equal to the square root of the ratio of the AUC (in the mouse) at the mouse LD_{10} to the entry dose AUC in humans can dramatically reduce the total number of escalation steps. At least two studies sponsored by the National Cancer Institute have successfully employed such escalation patterns modified on the basis of drug levels allowing for safe entry level doses 25 times higher than by standard procedures and estimated time savings of 12–24 months in the development process (Collins et al. 1990).

Such procedures for more rapid escalation, variations on them, and underlying assumptions are covered in some detail elsewhere (Collins et al. 1986, 1990; EORTC 1985, 1987; Davis et al. 1988). A proposed general scheme is summarized in Table 1, modified from the EORTC recommendations (1987). Certain practical points emerge with regard to minimizing variance and assuring safety. At the preclinical stage, toxicity and pharmacokinetic studies should ideally be performed on the same randomized group of mice; obviously, a sensitive assay to allow accurate determination of both the LD_{10} or other target AUC in mice or other species and whatever fraction of the animal dose is selected to begin in humans is required and, to assure quality control, ideally run in the same laboratory. Protein binding of certain drugs may differ between species, a factor which must be checked if a compound is highly protein bound. Toxic active metabolites pose special problems since the AUC only "corrects" for interspecies variation in the clearance of the parent drug and does not predict what proportion will be converted to what metabolite or excreted unchanged. Also, in cases where there is a non-linear relationship between dose and AUC, a set dose-escalation procedure would be unwise although pharmacokinetic monitoring in human subjects would be essential. Another aspect of being able to predict the human MTD based on an AUC measurement is that the information could feed back to preclinical studies to see if the desired pharmacologic effect is likely to be achieved at the MTD. If not, the compound in question is unlikely to be clinically useful (Davis et al. 1988).

The extent to which recommendations from the field of antitumor drug development apply in their specifics to psychotropic drugs may, at first glance, appear minimal. One view is that, in looking for a new psychotropic, one would only select compounds with a probable wide therapeutic index. This criteria would, however, have precluded selection of drugs such as lithium and tricyclic antidepressants for trials in humans. Obviously, there is no necessary connection between the therapeutic potential of psychotropics and toxicity as is the case for many antitumor drugs, but it is interesting that some of our major drugs have had a rather narrow therapeutic index. Thus, in the search for truly novel treatments for refractory patients, we must keep open the option of exploring relatively toxic compounds in humans that offer hope of real therapeutic advances. Although we may often need only aim for some maximal "desired" dose instead of MTD in our Phase I studies, we should be prepared to expeditiously develop certain compounds for human studies along the MTD approach. The point for our field is to note that novel approaches to Phase I trials are not impossible. A recent general review of Phase I studies (Posvar and Sedman 1989) emphasizes the possibilities of learning more from these, a point echoed by commentators from academia, industry, and the Food and Drug Administration (FDA) (Colburn 1990). The second, and most important, point concerns using AUC data in animals and humans to make judgments about the next step. This may be the only accessible measure to infer whether one is exerting the desired pharmacologic effect with a compound acting in the brain.

Current practice in psychopharmacology with regard to introducing compounds for the first time into humans is based on general rules of thumb, such as starting with 1/10th and even 1/5th the dose (on a mg/m^2 basis) that produces no toxicity in animals. One's confidence increases if the toxic doses are roughly the same across three species (usually rat, mouse, and dog). Initial escalating single dose studies can frequently be carried out in ten or fewer subjects. For many newer compounds toxicity is low and is first identified in animals as an inhibition of weight gain at very high doses, between two and three orders of magnitude above the pharmacologic dose. One notes the use of dose and not AUC. Interestingly, a soon-to-begin

Table 2. Fast-track drug development using PK/PD

Preclinical	PK: toxic in rodents
Phase I	PK: guided dose escalation PK and preliminary PD (Toxicity)
Phase II	Randomized concentration and controlled trial PK: guided dose-response trial

PK/PD, pharmacokinetics/pharmacodynamics; modified from a presentation of Peck (1990).

Phase I study, which has been targeted toward FDA approval rather than maximal pharmacologic information, involves i.v. administration of a highly selective α_2-antagonist, at most "includes" some blood samples for possible later determination of drug concentration, and requires seven escalation steps. All of this work will be done without necessarily obtaining any pharmacokinetic data. In this instance, acute increases of plasma norepinephrine are expected at pharmacologic doses, and these will be the pharmacodynamic end point.

Consider the dilemma for establishing an end point, however, if one were developing a compound which had as its target an effect such as retardation of the cytosolic to membrane translocation of some specific isozyme of protein kinase C (PKC) in discrete brain areas. For the sake of argument, assume no measurable toxic or *other* effects of the compound in animal models in vivo at doses which, following sacrifice, could be shown to maximally inhibit the PKC translocation in brain membrane preparations. Assume also that an investigator has reason to believe that it is important to know what effect this inhibition of PKC translocation would have in humans. How does he or she select a dose to test in humans?

One could consider a plan such as outlined in Table 2. The AUC predicted to be associated with the maximum "desired" dose could be used to suggest an average steady-state concentration which could then be tested for pharmacologic effects in some preclinical model. Means of administration would need to be identical to that planned for studies in humans, the most likely being repeat intravenous bolus or infusion and repeat oral ingestion. Duration of administration would depend on the clinical investigator's specification of the minimal time necessary in humans to provide evidence that something of interest (e.g., antidepressant effect) is occurring. If, for example, 3 weeks were desired, one would administer the compound over a 3 week period to produce the specified AUC in an animal, sacrifice the animal, and see if PKC translocation was maximally inhibited. Thus, one could have some confidence that the AUC achieved in humans would produce the desired biochemical effect over time and hence test the question of whether that particular action was associated with any detectable therapeutic, behavioral, or cognitive effect. More general application of concentration-controlled clinical trials has recently been recommended by the FDA (Peck 1990; Peck et al. 1990). In the hypothetical instance discussed here, a concentration-controlled trial would constitute a form of exploratory testing in humans of whether a specific biochemical manipulation has potentially therapeutic effects. The animal model would serve only to establish the safety and measurable pharmacokinetic parameters associated with producing the biochemical change in the desired (but inaccessible to measure in humans) brain compartment.

Obviously, we may ultimately have sufficient varieties of noninvasive brain imaging techniques to directly assess whether a biochemical effect is present in humans such as the dopamine receptor blockade which can be shown in human striatum utilizing positron emission tomography (PET) (Frade et al. 1988). It seems unlikely, however, that brain imaging techniques can be developed rapidly enough to test the large varieties of distinct biochemical manipulations emerging from the field of molecular pharmacology. Here we refer to PET data as a means of showing that there is a predictable relationship between plasma concentrations of a compound and, for instance, dopamine receptor occupancy.

It may seem unlikely that anyone would be willing to test a compound without either a good animal model or a sure marker of activity in humans, but that decision has been made more than once. A particularly provocative example is *S*-adenosyl-methionine (SAMe), which was tested in schizophrenics purely on the basis of theoretical speculations and was noted to be activating (Salvadorini et al. 1980) rather than therapeutic. The characteristics of the activation suggested that SAMe might be antidepressant, a speculation for which there is an increasing body of clinical evidence. Exogenous SAMe was originally observed to have minimal effects in animals except for psychostimulant potentiation (Sansone 1978) and only very recently was shown to potentiate norepinephrine-stimulated cAMP activity, first in vitro using rat brain slices, then ex vivo (Kellar et al., personal communication). Whether this biochemical effect is related to methylation remains to be determined. In any event, development moves forward in the absence of clear preclinical data. Moreover, to date, it has not been possible to demonstrate any physiologic or biochemical effect of SAMe in humans. An earlier observation of reduction in norepinephrine response on going from a lying to standing position (Sherer et al. 1986) now seems best explained as an ordering effect and not a result of SAMe.

At least from the point of view of clinical investigators interested in pathophysiology, it is worth having novel compounds to administer to humans to see if certain biochemical manipulations have therapeutic, adverse, or no effects in psychiatric terms. A new Alcoliol, Drug Abuse, and Mental Health Administration (ADAMHA) program includes development of such compounds which can be both tested as theoretical constructs and explored as therapeutic agents in a wide variety of psychiatric and substance abuse disorders. It is hoped that as part of this program new approaches to Phase I studies will emerge.

Not all novel CNS compounds will be devoid of some accessible marker of a pharmacologic effect; as noted in the above actual example of an α_2-antagonist, increases in plasma norepinephrine provide a convenient and appropriate index of desired biochemical activity. It would appear, however, that for those without a marker and which produce some novel CNS alteration only detectable in animal studies, we can best rely on AUC measures to show that we are in the desired dose range.

Clinical investigators have exerted considerable ingenuity in trying to find markers of effect. For instance, an established antagonist of α_2-adrenergic receptors, idazoxan, was initially assessed in humans by observing a shift to the right in the cardiovascular responses to an α_2-agonist (Elliot et al. 1984). Neuroendocrine responses in humans have been a particularly favored means of implicating CNS activity of a compound. It is possible to establish dose-response relationships between drug and release of a variety of hormones such as prolactin, growth hormone, ACTH, and cortisol presumably mediated by an effect on hypothalamic releasing factors. Obviously, this strategy is limited to drugs which include effects on these systems, but a surprising number of compounds do so. For instance, the potent triazolobenzodiazepine, alprazolam, increases growth hormone in a concentration dependent manner following intravenous administration (Osman et al. 1991). This does not appear to implicate any primary biochemical action beyond acting as an agonist at benzodiazepine receptors which sets off some unspecified cascade of events. The advantage of having an acute measurable pharmacodynamic output bearing some linear relationship to a particular primary biochemical event (e.g., stimulation of benzodiazepine receptors) is that combined pharmacokinetic/pharmacodynamic modeling can often identify where one is on a concentration/effect curve.

It seems reasonable to assume that many biochemical effects of novel compounds in the brain will follow a classic sigmoid relationship based on a single site of action and a saturable effect, an approach reflected in the application of the Hill equation to steady-state pharmacodynamic modeling by Wagner (1968). Linear, E_{max}, and sigmoid E_{max} models are used to fit steady-state plasma concentration and effect data. The models E_{max} and sigmoid E_{max} predict that as the concentration increases there will be a maximal effect beyond which a further increase in drug concentration will produce no further changes in effect.

The E_{max} model:

$$E = \frac{E_{max}Cp}{\mathrm{EC}_{50} + Cp}$$

where E is the effect, E_{max} is the maximum effect, Cp is the plasma drug concentration, and EC_{50} is the plasma concentration at 50% of E_{max}. From the E_{max} model, if Cp is $\ll$ than EC_{50}, the above equation reduces to a linear equation. This linear model does not predict a maximal response.

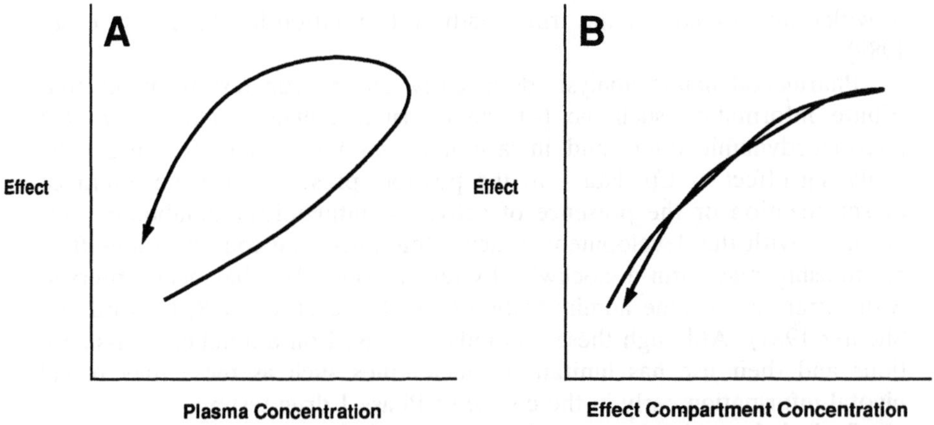

Fig. 1. Counterclockwise hysteresis loop (**A**) of a hypothetical drug with an equilibration time lag from the plasma to the site of its effect. The hysteresis loop "collapses" (**B**) when effect is plotted vs the estimated effect compartment concentration

Pharmacodynamic studies under steady-state conditions for *E*/*C*p are often times consuming and expensive. Early in drug testing potentially valuable information could be obtained from nonsteady-state studies. Although there are limitations to this approach, early understanding of the pharmacodynamics of a drug utilizing often routinely collected data may accelerate the drug testing process. Simultaneous modeling of single dose pharmacokinetic and pharmacodynamic data has been advocated (Fuseau and Sheiner 1984; Sheiner 1985; Unadkat et al. 1986; Verotta and Sheiner 1987). What is needed are plasma drug concentration, time, and drug effect data. For many drugs plasma concentration vs time and effect vs time curves do not overlap. Multiple factors may account for this (e.g., tolerance or formation of active metabolites). A time delay in drug transport from the plasma to the site of drug effect may produce such a pattern. Since it is usually not possible to measure the drug concentration at the site of its effect (*C*e), plasma concentration (*C*p) is usually used. In this case, when effect is plotted vs *C*p in time-ordered sequence, a counterclockwise hysteresis loop is observed (Fig. 1A).

Parametric and nonparametric methods have been used to estimate *C*e (Sheiner 1985). By substituting the estimated effect compartment levels for the plasma levels, the hysteresis loop "collapses" and takes on the shape of the pharmacodynamic concentration effect curve (Fig. 1B). A particularly impressive application of this approach is analysis of the counterclockwise hysteresis loop observed for an effect of verapamil (change in P-R interval) after a single i.v. dose. Nonsteady-state effect, plasma concentration, and time data were used in modeling estimated effect site concentrations and provided an estimate of the true steady-state relationship (Schwartz et al. 1989).

Pharmacodynamic analysis done early on in drug testing might contribute information such as: (a) the pharmacodynamic relationship, (b) pharmacodynamic inter- and intra-subject variability, and (c) cues – by analyzing effect vs *Cp* data – to the possible presence of acute tolerance or sensitization or the presence of active or antagonistic metabolites. For instance, with the development of acute tolerance, the concentration-effect relationship may form a clockwise hysteresis loop. This has been observed with intranasal cocaine administration (Van Dyke et al. 1978; Holford and Sheiner 1981). Although these methods are based on a number of assumptions and their use has limitations, techniques such as these may reveal pivotal information early in the course of Phase I drug testing.

Such information may reduce the need for sequential steady-state concentration-response studies to establish the EC_{50} and dose necessary to approach the maximum pharmacologic effect. Of course, in cases where there is a large population variance in sensitivity to a particular effect, there will be an equally large variation in the EC_{50} across individuals. For instance, the EC_{50} for infused norepinephrine to constrict basal veins in 15 unrelated subjects ranged from 1.4 to 110.2 ng/ml (Luthra et al. 1991). Nonetheless, if one is testing the potential of a novel compound in a few individuals, applying the approach described by Verotta and Sheiner (1987) provides an elegant method of approximating the concentration/effect relationship.

The major weakness of such indirect pharmacodynamic modeling is the unproven assumption that different effects in different areas of the brain, even when mediated by the same receptor type, will have the same EC_{50}. There are, for instance, preclinical studies that demonstrate different EC_{50}s, perhaps reflecting effects at different receptors after administration of compounds such as clonidine and apomorphine (Paalzow and Edlund 1979; Paalzow et al. 1985). To distinguish whether different effects reflect actions at different receptors or receptors linked to different functions is complex. The extent of preclinical studies one is willing to undertake is going to be influenced by the degree of application to clinical studies. What is being discussed here are possible ways in which combined pharmacokinetic/pharmacodynamic studies in animals would permit interpretation of plasma concentration data in humans.

The pharmacologic approaches discussed above are offered as a first step in moving from a state of relative paralysis in the testing of biochemically novel compounds in humans that do not give a "positive" indication of therapeutic potential in animal models. One can argue the pros and cons of how to select among such novel compounds, but the real test is whether significant behavioral or therapeutic effects are produced in humans. There are already many compounds with at least one known novel biochemical effect in animal brain which are nowhere near being tested in humans. Could the field agree on initial criteria of what would constitute the least expensive but adequate exploratory trial of a novel compound? Possible criteria might be:

1. Establish either a maximum "desired" dose or MTD in ten (or fewer) individuals (normal volunteers or patients as appropriate) using the most accelerated dose escalation whenever possible (see Table 1).
2. On the basis of the AUC data in humans used to carry out the dose escalation and the AUC in animals, target an average steady-state concentration predicted to produce a near maximal effect at the biochemical target site in the CNS.
3. On the basis of the above, select a dose in the same individual to give repeatedly to test for behavioral (in healthy volunteers) and therapeutic (in patients) effects for the desired time period.
4. In general, purely exploratory testing could be done with intravenous administration which avoids the sometimes arduous process of developing a reliable p.o. formulation (e.g., SAMe). A corollary is that preclinical toxicology, including for instance murine LD_{10}, would only need to be done using intravenous administration.

The underlying assumptions of such a schema are that small numbers of intensively studied individuals can provide meaningful therapeutic clues as well as evidence of pharmacologic effects. No one would question that small numbers of healthy volunteers (6–8) are sufficient to provide evidence of biochemical effects (if measurable) using each person as his or her own control. For instance, monoamine uptake and monoamine oxidase inhibitors can be counted on to produce their predicted pharmacologic effects in every individual if side effects do not limit the dose. Although what would constitute a sufficient therapeutic clue will vary according to the judgment of each investigator, one would probably be discouraged if one didn't see a positive effect in, say, at least one of the first five or six patients with refractory schizophrenia or depression.

Whatever the judgments with regard to magnitude or frequency of clinical effects, extensive early pharmacologic data should provide reassurance that any lack of improvement is not because too little compound was given to produce the CNS pharmacologic effect being tested. What is being discussed are strategies for testing the therapeutic potential of preselected CNS pharmacologic effects not of compounds that are serendipitously observed to produce potentially useful effects (e.g., angiotensin converting enzyme inhibitors). Standard approaches obviously work in the latter situations; however, they do not yield the level of pharmacokinetic and pharmacodynamic data which allows us to utilize the conceptual and methodologic advances touched on here. The field of neuroscience enjoys the position of being on the "cutting edge;" we should see to it that bringing the discoveries of basic neuroscience into the realm of clinical psychopharmacology is carried out in as innovative and scientifically guided manner as possible.

References

Colburn WA (1990) Controversy V: phase 1, first time in man studies. J Clin Pharmacol 30:210–222

Collins JM, Zaharko DS, Dedrick RL, Chabner BA (1986) Potential roles for preclinical pharmacology in phase 1 clinical trials. Cancer Treat Rev 70:73–80

Collins JM, Grieshaber CK, Chabner BA (1990) Pharmacologically guided phase 1 clinical trials based upon preclinical drug development. J Natl Cancer Inst 82: 1321–1326

Davis LE, Alberts DS, Plezia PM et al. (1988) Predictive model for plasma concentration versus time profiles of investigational anticancer drugs in patients. J Natl Cancer Inst 80:815–819

Delini-Stula A (1990) Clinical trials in Europe and the development of new psychotropics as viewed by European manufacturers. Pharmacopsychiatry 23(4):164–70

Dreyfus JF, Cremniter D, Guelfi JD (1989) Reflections on FDA and WHO recommendations concerning clinical trials. Psychiatry Psychobiol 4:117–122

Elliott HL, Jones RC, Vincent J, Lawire CB, Reid JL (1984) The alpha adrenoceptor antagonist properties of idazoxan in normal subjects. Clin Pharmacol Ther 36(2): 190–196

EORTC New Drug Development Committee (1985) EORTC guidelines for phase 1 trials with single agents in adults. Eur J Cancer Clin Oncol 21:1005–1007

EORTC Pharmacokinetics and Metabolism Group (1987) Pharmacokinetically-guided dose escalation in phase 1 clinical trials. Eur J Cancer Clin Oncol 23:1083–1087

Farde L, Wiesel F-A, Halldin C, Sedvall G (1988) Central D-2 dopamine receptor occupany in schizophrenic patients treated with antipsychotic drugs. Arch Gen Psychiatry 45:71–76

Fuseau E, Sheiner LB (1984) Simultaneous modeling of pharmacokinetics and pharmacodynamics with a nonparametric pharmacodynamic model. Clin Pharmacol Ther 35(6):733–741

Gariano RF, Groves PM (1989) A mechanism for the involvment of colocalized neuropeptides in the actions of antipsychotic drugs. Biol Psychiatry 26(3):303–314

Goldsmith MA, Slavik M, Carter SK (1975) Quantitative prediction of drug toxicity in humans from toxicology in small and large animals. Cancer Res 35:1354–1364

Goodwin FK, Sack RL (1974) Behavioral effects of a new dopamine-beta-hydroxylase inhibitor (fusaric acid) in man. J Psychiatr Res 22:211–217

Holford NHG, Sheiner LB (1981) Understanding the dose-effect relationship: clinical applications of pharmacokinetic-pharmacodynamic models. Clin Pharmacokinet 6:429–453

Kane J, Oaks G, Honigfeld G, Singer J, Hanover NJ, Meltzer H, Cleveland MD and the Clozaril Collaborative Study Group (1988) Clozapine for the treatment-resistant schizophrenic. Arch Gen Psychiatry 45(9):789–796

Luthra A, Borkowski KR, Carruthers SG (1991) Genetic aspects of variability in superficial vein responsiveness to norepinephrine. Clin Pharmacol Ther 49:355–361

Osman OT, Potter WZ (1991) Potentiation of dopamine in the treatment of refractory depression. In: Amsterdam JD (ed) Refractory depression. Raven, New York, p 41 (Advances in neuropsychiatry and psychopharmacology, vol 2)

Osman OT, DeVane CL, Greenblatt DS, Potter WZ (1991) Pharmacokinetic and dynamic correlates of intravenous alprazolam challenge. Clin Pharmacol Ther 50:656–662

Paalzow LK, Edlund PO (1979) Multiple receptor responses. A new concept to describe the relationship between pharmacological effects and pharmacokinetics of a drug: studies on clonidine in the rat and cat. J Pharmacokinet Biopharm 7:495–510

Paalzow LK, Paalzow GHM, Tfelt-Hansen P (1985) Variability in bioavailability: concentration versus effect. In: Rowland M et al. (eds) Variability in drug therapy: description, estimation, and control. Raven, New York, p 167

Peck C (1990) The randomized concentration-controlled clinical trial (CCT): an information-rich alternative to the randomized placebo-controlled clinical trial (PCT). Clin Pharmacol Ther 47(2):148

Peck C, Collins J, Harter J (1990) Incorporation of pharmacokinetic and pharmacodynamic intelligence into early drug development. Clin Pharmacol Ther 47(2):126

Posvar EL, Sedman AJ (1989) New drugs: first-time in man. J Clin Pharmacol 19: 961–966

Prien RS, Potter WZ (1990) NIMH workshop report on treatment of bipolar disorder. Psychopharmacol Bull 26:409–427

Salvadorini F, Galeone F, Saba P, Tognetti G, Mariani G (1980) Evaluation of S-adenosylmethionine (SAMe) effectiveness on depression. Curr Ther Res 27(6): 908–918

Sansone M (1978) Effects of S-adenysyl-L-methionine on the behavior of mice. In: Andreoli VM, Agnoli A, Fazio C (eds) Transmethylations and the central nervous system. Springer, Berlin Heidelberg New York, p 121

Schwartz JB, Verotta D, Sheiner LB (1989) Pharmacodynamic modeling of verapamil effects under steady-state and nonsteady-state conditions. J Pharmacol Exp Ther 251(3):1032–1038

Sheiner LB (1985) Modeling pharmacodynamics: parametric and nonparametric approaches. In: Rowland M et al. (eds) Variability in drug therapy: description, estimation, and control. Raven, New York, pp 139–152

Sherer MA, Cantoni GL, Golden RN, Rudorfer MV, Potter WZ (1986) Effects of S-adenosyl-methionine on plasma norepinephrine, blood pressure, and heart rate in healthy volunteers. Psychiatry Res 17:111–118

Shopsin B, Friedman E, Gershon S (1976) Parachlorophenylalanine reversal of tranylcypromine effects in depressed patients. Arch Gen Psychiatry 33:811–819

Sjoerdsma A, Lovenberg W, Engelman K, Carpenter WT, Wyatt RJ, Gessa GL (1970) Serotonin now: clinical implications of inhibiting its synthesis with para-chlorophenylalanine. J Intern Med 73:607–629

Taylor DP, Allen LE, Becker JA, Crane M, Hyslop DK, Riblet LA (1984) Changing concepts of the biochemical action of the anxioselective drug buspirone. Drug Dev Res 4:95–108

Unadkat JD, Bartha F, Sheiner LB (1986) Simultaneous modeling of pharmacokinetics and pharmacodynamics with non-parametric kinetic and dynamic models. Clin Pharmacol Ther 40(1):86–93

Van Dyke C, Jatlow P, Ungerer J, Barash PG, Byck R (1978) Oral cocaine: plasma concentrations and central effects. Science 200:211–213

Verotta D, Sheiner LB (1987) Simultaneous modeling of pharmacokinetics and pharmacodynamics: an improved algorithm. Comput Appl Biosci 3(4):345–349

Wagner JG (1968) Kinetics of pharmacologic response. I. Proposed relationships between response and drug concentration in the intact animal and man. J Theor Biol 20: 171–201

Neuroleptics and Diagnostic Heterogeneity in Relation to Drug Evaluation

F.-A. WIESEL

1 Introduction

The opinion that schizophrenia is a heterogenous disease goes back to E. Bleuler who in his monograph *Dementia Praecox oder Gruppe der Schizofrenien* (Bleuler 1911) proposed the term schizophrenia in his psychopathological descriptions of patients with dementia praecox. In his textbook *Lehrbuch der Psychiatrie* he writes: "*Wenn wir auch eine natürliche innere Einteilung noch nicht machen können, so erscheint uns die Schizophrenie doch nicht als eine Krankheit im engeren Sinne, sondern als eine Krankheitsgruppe, etwa analog der Gruppe der Organischen, die in Paralyse, senile Formen usw. zerfällt. Man sollte deswegen eigentlich von Schizophrenien in der Mehrzahl sprechen*" (Since we cannot divide schizophrenia on objective grounds, schizophrenia seems not to be one disease, but rather a group of disorders, more like the organic psychoses – paralysis, dementia. One should conceive of schizophrenia in plural.) (Bleuler 1916) However, in previous research most investigators have conceived schizophrenia as a uniform disease with Kraepelin's subtypes, i.e., catatonic, paranoid, and hebephrenic schizophrenia. Over the years several different diagnostic systems have been developed and used in schizophrenia research. This means that different criteria for selection of patients in research have been used, suggesting that quite different patient categories have been studied. Thus Brockington et al. (1978), using 10 diagnostic systems in the study of 119 psychotic patients, found that the number of patients with a diagnosis of schizophrenia ranged between 4% and 45%. Similar findings have been reported by other investigators (Strauss and Gift 1977). However, diagnostic heterogeneity does not seem to have influenced the overall efficiency of neuroleptics in the acute treatment of patients with schizophrenia. This is in accordance with the fact that neuroleptics are antipsychotic and not anti-schizophrenic compounds. In evaluation of drug treatment, it is common to pool studies to obtain high patient numbers but if different diagnostic systems for patient selection have been used, this may obscure different drug treatment profiles. This is further accentuated by the technique of

Department of Psychiatry, Uppsala University, Ulleråker, 750 17 Uppsala, Sweden calculating equivalent drug doses which will favor broad clinical effects on behalf of possible specific clinical profiles of the respective neuroleptic compound.

Definite progress in psychiatric research came with the development of DSM-III (1980) for diagnosis. This system has reached wide acceptance and therefore makes it possible to perform more appropriate comparisons among studies. However, the use of one system does not preclude the lumping of several diseases into one diagnostic category. To obtain more knowledge about the profile of a compound, one may select patients according to several different diagnostic systems or use a broad definition for selection, later making a diagnosis with several systems which may deepen our knowledge of the therapeutic profile of a compound. The potential usefulness of such a strategy is suggested from a study in which prolactin levels in serum were measured (Keks et al. 1990). Eleven different diagnostic systems for schizophrenia were used and four of these (DSM-III, Feighner, RDC, and Taylor and Abrams) selected patients with lower basal prolactin concentrations than in the controls. The four systems excluded schizophrenic patients with elevation or depression of affect. This finding directly points to the relevance of taking into account the diagnostic system used when comparing different studies. There are other important selection mechanisms more seldom discussed such as which patients are willing to be an inpatient and to take part in a drug trial or are too sick to participate. These factors may vary from time and space.

The importance of diagnostic heterogeneity in drug evaluation is relevant for discussion at three different levels – etiology, pathophysiology, and phenomenology.

2 Etiology

For schizophrenic symptoms there are several pathogenetic mechanisms such as neurodegenerative diseases (Huntington's chorea) and metabolic diseases (systemic lupus erythematosus), toxic factors (amphetamines), psychological factors, and idiopathic factors. For idiopathic schizophrenia there is some indirect evidence of a genetic cause. Genetic heterogeneity is probable and indicated by the finding of schizophrenia to be linked to one region of chromosome 5 in one study but not in other pedigrees (Sherrington et al. 1988; Kennedy et al. 1988). It is obvious that evaluation of treatment should be made in relation to the genetic aberration of the disease when possible. However, today one can only state that individuals with familial schizophrenia probably respond to neuroleptic treatment in a similar way as those with sporadic schizophrenia. Other possible etiological factors to be discussed are obstetric complications and virus infections. These factors may by themselves or together with genetic changes result in a pathophysiological disturbance and the disease. It is not known whether patients in these possible categories respond differently to neuroleptic treatment. Recently a disturbed tyrosine transport across cell membranes in patients with schizophrenia was found (Hagenfeldt et al. 1987; Wiesel et al. 1991). This transport disturbance may be a pathogenetic mechanism but it probably does not influence treatment response.

3 Pathophysiology

In 1976 Crow and coworkers rediscovered that chronic patients with schizophrenia may have enlarged ventricles (Johnstone et al. 1976). Later Crow divided patients with schizophrenia into two categories: type I, with positive symptoms, normal ventricles, a good response to neuroleptic treatment, and an increased number of dopamine receptors; and type II, with affective flattening, enlarged ventricles, sometimes intellectual impairment, and a poor neuroleptic response (Crow 1980). Brain morphological changes have been taken as an evidence of at least two subgroups of schizophrenia with different etiology. On the other hand, the observed anatomical deviations may be the top of an iceberg and the cause for the changes may be at hand for all schizophrenics. In a statistical analysis of over 600 patients investigated by computed tomography, Weinberger (1990) reported that the data were best described by a unimodel of distribution. Several investigators have studied the neuroleptic response in relation to the occurrence of ventricular changes. The results are not unequivocal and in a review by Gattaz et al. (1990) eight studies were found to support the view that ventricular enlargement was related with a poor response to neuroleptic treatment but four studies did not. It seems as if patients with ventricular enlargement do respond to neuroleptic treatment but more slowly or to a lesser degree than patients without morphological changes. This means that if patients both with and without ventricular changes participate in a study, the variance of drug effects will increase. The hypothesis that one type of schizophrenia should involve an increase of D_2 dopamine receptors and also have a good response to neuroleptic treatment is attractive. However, neuroleptically naive patients do not seem to have an increased number of D_2 dopamine receptors (Farde et al. 1990). The increase observed in deceased patients may therefore be due to previous drug treatment or to other conditions during the course of the disease. However, measurements of homovanillic acid (HVA) levels in plasma give some support for the opinion that dopaminergic mechanisms are involved in the neuroleptic treatment response. Thus there are several reports demonstrating that patients with a good outcome have a decline of plasma HVA over time (Bowers et al. 1986; Chang et al. 1988; Alfredsson and Wiesel 1990). These results may be interpreted as pathophysiological differences in dopaminergic function between patients which influence the therapeutic effect of neuroleptic treatment.

Glutamate in plasma may also be an indicator of different pathophysiological mechanisms in schizophrenia. Glutamate is an excitatory transmitter in CNS (see Fonnum 1984) which interacts reciprocally with dopamine in striatum (Roberts et al. 1982; Cheramy et al. 1986). There is a glutamate hypothesis which states that there is a hypofunction of central glutamatergic neurons in schizophrenia (Kornhuber et al. 1984; Carlsson and Carlsson 1990). In a study we measured glutamate levels in serum before and during sulpiride treatment in patients with schizophrenia (DSM-III-R) (Alfredsson and Wiesel 1990). The patients were divided into responders and nonresponders after 6 weeks of treatment according to the global rating of psychosis. Patients with more than a 50% decrease of the scores were considered responders, otherwise nonresponders. It was found that the glutamate levels were significantly lower before treatment in the responders than in the nonresponders. During treatment the glutamate level increased in the responders, while it decreased in the nonresponders. There was also a correlation between the increase of glutamate during treatment and the clinical improvement. In the responders also a decline in HVA levels was found. The fact that in responders HVA levels declined and glutamate levels increased during treatment indicates that a good response to neuroleptic treatment requires an interplay between dopaminergic and glutamatergic mechanisms. A pathophysiological mechanism in nonresponders may be a disturbance of the glutamatergic system involved in the interplay between neuronal mechanisms for dopamine and glutamate. However, the biochemical findings do not preclude pathogenetic homogeneity by analogy with the former reasoning for morphological changes.

Positron emission tomographic studies indicate that patients with schizophrenia have a lower glucose metabolism than normal individuals (see Wiesel 1989). Whether changes in glucose metabolism interfere with the neuroleptic response is not known, but a decrease in metabolism does not seem to preclude a good neuroleptic response (Wik et al. 1989).

4 Phenomenology

Subtyping of schizophrenia on phenomenological grounds into catatonic, paranoid, and hebephrenic schizophrenia was made by Kraepelin. There is no clear evidence that this classical subtyping of schizophrenic patients is of significant importance in the outcome of drug treatment. In clinical psychiatry the concept of type I and type II schizophrenia was initially met with great enthusiasm and considered to be a more relevant subtyping. However, the basis for the original classification of type I and II schizophrenia has only a limited support in research data. From Crow's categorization the concept of positive and negative symptoms was further developed and special rating scales have been introduced (Andreasen 1982). In a prospective, double-blind longitudinal study by Kay and Singh (1989) both positive and negative symptoms were found to respond to neuroleptic treatment with a marginally greater effect on positive features. Similar findings have also been reported by Angst et al. (1989) using another rating scale for negative symptoms. It seems as if responders, partial responders, and nonresponders have a similar response or lack of response on the whole symptom spectrum. Recently it was demonstrated that patients with a schizophreniform disorder (DSM-III) had a more rapid response to neuroleptic treatment than patients with schizophrenia (DSM-III) (McDermott et al. 1991). This finding was suggested to demonstrate diagnostic heterogeneity in schizophrenia. However, the most important factor for treatment outcome seemed to be duration of disease rather than diagnosis. An alternative explanation is also given by the investigators whereby a schizophreniform disorder may be looked upon as a less severe form of schizophrenia.

About 20%–30% of patients with schizophrenia have only a marginal effect of neuroleptic treatment and could be described as resistant to neuroleptic treatment. During the 1970s it was thought that a substantial proportion of these patients did not respond to treatment for pharmacokinetic reasons. However, pharmacokinetics cannot explain the major group of treatment-resistant patients. With positron emission tomography it is possible to measure dopamine receptor blockade by neuroleptics in drug-treated patients (Farde et al. 1988). Such studies have demonstrated that patients responding to treatment have a substantial blockade of their D_2 dopamine receptors (Wiesel et al. 1990). However, treatment-resistant patients seem also to have a substantial D_2 receptor blockade (Wolkin et al. 1989). Thus neither pharmacokinetics nor pharmacodynamics of classial neuroleptics can explain treatment failure. Clozapine, in contrast to the classical neuroleptics and the benzamides, blocks the D_2 dopamine receptors to a lower extent than the other compounds (Wiesel et al. 1990). This finding, together with the treatment results of clozapine, demonstrating a significant effect on the whole spectrum of psychiatric symptoms in treatment-resistant patients is of great importance (Kane et al. 1988). It points to the fact that we have true treatment heterogeneity and that there must be several pharmacodynamic ways to influence a schizophrenic psychosis. Considering the difficulties in demonstrating superiority among different neuroleptics in the treatment of patients with schizophrenia (besides side effects), drug development and evaluation should focus on the treatment-resistant patients. The finding of treatment heterogeneity must also be taken into account in schizophrenia research on pathogenetic and pathophysiological mechanisms. The hope of the future is in molecular genetics, which is the only way to solve the question of diagnostic heterogeneity in schizophrenia.

Acknowledgements. Ms. A. Liberg is gratefully acknowledged for preparing the manuscript. This study was supported by grants from the Swedish Medical Research Council (Nr 8318).

References

Alfredsson G, Wiesel F-A (1990) Relationships between clinical effects and monoamine metabolites and amino acids in sulpiride-treated schizophrenic patients. Psychopharmacology (Berl) 101:324–331

Andreasen NC (1982) Negative symptoms in schizophrenia. Arch Gen Psychiatry 39: 784–788

Angst J, Stassen HH, Woggon B (1989) Effect of neuroleptics on positive and negative symptoms and the deficit state. Psychopharmacology (Berl) 99:S41–S46

Bleuler E (1911) Dementia praecox oder Gruppe der Schizophrenien. Deuticke, Leipzig

Bleuler E (1916) Lehrbuch der Psychiatrie. Springer, Berlin

Bowers MB Jr, Swiger ME, Jatlow PI, Hoffman FJ, Giocoechea N (1986) Early neuroleptic response in psychotic men and women: correlation with plasma HVA and HMPG. Compr Psychiatry 27:181–185

Brockington IF, Kendell RE, Leff JP (1978) Definitions of schizophrenia: concordance and prediction of outcome. Psychol Med 8:387–398

Carlsson M, Carlsson A (1990) Schizophrenia: a subcortical neurotransmitter imbalance syndrome? Schizophr Bull 16(3):425–432

Chang W-H, Chen T-Y, Lee C-F, Hung J-C, Hu W-H, Yeh E-K (1988) Plasma homovanillic acid levels and subtyping of schizophrenia. Psychiatry Res 23:239–244

Cheramy A, Romo R, Godeheu C, Baruch P, Glowinski J (1986) In vivo presynaptic control of dopamine release in the cat caudate nucleus-II. Facilitatory or inhibitory influence of L-glutamate. Neuroscience 19:1081–1090

Crow TJ (1980) Molecular pathology of schizophrenia: more than one disease process? Br Med J 66–68

Farde L, Wiesel F-A, Halldin C, Sedvall G (1988) Central D2-dopamine receptor occupancy in schizophrenic patients treated with antipsychotic drugs. Arch Gen Psychiatry 45:71–76

Farde L, Wiesel F-A, Stone-Elander S, Halldin C, Nordström A-L, Hall H, Sedvall G (1990) D2-Dopamine receptors in neuroleptic-naive schizophrenic patients – a PET-study with (^{11}C)raclopride. Arch Gen Psychiatry 47:213–219

Fonnum F (1984) Glutamate: a neurotransmitter in mammalian brain. J Neurochem 42:1–11

Gattaz WF, Kohlmeyer K, Gasser T (1990) Computer tomographic studies in schizophrenia. In: Häfner H, Gattaz WF (eds) Search for the causes of schizophrenia, vol 2. Springer, Berlin Heidelberg New York, pp 242–256

Hagenfeldt L, Venizelos N, Bjerkenstedt L, Wiesel F-A (1987) Decreased tyrosine transport in fibroblasts from schizophrenic patients. Life Sci 41:2749–2757

Johnstone EC, Crow TJ, Frith CD, Husband J, Kreel L (1976) Cerebral ventricular size and cognitive impairment in chronic schizophrenia. Lancet 2:924–926

Kane J, Honigfeld G, Singer J, Meltzer H, Clozaril Collaborative Study Group (1988) Clozapine for the treatment-resistant schizophrenic. A double-blind comparison with chlorpromazine. Arch Gen Psychiatry 45:789–796

Kay SR, Singh MM (1989) The positive-negative distinction in drug-free schizophrenic patients. Arch Gen Psychiatry 46:711–718

Keks NA, Copolov DL, Kulkarni J, Mackie B, Singh BS, McGorry P, Rubin RT, Hassett A, McLaughlin M, van Riel R (1990) Basal and haloperidol-stimulated prolactin in neuroleptic-free men with schizophrenia defined by 11 diagnostic systems. Biol Psychiatry 27:1203–1215

Kennedy JL, Giuffra LA, Moises HW, Cavalli-Sforza LL, Pakstis AJ, Kidd JR, Castiglione CM, Sjögren B, Wetterberg L, Kidd KK (1988) Evidence against linkage of schizophrenia to markers on chromosome 5 in a northern Swedish pedigree. Nature 336:167–170

Kornhuber HH, Kornhuber I, Kim JS, Kornhuber ME (1984) Zur biochemischen Theorie der Schizophrenie (A biochemical theory of schizophrenia). Nervenarzt 55:602–606

McDermott BE, Sautter FJ, Garver DL (1991) Heterogeneity of schizophrenia: relationship to latency of neuroleptic response. Psychiatry Res 37:97–103
Roberts PJ, McBean GJ, Sharif NA, Thomas EM (1982) Striatal glutamatergic function: modifications following specific lesions. Brain Res 235:83–91
Sherrington R, Brynjolfsson J, Petursson H, Potter M, Dudleston K, Barraclough B, Wasmuth J, Dobbs M, Gurling H (1988) Localization of a susceptibility locus for schizophrenia on chromosome 5. Nature 336:164–167
Strauss JS, Gift TE (1977) Choosing an approach for diagnosing schizophrenia. Arch Gen Psychiat 34:1248–1253
Weinberger DR (1990) Brain anatomy in schizophrenia. Discussion. In: Häfner H, Gattaz WV (eds) Search for the causes of schizophrenia, vol 2. Springer, Berlin, Heidelberg New York, pp 275–281
Wiesel F-A (1989) Positron-emission tomography in psychiatry. Psychiatr Dev 1:19–47
Wiesel F-A, Farde L, Nordström A-L, Sedvall G (1990) Central D1- and D2 receptor occupancy during antipsychotic drug treatment. Proc NeuroPsychopharmacol Biol Psychiatry 14:759–767
Wiesel F-A, Blomqvist G, Venizelos N, Bjerkenstedt L, Halldin C, Hagenfeldt L, Sjögren I (1991) Altered transport of tyrosine across the blood brain barrier in patients with schizophrenia. Biol Psychiatry 2:337–340
Wik G, Wiesel F-A, Sjögren I, Blomqvist G, Greitz T, Stone-Elander S (1989) Effects of sulpiride and chlorpromazine on regional cerebral glucose metabolism in schizophrenic patients as determined by positron emission tomography. Psychopharmacology (Berl) 97:309–318
Wolkin A, Barouche F, Wolf AP, Rotrosen J, Fowler JS, Shiue C-Y, Cooper TB, Brodie JD (1989) Dopamine blockade and clinical response: evidence for two biological subgroups of schizophrenia. Am J Psychiatry 146:905–908

Residual and Negative Symptoms in Treatment with Neuroleptics

J.M. Kane

1 Introduction

The term "negative" symptoms is most frequently attributed to the neurologist Hughlings Jackson; however, other individuals also attempted to conceptualize this aspect of phenomonology in schizophrenia (Reynolds 1858). Kraepelin (1919) and Bleuler (1950) considered blunted affect and emotional withdrawal as core features of this illness. Though the presence of apathy, anergia, alogia and blunted affect have always been considered as frequent aspects of schizophrenia, they have received varying attention and weight in different eras as criteria for diagnosis. To some extent this reflects the difficulty in reliably defining and measuring them, in contrast to positive symptoms. There is currently a renewed interest in negative symptoms because of their potential value in helping to subclassify patients in ways which might be useful from both a prognostic and pathophysiologic perspective. In addition, increasing efforts to develop antipsychotic compounds either with a broader or novel spectrum of activity have focused more attention on residual and negative symptoms. Since these are the symptoms that may remain most salient after optimal neuroleptic treatment, they contribute enormously to the chronic disability associated with schizophrenia.

2 Assessment of Negative Symptoms

Negative symptoms have generally been included in widely utilized rating scales such as the Brief Psychiatric Rating Scale (BPRS) (Overall and Gorham 1964), but interrater reliability has not always been easy to achieve and many clinicians and researchers feel that a broader array of items is necessary to adequately characterize and quantify these dimensions. As a result instruments such as the Manchester Scale (Krawiecka et al. 1977), the Scale for the Assessment of Negative Symptoms (SANS) (Andreasen and

Department of Psychiatry, Hillside Hospital, Long Island Jewish Medical Center, 75-59, 263rd Street, Glen Oaks, NY 11004, USA

Olsen 1982; Andreasen 1983) and the Positive and Negative Symptom Scale (PANSS) (Kay et al. 1989) have been widely used in recent years. There is a relative degree of consensus that flat affect, poverty of speech, avolition, apathy, and anhedonia should be considered negative symptoms, whereas delusions and hallucinations should be considered positive symptoms. Thought disorder, bizarre behavior, and inappropriate affect have been variably categorized by different investigators as positive at times and as negative at times. There is evidence (Liddle 1987; Liddle and Barnes 1990) suggesting that these symptoms constitute a third factor.

3 Subtyping Schizophrenia Based on Negative Symptoms

Crow (1980) further stimulated research on negative symptoms when he proposed two syndromes in schizophrenia: Type I, consisting of positive symptoms such as delusions and hallucinations, occurring in the context of acute schizophrenia with good response to dopamine receptor antagonists, better prognosis, and lack of intellectual impairment; and type II, conceptualized as involving negative symptoms (e.g., affective flattening, poverty of speech, and diminished drive), and being characterized by poor treatment response, cognitive impairment, and a higher proportion of abnormal findings on brain imaging. Subsequently (Crow 1985), the syndrome was expanded to include behavioral deterioration and abnormal involuntary movements not solely attributable to chronic neuroleptic exposure.

Numerous attempts have been made to further characterize a "negative" subtype in terms of premorbid adjustment, age at onset, response to treatment, neurologic soft signs, eye movements, cognitive function, structural and functional brain imaging, etc. Hopefully this line of investigation will prove fruitful in leading to further understanding of the probable etiologic and pathophysiologic heterogeneity of schizophrenia.

4 Differentiating Negative from Depressive Symptoms

From a clinical perspective it is important to differentiate putative negative symptoms from depression and from aspects of neuroleptic drug side effects. Anhedonia, poverty of speech, and emotional and social withdrawal can be manifestations of a depressive episode. A number of studies have examined cohorts of patients to attempt to discriminate negative from depressive features. In most studies significant correlations between depressive symptoms and negative symptoms have not been found; however, this relationship would depend heavily on the extent of depressive symptoms. Specific attention should be given to schizophrenic patients with a depressive episode to determine the extent to which its features would be distinguishable from negative symptoms. The subjective or cognitive aspects of depression (i.e., depressed mood, guilt, and suicidal ideation) may be critical in this context. Lindenmayer et al. (1986; Lindenmayer and Kay 1989) did report a positive relationship between depression and affective impairment in acute schizophrenic patients, suggesting some overlap between depressive and negative symptomatology. It is quite likely that age, treatment status, phase of illness, and assessment procedures may be important factors to consider in examining this relationship. Siris et al. (1988) examined patients specifically selected for a syndrome of postpsychotic depression. Twenty-three of 46 such patients (50%) also fulfilled the investigators' criteria for a negative syndrome. However, these patients did not differ in terms of severity of depressive symptoms from those who did not meet negative syndrome criteria, suggesting that it is not merely the level of depressive symptomatology which accounts for this overlap. In a double-blind, placebo-controlled trial of imipramine (used in conjunction with neuroleptic treatment) it was also shown that antidepressant response did not necessarily serve to discriminate between depressive or negative symptoms.

5 Differentiating Negative Symptoms from Drug-Induced Parkinsonism

Currently available antipsychotic medications produce varying degrees of extrapyramidal side effects. Though further development of atypical compounds such as clozapine may ultimately reduce the incidence of this class of adverse effects, at present they remain a frequent complication of both acute and long-term neuroleptic treatment. It is clear from a variety of different perspectives that negative symptoms per se are not primarily side effects of antipsychotic drug treatment. First they were observed to be an important component of schizophrenic psychopathology long before the introduction of neuroleptic drugs, and, secondly, some aspects of the negative symptoms are responsive to neuroleptic drugs (Goldberg 1985). In addition, even employing modern-day diagnostic criteria, negative symptoms are frequently seen in drug-naive, first-episode schizophrenic patients (Lieberman et al. 1991).

At the same time, however, neuroleptic drugs are capable of producing psychomotor retardation, akinesia, and blunted affect which may exacerbate preexisting negative symptoms or produce a clinical picture which may be mistaken for the negative syndrome. Clearly, if neuroleptics can improve some aspects of negative symptoms while at the same time producing adverse effects which can to some extent mimic negative symptoms, this poses a challenge to cross-sectional assessments as well as to clinical trials. These drug effects can continue to be apparent even in the maintenance phase of treatment as illustrated by double-blind antiparkinsonian medication discontinuation studies (Rifkin et al. 1978) and studies involving substantial reduction in maintenance neuroleptic dosage (Kane et al. 1983).

This complicates the assessment of negative symptoms in neuroleptic-treated patients. In addition, when antipsychotic compounds are compared with regard to efficacy for negative symptoms, the role of drug-induced parkinsonism may be critical. This issue will be reviewed in more detail subsequently.

Given these concerns, the assessment and differential diagnosis of negative symptoms becomes critical. Objective measures which could help in facilitating differential diagnosis would be highly desirable. A potential example of this would be Alpert's (1991) use of voice analysis. His data suggest that schizophrenic patients with flat affect have different speech characteristics than patients with major depressive disorder who are rated as showing flat affect on negative symptom scales and that neuroleptics appear to affect measures of speech productivity and expressiveness rather than rate. More work needs to be done to fully explore the potential of such an approach, but it is cited as an example of possible strategies.

The use of antiparkinsonian medication trials, neuroleptic dosage reduction, or complete neuroleptic withdrawal are also strategies to be employed in this context, but it is necessary to allow sufficient time to assess their impact. It is important to keep in mind that in some studies withdrawal of neuroleptics has also been shown to lead to an increase of both positive and negative symptoms (Brier et al. 1987).

6 Pharmacologic Treatment of Negative Symptoms

Given the prevalence and impact of negative symptoms on social and vocational functioning, efforts to improve treatment response in this area are becoming an increasing focus of new treatment strategies and new drug development. Assessing the effects of specific pharmacologic treatments for negative symptoms is complicated by the fact that some negative symptoms may respond if they occur in the context of an acute exacerbation of positive symptoms as well. Some investigators have suggested that negative symptoms in some contexts may be secondary to positive symptoms and respond concurrently with positive symptom response to neuroleptics (Goldberg 1985). Others have argued that even in the treatment of an acute exacerbation of positive symptoms, the response of negative symptoms to neuroleptics is at least partially independent.

The response of negative symptoms may also vary depending upon the phase of illness. Ventura et al. (1991) recently reported preliminary data from a cohort of first-episode patients, suggesting that over the first 3 years of treatment there was a tendency for positive symptoms to get worse, but for negative symptoms to show no consistent increase. In fact, almost half of the patients with negative symptoms showed a decrease in negative symptoms over time.

Carpenter et al. (1985) have argued that the deficit or residual negative symptoms which remain after the treatment of an acute exacerbation should be identified as core features of the schizophrenic illness and considered primary negative symptoms. Clearly, there are a variety of conceptual and methodologic issues which need to be addressed in assessing the impact of pharmacologic agents.

In general, most clinical trials of different neuroleptics have not shown significant superiority of one drug or drug class over another in the treatment of negative (or positive) symptoms. There has been some suggestion that different classes of drugs may be superior in the treatment of negative symptoms. Several investigators (Kolivakis et al. 1974; Chouinard and Annable 1979; Haas and Beckmann 1982; Lapierre and Lavallee 1975; Lapierre 1978) have suggested that the diphenylbutylpiperidines (pimozide, clorpimozide, fluspirilene, and penfluridol) might be superior in the treatment of negative symptoms.

Although taken together these studies do suggest some superiority for this class of compounds, the overall impression is not one of substantial differences as compared to other drugs. A major concern in these and other studies is the issue of dose equivalency and whether one group is experiencing more extrapyramidal side effects than another. Despite efforts to rate or prevent parkinsonian side effects, subtle differences between groups may not be apparent though they may influence the behavioral ratings.

Clozapine (Kane et al. 1988) has been shown to have significantly greater effect on positive and negative symptoms in comparison to chlorpromazine plus benztropine. These differences were observed in a group of patients selected for the presence of positive symptoms which were not responsive to traditional antipsychotics. A study of clozapine in patients with predominant negative symptoms has not yet been carried out.

Various other pharmacologic agents besides antipsychotic drugs have been employed in the treatment of negative symptoms. Drugs which enhance dopaminergic transmission, e.g., L-dopa and amphetamine, have been reported to be of some use when combined with neuroleptic drugs (Inanaga et al. 1972; Gerlach and Luhdrof 1975; Cesarec and Nyman 1985; Angrist et al. 1980; Van Kammen and Boronow 1988). Some improvement in negative symptoms has also been reported with propranolol (Sheppard 1979; Eccleston et al. 1985), alprazolam (Wolkowitz et al. 1986, 1991) and tranylcypromine (Bucci 1987).

7 Conclusion

Considerable efforts are now underway to develop antipsychotic compounds which might differ from traditional neuroleptics in their propensity to produce extrapyramidal side effects and/or to improve negative symptoms. Compounds with a variety of different preclinical profiles are now in various stages of clinical trails, and it is hoped that over the next several years a better appreciation of the relevance of different receptor binding profiles to specific clinical effects will be forthcoming. However, at the same time the problems discussed previously must be addressed in order to develop methodologic strategies that will allow meaningful conclusions.

References

Alpert M (1991) Vocal acquistic correlates of flat affect: contrast with other negative signs and depression. Schizophr Res 4:247–248

Andreasen NC (1983) The scale for the assessment of negative symptoms (SANS). University of Iowa Press, Iowa

Andreasen NC, Olsen S (1982) Negative and positive schizophrenia: definition and validation. Arch Gen Psychiatry 39:789–793

Angrist B, Rotrosen J, Gershon S (1980) Differential effects of amphetamine and neuroleptics on negative versus positive symptoms in schizophrenia. Psychopharmacology (Berl) 72:17–19

Barnes TRE, Liddle PF (1990) The symptoms of chronic schizophrenia. Br J Psychiatry 157:558–561

Bleuler E (1950) Dementia praecox or the group of schizophrenias. International Universities Press, New York

Brier A, Wolkowitz OM, Doran AR et al. (1987) Neuroleptic responsivity of negative and positive symptoms in schizophrenia. Am J Psychiatry 144:1549–1555

Bucci L (1987) The negative symptoms of schizophrenia and the monoamine oxidase inhibitors. Psychopharmacology (Berl) 91:104–108

Carpenter WT Jr, Heinrichs DW, Alphs LD (1985) Treatment of negative symptoms. Schizophr Bull 11:440–452

Cesarec Z, Nyman AK (1985) Differential response to amphetamine in schizophrenia. Acta Psychiatr Scand 71:523–528

Chouinard G, Annable L (1979) Pimozide in the treatment of acute schizophrenia. Paper presented at the American Psychiatric Association Annual Meeting, Chicago

Crow TJ (1980) Molecular pathology of schizophrenia: more than one dimension of pathology? Br Med J 143:66–68

Crow TJ (1985) The two-syndrome concept: origins and current status. Schizophr Bull 11:471–486

Eccleston D, Fairbain AF, Hassanyeh F et al. (1985) The effect of propranolol and thioridazine on positive and negative symptoms of schizophrenia. Br J Psychiatry 147:623–630

Gerlach J, Luhdrof K (1975) The effect of L-dopa on young patients with simple schizophrenia treated with neuroleptic drugs. Psychopharmacology (Berl) 44:105–110

Goldberg SC (1985) Negative and deficit symptoms in schizophrenia do respond to neuroleptics. Schizophr Bull 11:453–456

Haas S, Beckmann H (1982) Pimozide versus haloperidol in acute schizophrenia: A double-blind controlled study. Pharmacopsychiatry 15:70–74

Inanaga K, Inouee K, Tachibana H et al. (1972) Effect of L-dopa in schizophrenia. Folia Psychiatr Neurol Jn 26:145–157

Kane J, Rifkin A, Woerner M et al. (1983) Low dose neuroleptic treatment of outpatient schizophrenics: preliminary results for relapse rates. Arch Gen Psychiatry 4:893–896

Kane J, Honifgeld G, Singer J, Meltzer H and the Clozaril Collaborative Study Group (1988) Clozapine for the treatment-resistant schizophrenic: a double-blind comparison with chlorpromazine. Arch Gen Psychiatry 45:789–796

Kay SR, Opler LA, Lindenmayer JP (1989) The positive and negative syndrome scale (PANSS): rationale and standardization. Br J Psychiatry (Suppl) 7:59–65

Kolivakis T, Azian H, Kingstone E (1974) A double-blind comparison of pimozide and chlorpromazine in the maintenance of chronic schizophrenic patients. Curr Ther Res 16:998–1004

Kraepelin E (1919) Dementia praecox and paraphrenia. Krieger, New York

Krawiecka M, Goldberg D, Vaughan MA (1977) Standardized psychiatric assessment for rating chronic patients. Acta Psychiatr Scand 55:299–308

Lapierre YD (1978) A controlled study of penfluridol in the treatment of chronic schizophrenia. Am J Psychiatry 135:956–959

Lapierre YD, Lavallee J (1975) Pimozide and the social behaviors of schizophrenics. Curr Ther Res 18:181–188

Liddle PF (1987) The symptoms of chronic schizophrenia. A re-examination of the positive-negative dichotomy. Br J Psychiatry 151:145–151

Lieberman JA, Jody D, Alvir JMJ, Borenstein M, Mayerhoff DI (1991) Negative symptoms in schizophrenia: relationship to positive symptoms and outcome. In: Maneros A, Andreasen NC, Tsuang M (eds) Netative Versus Positive Schizophrenia. Springer, Berlin Heidelberg New York, pp 109–125

Lindenmayer JP, Kay SR (1989) Depression, affect and negative symptoms in schizophrenia. Br J Psychiatry 155 (Suppl):108–114

Lindenmayer JP, Kay SR, Friedman C (1986) Negative and positive schizophrenic syndromes after the acute phase: a prospective follow-up. Compr Psychiatry 27:276–286

Overall JE, Gorham D (1964) The brief psychiatric rating scale. Psychol Rep 10:799–812

Reynolds JR (1858) On the pathology of convulsions with special reference to those of children. Liverpool Med Chir J 2:1–14

Rifkin A, Quitkin F, Kane JM et al. (1978) Are prophylactic antiparkinsonian drugs necessary? A controlled study of procyclidine withdrawal. Arch Gen Psychiatry 35:483–389

Sheppard GP (1979) High dose propranolol in schizophrenia. Br J Psychiatry 134:47–476

Siris SG, Adan F, Cohen M et al. (1988) Post-psychotic depression and negative symptoms: an investigation of syndromal overlap. Am J Psychiatry 145:1532–1537

Siris SG, Adan F, Cohen M, Mandeli J, Aronson A, Casey E (1988) Post-psychotic depression and negative symptoms: An investigation of syndromal overlap. Am J Psychiatry 145:1532–1537

Van Kammen DP, Boronow JJ (1988) Dextro-amphetamine diminishes negative symptoms in schizophrenia. Int Clin Psychopharmacol 3:111–121

Ventura J, Nuechterlein K, Green M, Mintz J (1991) Characterization of positive and negative symptoms in the early course of schizophrenia. Schizophr Research 4:270–271

Wolkowitz OM, Pickar D, Doran AR et al. (1986) Combination alprazolam-neuroleptic treatment of the positive and negative symptoms of schizophrenia. Am J Psychiatry 143:85–87

Wolkowitz OM, Turetsky N, Reus VI et al. (1991) Benzodiazepine responsivity in schizophrenia. Schizophr Res 4:296

Clinical Dosing of Neuroleptics

R.J. BALDESSARINI, B.M. COHEN, and M.H. TEICHER

1 Introduction

The antipsychotic, or neuroleptic, drugs were introduced in the early 1950s (Laborit et al. 1952) and, since then, they and other effective and well accepted psychotropic agents have had a revolutionary impact on the theory and practice of contemporary psychiatry worldwide (Baldessarini 1985, 1990a). Despite their exposure to intensive study and clinical application for four decades, many fundamental aspects of the clinical pharmacology of the neuroleptics remain remarkably poorly informed by research data. The present overview considers relationships between dose or plasma concentrations and the effects of this class of commonly used agents. Optimal dosing for maximum efficacy and safety of most antipsychotic drugs largely escaped serious scientific scrutiny until surprisingly recently. Since 1980, a substantial body of appropriately designed, randomized, double-blind studies of the clinical benefits and side effects of some antipsychotic agents has been carried out with acutely and chronically psychotic patients treated for periods ranging from several hours to several months (Baldessarini et al. 1988, 1990). In addition, there have been studies of relationships between plasma concentrations of neuroleptic agents and their effects which complement studies of dose-effect relationships.

2 Short-Term Studies of Neuroleptic Dose–Effect Relationships

By the early 1980s, particularly in the USA, there was a tendency to use neuroleptic agents aggressively, with rapidly increasing doses, in the early treatment of acutely psychotic and manic patients in the hope of inducing a more rapid and cost-effective response. This trend was most apparent with the agents of high potency, which were used in doses up to 6.5 times the

Departments of Psychiatry and Neuroscience Program, Harvard Medical School, Boston, MA, and Laboratories for Psychiatric Research, Psychotic Disorders Program, and Developmental Biopsychiatry Program, McLean Hospital, Belmont, MA 02178, USA

Table 1. High vs moderate doses of neuroleptics in acute psychosis

Condition	Mean dose (CPZ-eq mg/24 h)	Improvement (% change)
Doses ≤ median	311 ± 31	56.2 ± 4.8
Doses > median	3613 ± 1757	50.2 ± 4.4
Ratio	11.6	1.12

Data are based on 19 studies involving 24 groups, divided at the median daily dose (600 mg CPZ-eq), in references cited elsewhere (Baldessarini et al. 1988, 1990). Data are means ± SEM; difference is not significant by *t*-test ($p > 0.25$).

equivalent amount of chlorpromazine (CPZ), as a standard agent of low potency, or in doses as high as the equivalent of 4–5 grams of CPZ daily (Baldessarini et al. 1984).

In our recent reviews, we found 19 controlled clinical trials involving random prospective assignment of acutely psychotic schizophrenic or manic patients to dissimilar controlled doses of a neuroleptic agent, with nominally double-blind assessment (see Baldessarini et al. 1988, 1990). When the results of these studies were evaluated in terms of percentage change in initial psychopathology ratings, there were only insignificant differences between doses. Based on an analysis of 33 possible pairings of high vs moderate dosage groups (mean ± SEM = 466 ± 47 and 2384 ± 1349 mg CPZ-equivalent [CPZ-eq] per day – a 5.1-fold difference, usually given as a high-potency agent), the mean change was 46.8% ± 4.7% at moderate doses vs 53.3% ± 4.7% at high doses ($p > 0.25$). In an alternative analysis, the data were divided at the median daily dose (600 mg CPZ-eq), with an even greater difference in average dose (11.6-fold) but, again, little difference in the average degree of clinical improvement by dosage group (Table 1). Similar conclusions were reached by assessing the proportion of patients considered to have "responded" in a clinically significant manner (Baldessarini et al. 1988). For example, in comparing 22 paired groups, we found the mean percent responding to be 34.1% ± 3.6% at a moderate mean daily CPZ-eq dose of 506 ± 114 mg, and 43.3% ± 3.8% at 2035 ± 782 mg.

The short-term studies just summarized involved durations ranging from 1 h to 45 days, making their pooling and interpretation hazardous. Nevertheless, comparing results at different times also failed to reveal appreciable or consistent differences between high and moderate doses. This conclusion was reached when results for 1–24 h were compared with results from 2–10 days (Baldessarini et al. 1988) or in a further comparison of results within the first 24 h of treatment and at 2, 10, or 45 days (not previously reported).

Evaluation of these studies is further complicated by the inclusion of *multiple* fixed doses within only a few individual studies, which might serve as a basis for a dose-effect analysis to compute ED_{50} values or estimate the magnitude of maximum benefit. Typical levels of benefit reported by 4–6 weeks in other reports in this series were up to 65%–70% of patiens "responding," but with variable degrees of change in initial symptom–severity ratings between studies. Data pooled from three studies involving effects of several doses of haloperidol (ranging from zero, or 2.5, to 40 mg, IM) suggested that the maximum initial benefit (found at 12–15 mg) was as great as 50% reduction in initial psychopathology ratings within the first hours of starting treatment; doses >20 mg were associated with somewhat *inferior* results (Baldessarini et al. 1988). Such improvements in ratings within the first day might reflect sedative or other nonspecific central depressant effects of large doses of neuroleptic agents and not "true antipsychotic" effects. This is a difficult distinction to make, and it may be limited in practical importance. Indeed, there is growing evidence that use of sedative agents, such as potent benzodiazepines, can reduce the need for neuroleptics, or even effectively and safely replace them in the short-term management of acutely psychotic or manic patients (Lerner et al. 1979; Chouinard et al. 1983; Modell et al. 1985; Cohen and Lipinski 1986; Garza-Trevino et al. 1989).

Taken together, these short-term observations strongly suggest, not only that there was no consistent added overall benefit to raising doses of potent neuroleptic agents more than 10-times above standard doses over 4–6 weeks of treatment of acute psychotic illness, but that the *rate* of improvement (percent change per day or per week) also did not appear to increase with increased doses. This literature also highlights shortcomings in the scientific basis for contemporary clinical use of antipsychotic agents that still remain 40 years after the introduction of CPZ. These have considerable clinical and economic importance in planning safe, efficacious, and cost-effective treatment programs for psychotic patients. Limitations of knowledge include a scarcity of dose-effect data for most neuroleptics, and even more limited information on comparisons of widely ranging doses as a function of time, or comparisons of a neuroleptic with a sedative or placebo over time (Keck et al. 1990).

3 Long-Term Studies of Neuroleptic Dose–Effect Relationships

In addition to the recent experimental study of high vs moderate doses of potent neuroleptic agents in the short-term treatment of acutely psychotic patients, there is a substantial body of investigations aimed at similar assessments longer-term in chronically psychotic, presumably schizophrenic, patients. A representative early study which explored relatively high doses of fluphenazine found little additional benefit to increasing daily doses above 20–30 mg, especially if a more moderate dose were continued for 4 weeks (Quitkin et al. 1975). Similar conclusions were reached by Aubree and

Table 2. High vs moderate neuroleptic doses in maintenance treatment of chronically psychotic patients

Measure	Value
Studies (*n*)	23
Patient-subjects (*n*)	2346
Mean duration (months)	5.84 ± 0.7
Mean daily moderate dose (mg CPZ-eq)	399 ± 85
Mean daily high dose (mg CPZ-eq)	5215 ± 2169
Net proportion with some clinical benefit high > moderate dose	10.0%
Proportion with side-effect risk high > moderate dose	95.0%

Data are means ± SEM, based on references cited elsewhere (Baldessarini et al. 1988, 1990); 32% of the studies suggested superiority of the higher dose, 22% found the opposite, and 46% found no difference.

Lader (1980) in their review of 11 long-term neuroleptic maintenance studies involving over 700 schizophrenic patients. They found little evidence of a gain in benefit between average daily doses of 600 mg and more than 9 grams CPZ-eq (usually given as high-potency agents), but a 64% increased risk of neurological side effects. In more recent reviews of this topic, we found 33 studies providing pertinent long-term data (Baldessarini et al. 1988, 1990); their salient findings are summarized in Table 2.

These trials have involved more than 2000 schizophrenic patients studied under scientifically appropriate conditions for approximately 6 months, with moderate mean CPZ-eq daily doses of about 400 mg compared with high doses above 5 grams. The results of these studies are difficult to evaluate quantitatively, but only a minority (32%) gave an indication of some added benefit at the higher dose given in each trial, while another similar proportion (22%) suggested superiority of the lower dose, and nearly half (46%) found no clear difference in antipsychotic effect. In sharp contrast, nearly every study found increased risk or severity of side effects at the higher doses. These results add to the conclusion that doses above the equivalent of 300–600 mg of CPZ daily, or 5–15 mg of fluphenazine or haloperidol, are unlikely to gain appreciable benefit but do carry increased risks of side effects, particularly involving the central nervous system. Like the short-term studies, these are usually limited by a lack of prospective assignment to a broad range of doses within individual trials with which to construct credible dose-effect relationships, by the lack of considering low vs moderate doses, by the paucity of studies of agents other than phenothiazine (80% of agents evaluated long-term), and by the limited sensitivity or effect size to be found in studies of chronically ill patients.

A few studies of two or more low and moderate doses of neuroleptics have appeared in recent years (Baldessarini et al. 1988, 1990). In one of the best designed and longest of these, Kane (1985) and Kane et al. (1983), found a clear dose-effect relationship after 1 year of double-blind evaluation of schizophrenic patients assigned to a narrow range of usual biweekly doses of fluphenazine decanoate (mean, about 31.2 mg), or to material diluted by five- (6.2 mg) or 10-fold (3.1 mg/2 weeks). The 1 year rates of "survival" in a clinically stable state were 88%, 72%, and 44%, respectively, for these descending dosage groups. Since comparable 1 year survival rates with an inactive placebo have been in the range of 10%–25%, even the lowest dose – equivalent to approximately 50 mg/day of oral CPZ – gave a substantial benefit above that expected from a placebo.

In a more quantitative analysis of the data from this study as well as several others (Rifkin et al. 1977; Hogarty et al. 1976, 1979; Kane et al. 1983; Hogarty 1984; Marder et al. 1984), we found evidence of a biphasic dose-response relationship, as was also suggested by the acute haloperidol studies already discussed above. A basic assumption in approaching such data is that conditions of *random assignment* of patients obtained across the range of doses, as was assured in the reports evaluated. The pooled data fit a model based on the interaction of positive (beneficial) and putative negative (worsening) functions, with computed ED_{50} values of 2 and 45 mg of intramuscularly injected fluphenazine decanoate per 2 weeks, respectively (Teicher and Baldessarini 1985; Baldessarini et al. 1988). The lower computed value for beneficial effects, of only 2 mg/2 weeks, seems remarkably small and somewhat theoretical. Clinicians are more interested in optimal doses, with maximal benefit:risk ratios. Even these were found in this analysis to be relatively moderate and narrow (in the range of about 10–30 mg/2 weeks), while biweekly doses above 30 mg were associated with diminishing benefit, so that 1-year "survival" fell from ⩾90% to ca 60% between 30 and 40 mg. It is interesting that many studies of correlations between plasma concentrations of neuroleptic agents and clinical benefit also suggest similar biphasic concentration-response relationships or, at least, a lack of consistently greater benefit a higher levels (Baldessarini et al. 1988).

While a full explanation of these intriguing observations remains to be found, a plausible factor contributing to the finding of inferior benefit at higher doses or tissue levels of neuroleptic drug may be the negative impact of neurological side effects, such as akathisia and akinesia, both as actual clinical effects and, more technically, as they influence ratings on typical clinical symptom rating scales used in such studies (Marder et al. 1984, 1987; Van Putten et al. 1990). Further testing of the implication that *lowering* doses of a neuroleptic might lead to improved benefit and greater comfort to patients awaits additional research, although there is some experience to suggest that this may actually occur clinically in some patients, short-term (Van Putten et al. 1985; Cohen et al. 1989).

Table 3. Dose, steady-state plasma concentrations of haloperidol and antipsychotic response

Study	Dose (mg/day)	Plasma [haloperidol] (ng/ml)		Responding at optimal levels
		Full range	Optimal range	
Garver et al. (1984)	6–24	2–19	3–11	7/14
Mavroidis et al. (1985)	6–24	2–8.5	4–11	5/14
Potkin et al. (1985)	10–28	1–74	4–26	15/44
Van Putten et al. (1985)	5–25	1–24.5	2–12	42/67
Smith et al. (1985)	10–25	2–23	6.5–16.5	25/33
Santos et al. (1989)	15–30	1–59	10–25	20/30
Means/totals	9–26	1.5–36.3	4.9–16.5	124/202 (61.4%)

Data are based on reanalyses of data in the studied cited and indicate that over 60% of patients responded at drug levels of 5–16.5 ng/ml.

4 Additional Evidence Concerning Dose or Blood Level vs Response Relationships

Despite a good deal of effort to apply various chemical and biological assays of plasma concentrations of psychotropic agents for nearly two decades in order to guide clinical treatment, the yield from these studies has been surprisingly small. With the clear exception of lithium ion, several antidepressants (notably, nortriptyline), and perhaps haloperidol among the neuroleptics, there is very little certainty about optimal drug concentrations which can yield substantial benefit with limited risk of toxicity (Baldessarini 1985, 1991; Baldessarini et al. 1988, 1991).

A representative sampling of data obtained from appropriately designed studies, involving a fairly broad range of *fixed* doses of haloperidol in psychotic patients with sufficiently acute symptoms as to have some chance to respond is summarized in Table 3. Assay of plasma concentrations of haloperidol has been favored in studies of this kind due its relatively simple metabolism, mainly to inactive by-products. There has been a great deal of discussion of appropriate mathematical analyses of data of this kind, and a debate as to whether the data are more consistent with a linear or rising-and-falling curvilinear relationship between drug level and clinical effects, or whether the relationship is so weak as to preclude meaningful generalizations about optimal concentrations. Typical concentrations encountered at standard clinical doses of haloperidol range from <1 to >50 ng/ml. If portions of this range are taken which account for most patients who show appreciable antipsychotic response within each study, an average of approximately "optimal" drug concentrations so-estimated ranges from about 5 to 16 ng/ml (Table 3). Correlations of drug concentrations vs dose also are good with haloperidol ($r > 0.9$), so that one can predict plasma levels of approximately 5–15 ng/ml with daily doses of 10–15 mg.

Independent evidence that such concentrations, attained at typical clinical doses of antipsychotic agents, may be biologically meaningful is forthcoming from recent positron emission tomographic (PET) brain scanning studies of occupation of dopaminergic D_2 receptor sites, labeled with tracer doses of neuroleptic radioligands, in the extrapyramidal basal ganglia of psychotic patients. Such methods provide striking evidence that daily doses in the range of 100–300 mg CPZ-eq (Farde et al. 1988, 1992), as well as plasma concentrations of haloperidol (ca 5–15 ng/ml) considered to be approximately optimal based on clinical evidence already considered, are those required to obtain $\geqslant$85% occupancy of D_2 dopamine receptors in the human basal ganglia (Cannon et al. 1988; Wolkin et al. 1989). Presumably such levels of receptor occupancy are relevant to pharmacological and clinical effects of the neuroleptics. This assumption is supported further by considering the implications of seeking even higher levels of occupancy (say, 99%), for which the hyperbolic-asymptotic nature of the function relating plasma drug level and D_2 receptor occupancy (Wolkin et al. 1989) would call for clinically unrealistic doses of haloperidol.

One reason that it has been difficult to find clear relationships between plasma concentrations of typical neuroleptics, including haloperidol, and their clinical effects may be that relationships between plasma concentrations and either cerebral concentrations or pharmacological effects are more complex than had been appreciated. For example, recent observations challenge traditional two-compartment pharmacokinetic models of how certain neuroleptic drugs are distributed and eliminated. While the nominal elimination half-life of haloperidol, for example, had been believed to be approximately 20–24 h in laboratory animals and humans, this impression may reflect the limited sensitivity of older drug assay methods, which could rarely follow plasma concentrations into the sub-ng/ml range for more than a few days after acute dosing. It now seems that haloperidol almost certainly has a complex, multiphasic elimination, with an apparent near-terminal plasma half-life on the order of a week in human subjects (Hubbard et al. 1987). There are similarly prolonged tissue levels and antidopaminergic actions of this agent in rat brain (Campbell et al. 1985; Cohen et al. 1991, 1992), suggesting that it may take at least several weeks to come back to a physiological baseline after even a single moderate dose of this agent. These observations have found further support in recent applications of PET scanning to estimate the timecourse of recovery of access of a positron-emitting radioligand to brain D_2 dopaminergic receptors of the basal ganglia after a single clinical dose of an agent such as haloperidol. Such recovery times may be *even slower* than are estimated by elimination rates from plasma using very sensitive analytical methods (Farde et al. 1988). Other agents, including some phenothiazines (fluphenazine, for example), follow more traditional elimination kinetics and may exit within several days.

However, they can induce physiological changes (such as acute dopaminergic supersensitivity) which may still require several weeks to return to baseline values (Cohen et al. 1991, 1992).

A prudent generalization arising from this work is that standard plasma pharmacokinetics assessments cannot be assumed to apply reliably to the timing of distribution and elimination of some neuroleptic agents in the brain. In addition to the use of PET scanning to study the pharmacokinetics and pharmacodynamics of neuroleptics at D_2 receptor sites in human brain tissue, the application of magnetic resonance spectroscopy to detect fluorine-containing neuroleptic compounds (such as trifluoperazine or fluphenazine) through detectors placed on the human head recently has been shown to be feasible (Komoroski et al. 1990). These methods may facilitate clinical comparisons of plasma vs brain disposition of neuroleptic agents.

5 Conclusions

The research reviewed above supports the strong impression that doses of neuroleptic agents initially considered standard in American psychiatry and maintained in most European and other countries are adequate for the great majority of psychotic patients. The later use of very high doses of neuroleptic agents, rapidly applied, has largely been abandoned in US centers in recent years. Thus, recent surveys of contemporary practices in representative American psychiatric hospitals indicate that average daily doses equivalent to 200–300 mg of CPZ are now usual (Gelenberg et al. 1988; Vuckovic et al. 1990).

This trend appears to reflect growing appreciation of the research reviewed here, but also a high level of medical-legal concern about long-term neurological risks that increasingly appear to be associated with high, prolonged dosing with neuroleptics (Baldessarini 1988; Casey and Gardos 1986). In addition, the now-frequent combination of sedative agents with moderate doses of neuroleptic agents, especially in the initial management of acutely disturbed psychotic and manic patients, has contributed to increased conservatism in the use of neuroleptics in the United States. There also has been growing interest in differential diagnosis of psychotic disorders, some narrowing of clinical indications for neuroleptic therapy, and increasing use of mood-altering and anticonvulsant agents as alternatives to neuroleptics for many patients with conditions other than schizophrenia (Baldessarini 1985, 1990b, 1993; Cohen and Lipinski 1986; Baldessarini et al. 1991).

Contemporary practice in the long-term application of maintenance neuroleptic treatment in chronically psychotic patients who require it also has been modified toward greater flexibility of dosing to meet changing clinical needs. Research on attempts to find minimum effective doses or to explore intermittent long-term dosing, indicates that such strategies, inflexibly applied, can carry increased risks of morbidity or acute relapses (Carpenter et al. 1987; Herz et al. 1991). Nevertheless, standard treatment with antipsychotic agents appears, appropriately, to be moving toward the use of minimal doses as much as possible and adding moderate increases at times of stress of reemerging acute symptoms.

References

Aubree JC, Lader MH (1980) High and very high dosage antipsychotics: a critical review. J Clin Psychiatry 41:341–350

Baldessarini RJ (1985) Chemotherapy in psychiatry: principles and practice, 2nd edn. Harvard University Press, Cambridge

Baldessarini RJ (1988) A summary to current knowledge of tardive dyskinesia. Encephale 14:363–368

Baldessarini RJ (1990a) The future of psychiatric research and academic psychiatry. McLean Hosp J 15:53–68

Baldessarini RJ (1990b) Drugs and the treatment of psychiatric disorders. In: Gilman AG, Goodman LS, Rall TW, Murad F (eds) Goodman and Gilman's the pharmacologic basis of therapeutics, 8th edn. Pergamon, New York, pp 383–435

Baldessarini RJ (1993) Overview of modern psychopharmacology. In: Baldessarini RJ (ed) Chemotherapy in psychiatry: principles and practice, 3rd edn. Harvard University Press, Cambridge

Baldessarini RJ, Katz B, Cotton P (1984) Dissimilar dosing with high-potency and low-potency neuroleptics. Am J Psychiatry 141:748–752

Baldessarini RJ, Cohen BM, Teicher MH (1988) Significance of neuroleptic dose and plasma level in the pharmacological treatment of psychoses. Arch Gen Psychiatry 45:79–91

Baldessarini RJ, Cohen BM, Teicher MH (1990) Pharmacological treatment. In: Levy ST, Ninan PT (eds) Schizophrenia – treatment of acute psychotic episodes. American Psychiatric Press, Washington, pp 61–118

Baldessarini RJ, Fleischhacker W, Sperk G (1991) Chemotherapie in Psychiatrie. Thieme, Stuttgart

Campbell A, Baldessarini RJ, Kula NS (1985) Prolonged antidopamine actions of single doses of butyrophenones in the rat. Psychopharmacology (Berl) 87:161–166

Cannon D, McMillan D, Newton J, Fody EP, Metzer WS, Claybrook M, Couch L, Piage SR (1988) Serum haloperidol and neuroleptic receptor levels in chronic psychosis. Ann Clin Lab Sci 18:378–383

Carpenter WT Jr, Heinrichs DW, Hanlon TE (1987) A comparative trial of pharmacologic strategies in schizophrenia. Am J Psychiatry 144:518–521

Casey DE, Gardos G (eds) (1986) Tardive dyskinesia and neuroleptics APA, Washington

Chouinard G, Young SN, Annable L (1983) Antimanic effect of clonazepam. Biol Psychiatry 18:451–466

Cohen BM, Lipinski JF (1986) Treatment of acute psychosis with non-neuroleptic agents. Psychosomatics S27:7–16

Cohen BM, Benes FM, Baldessarini RJ (1989) Atypical neuroleptics: dose-response relationships, and treatment-resistant psychosis. Arch Gen Psychiatry 46:381–383

Cohen BM, Baldessarini RJ, Campbell A, Tsuneizumi T, Babb S (1991) Persistence of antipsychotic drug effects and tissue levels. In: Schulz SC, Tamminga CA (eds) Schizophrenia research. Raven, New York, pp 277–284 (Advances in neuropsychiatry and psychopharmacology, vol 2)

Cohen BM, Tsuneizumi T, Baldessarini RJ, Campbell A, Babbs S (1992) Differences between antipsychotic drugs in persistence of brain levels and behavioral effects. Psychopharmacology 108:338–344
Farde L, Wiesel F-A, Halldin C, Sedvall G (1988) Central D_2-dopamine receptor occupancy in schizophrenic patients treated with antipsychotic drugs. Arch Gen Psychiatry 45:71–76
Farde L, Nordström AL, Wiesel FA, Pauli S, Halldin C, Sedvall G (1992) Positron emission tomographic analysis of central D_1 and D_2 dopamine receptor occupancy in patients treated with classical neuroleptics and clozapine. Arch Gen Psychiatry 49: 538–544
Garver DL, Hirschowitz J, Glicksteen GA, Kanter DR, Mavroidis ML (1984) Haloperidol plasma and red blood cells levels and clinical antipsychotic response. J Clin Psychopharmacol 4:133–137
Garza-Trevino ES, Hollister LE, Overall JE, Alexander WF (1989) Efficacy of combinations of intramuscular antipsychotic and sedative-hypnotics for control of psychotic agitation. Am J Psychiatry 146:1598–1601
Gelenberg AJ, Bellinghausen B, Wojcik JD, Falk WE, Sachs G (1988) A prospective survey of neuroleptic malignant syndrome in a short-term psychiatric hospital. Am J Psychiatry 145:517–518
Herz MI, Glazer WM, Mostert MA, Sheard MA, Szymanski HV, Hafez H, Mirza M, Vana J (1991) Intermittent vs maintenance medication in schizophrenia. Arch Gen Psychiatry 48:333–339
Hogarty GE (1984) Depot neuroleptics: the relevance of psychosocial factors: a United States perspective. J Clin Psychiatry 45:36–42
Hogarty GE, Ulrich RF, Mussare F, Aristigueta N (1976) Drug discontinuation among long-term successfully maintained schizophrenic outpatients. Dis Nerv Syst 37:494–500
Hogarty GE, Schooler NR, Ulrich RF, Mussare F, Ferro P, Herron E (1979) Fluphenazine and social therapy in the aftercare of schizophrenic patients. Arch Gen Psychiatry 36:1283–1294
Hubbard JW, Ganes D, Midha KK (1987) Prolonged pharmacologic activity of neuroleptic drugs. Arch Gen Psychiatry 44:99–100
Kane JM (1985) Antipsychotic drug side effects: their relationship to dose. J Clin Psychiatry 46(5/2):16–21
Kane JM, Rifkin A, Woerner M, Reardon G, Sarantoakis S, Schiebel D, Ramos-Lorenzi J (1983) Low-dose neuroleptic treatment of outpatient schizophrenics. Arch Gen Psychiatry 40:893–896
Keck PE, Cohen BM, Baldessarini RJ, McElroy SL (1989) Time course of antipsychotic effects of neuroleptic drugs. Am J Psychiatry 146:1289–1292
Komoroski RA, Newton JEO, Karson C, Cardwell D, Sprig J (1990) Detection of psychoactive drugs in vivo in humans using ^{19}F NMR spectroscopy. Biol Psychiatry 29:711–714
Laborit H, Huguenard P, Alluaume R (1952) Un nouveau stabilisateur vegetatif, le 4560 RP. Presse Med 60:206–208
Lerner Y, Lwow E, Levitan A, Belmaker RH (1979) Acute, high-dose parenteral haloperidol treatment of psychosis. Am J Psychiatry 136:106–1064
Marder SR, Van Putten T, Mintz J, McKenzie J, Lebell M, Faltico G, May PRA (1984) Costs and benefits of two doses of fluphenazine. Arch Gen Psychiatry 41:1025–1029
Marder SR, Van Putten, T, Mintz J, Lebell M, McKensie J, May PRA (1987) Low- and conventional-dose maintenance therapy with fluphenazine decanoate: two-year outcome. Arch Gen Psychiatry 44:518–521
Mavroidis ML, Garver DL, Kanter DR, Hirschowitz J (1985) Plasma haloperidol levels and clinical response: confounding variables. Psychopharmacol Bull 21:62–65
Modell JG, Lenox RH, Weiner S (1985) Inpatient clinical trial of lorazepam for the management of manic agitation. J Clin Psychopharmacol 5:109–113

Potkin SG, Shen Y, Zhou D, Pardes H, Shu L, Phelps B, Poland R (1985) Does a therapeutic window for plasma haloperidol exist? Preliminary Chinese data. Psychopharmacol Bull 21:59–61
Rifkin A, Quitkin F, Robiner DJ, Klein DF (1977) Fluphenazine decanoate, fluphenazine hydrochloride given orally, and placebo in remitted schizophrenics. I. Relapse rates after one year. Arch Gen Psychiatry 34:43–47
Quitkin F, Rifkin A, Klein DF (1975) Very high dosage vs. standard dosage fluphenazine in schizophrenia. Arch Gen Psychiatry 32:1276–1281
Santos JL, Cabranes JA, Almogueraz I, Ramos JA, Vazquez C, Angeles F (1989) Clinical implications of determination of plasma haloperidol levels. Acta Psychiatr Scand 79:348–354
Smith RC, Baumgartner R, Shvartsburd A, Ravichandran GK, Vroulis G, Mauldin M (1985) Comparative efficacy of red cell and plasma haloperidol as predictors of clinical response in schizophrenia. Psychopharmacology (Berl) 85:449–455
Teicher MH, Baldessarini RJ (1985) Selection of neuroleptic dosage. Arch Gen Psychiatry 42:636–637
Van Putten T, Marder SR, Mintz J, Poland RE (1985) Haloperidol plasma levels and clinical response: a therapeutic window relationship. Psychopharmacol Bull 24:172–175
Van Putten T, Marder SR, Mintz J (1990) A controlled dose comparison of haloperidol in newly admitted schizophrenic patients. Arch Gen Psychiatry 47:754–758
Vuckovic A, Cohen BM, Keck PE Jr, Shedlack KJ (1990) Neuroleptic dosage regimens in psychotic inpatients: a retrospective comparison. J Clin Psychiatry 51:107–109
Wolkin A, Brodie JD, Barouche F, Rotrosen J, Wolf AP, Smith M, Fowler J, Cooper TA (1989) Dopamine receptor occupancy and plasma haloperidol levels. Arch Gen Psychiatry 46:482–483

Diagnostic Heterogeneity in Relation to Drug Evaluation: Antidepressants

E.S. Paykel

1 Introduction

This paper will review the evidence that different subgroups of depressives are responsive to different classes of antidepressants and will use this to draw conclusions as to suitable samples for evaluation of new antidepressants. The evidence is complex and has been accumulated over many years. The conclusions for new antidepressant studies are much simpler.

2 Classifications of Depression

The classification of depression has been a fruitful field for scholastic disputes in psychiatry. Broadly speaking, two major classifications have proved to be of lasting value: the distinction between bipolar and unipolar disorder and that between psychotic and neurotic (or endogenous and non-endogenous) disorders.

2.1 Unipolar and Bipolar Illness

The separation between bipolar affective disorders, with a history of mania, and unipolar disorders, showing depression alone, is comparatively recent. Kraepelin and his successors assumed that all affective psychoses were manic depressive, and official classifications followed suit. It was Perris (1966) and Angst (1966) who delineated the separation. Genetically, bipolar patients have a stronger family history, and it is virtually only bipolar patients whose relatives show bipolar disorder, although about half the family members in fact have unipolar disorder. The sex incidence is more nearly equal in bipolars; age at onset tends to be earlier and course more recurrent (Andreasen 1982; Perris 1992). There is clear evidence of better response to lithium and precipitation of manic episodes by tricyclic

---

Department of Psychiatry, University of Cambridge, Addenbrooke's Hospital, Cambridge CB2 2QQ, UK

antidepressants, but not much other evidence of differential response to antidepressants. There is less convincing evidence of other biological abnormalities.

2.2 Psychotic/Neurotic Distinction

Only a relatively small proportion of all depressions, perhaps around 10%, are bipolar. Reflecting this, most development of new antidepressants concentrates on unipolar depressions, as will this review. We are still left with the problem of how to divide up the large unipolar remainder. Here, the well-tried psychotic/neurotic or endogenous/non-endogenous distinction is still of value.

Terminology is unsatisfactory. Strictly, psychotic refers to the presence of severe illness with delusions, hallucinations and lack of insight; endogenous to the absence of psychological precipitants. However, the two concepts have tended to become fused with linkage between three elements: symptom picture, precipitant stress and personality (Rosenthal and Klerman 1966). The symptom picture of endogenous depression, also now referred to as melancholia or somatic syndrome, is said to be one of more severe illness, without short-term mood fluctuations in response to concurrent environmental changes; with severe guilt or pessimism which may reach delusional intensity; with psychomotor retardation or agitation; more severe somatic disturbances, such as insomnia, anorexia or weight loss; with early morning wakening and diurnal morning worsening.

The concept received considerable empirical confirmation in a large number of multivariate statistical studies published in the 1960s and 1970s (Kendell 1976). Boundaries between the two groups are at best fuzzy and there are many mixed cases.

The most consistent biological correlate is dexamethasone nonsuppression (Carroll et al. 1981), but other neuroendocrine abnormalities have been reported, such as blunted growth hormone response to clonidine (Checkley et al. 1984). A number of recent studies have shown that absence of life stress and presence of the endogenous symptom pattern are only weakly associated (Paykel et al. 1984). The endogenous symptoms appear to be the more informative aspect for response to physical treatment and for neuroendocrine correlates.

Two other types of depression which appear in the recent literature, dysthymia and atypical depression will be discussed in due course.

3 DSM-III and ICD 10

The two new competing official diagnostic classifications are DSM-III (currently under revision to DSM-IV) and the International Classification of

Table 1. Mood disorders (DSM-III-R)

Bipolar disorders	Depressive disorders
Bipolar disorder[a]	Major depression[a]
Mixed	Single episode
Manic	Recurrent
Depressive	Dysthymia
Cyclothymia	(Primary, secondary)
Bipolar disorder n.o.s.	(Early, late onset)
	Depressive disorder n.o.s.

n.o.s., not otherwise specified.
[a] Additional specifications for severity, psychotic, in remission, melancholia, seasonal.

Diseases, 10th revision (ICD 10). Both manage to be more complex than the simple schema just outlined. The classification of mood disorders in DSM-III-R (American Psychiatric Association 1987) is shown in Table 1. There is a separate category for bipolar disorders. A new term, major depression, is used for non-bipolar depressions. Neurotic depression disappeared from DSM-III, but the endogenous and psychotic classifications are partly preserved by subcategories of psychotic depression for depression with delusions and hallucinations, and of melancholia for depression with the endogenous pattern. Two other depressive disorders are included which might have been regarded as personality types: cyclothymia and dysthymia. Dysthymic disorder was a new invention in DSM-III to describe a pattern of persistent fluctuating mild depression that might be virtually life-long with short intermissions. This might previously have been regarded as characterological depression or one type of chronic neurotic depression. The concept is useful, although recent studies indicate that most dysthymics also develop major depression.

The ICD was unsatisfactory in ICD-9 with respect to affective disorders with many alternative subcategories and lax definitions. ICD-10, set out in Table 2, makes some radical changes. There are separate major categories for mania, bipolar affective disorder, depression, recurrent depressive disorder, persistent affective states (cyclothymia and dysthymia) and other affective episodes. Manic and depressive episodes can be subclassified. The separations of single manic attacks and of single and recurrent depressive disorders are of doubtful value, since there is good evidence that manic episodes are part of bipolar disorder, and on follow-up at least 50% of single depressive disorders become recurrent. The subclassification of depression allows separation of endogenous (somatic) and psychotic symptoms.

Table 2. ICD-10 affective disorders section[a] (main categories and main subcategories)

Manic episode
Hypomania
Mania
Without psychotic symptoms
With psychotic symptoms
Bipolar affective disorder
Current episode
Hypomania
Mania (subtypes as manic episode)
Depression (subtypes as depressive episode)
Mixed
Depressive episode
Mild severity
Without somatic symptoms
With somatic symptoms
Moderate severity
Without somatic symptoms
With somatic symptoms
Severe
Without psychotic symptoms
With psychotic symptoms
Recurrent depressive disorder
Current episode as depressive disorder
Persistent affective disorder
Cyclothymia
Dysthymia
Other mood (affective) disorders
Unspecified mood (affective) disorder

[a] Abridged version from ICD-10 (World Health Organization 1992).

4 Drug Response

4.1 Criteria for Evaluating Differential Drug Response

In evaluating differential drug response, we need first to consider the methodological requirements for conclusive studies. The essential test for specificity is the controlled trial. Many studies in the past have adopted a design in which depressed patients are treated with a single antidepressant, and then examined by some statistical technique to see what initial characteristics distinguish those who have done well and badly on the treatment. This design is not adequate. In any patient who improves on treatment, a number of different elements may contribute to the response. First, it may have been spontaneous, reflecting the natural history of the disorder. Spontaneous remission is probably not uncommon. It is clear from historical accounts that severe melancholia in the nineteenth century did in due course remit, although slowly. Milder depressions often remit without ever being recognised or treated.

Secondly, many other treatment processes are also at work in a patient who receives an antidepressant, such as the social effects of ventilation, support and hospital admission already referred to, and the effect of receiving an inert placebo. The limited evidence available (Paykel et al. 1975) suggests that the effects of the placebo itself are in fact quite weak, but the effects of other nonspecific treatment factors are probably quite powerful. Hospitalised patients with psychotic depression often improve markedly after admission with the supportive nursing environment, while drugs are still being withheld for research studies. The specific effects of the drugs are not very large. In placebo-controlled trials in depression, as a rule only 20%–30% more recoveries occur on active treatment than on placebo.

When predictor analyses of response only examine the change in a group of subjects given the single treatment under investigation, improvement is an amalgam of the above factors, and it is not possible to say to which element significant predictors are related. If one wants to say that a certain treatment is indicated for a specific patient, one needs to focus on the specific therapeutic benefit due to the treatment, i.e., the magnitude of the difference between improvement on this drug and on placebo or alternative treatment, and to show that this difference is greater in the patient group under consideration than those of other treatments. This requires a controlled trial against placebo or an alternative treatment. Probably the best technique is the factorial design where interactions of diagnosis and treatment effects can be sought, in two-way analyses of variance (Paykel 1988).

Irrespective of treatment, the general rule appears to be that those subjects who have already had long illnesses tend to improve less and also to benefit less from specific treatments. Those who have already had many episodes tend to have future recurrences (Coryell and Winokur 1992). Some years ago Leff (1973), based on experience in schizophrenia, suggested that patients with intermediate prognosis might be the best subjects for treatment trials as having the greatest potential variability to be affected by treatment. Those with good prognosis would do well irrespective of treatment; those with poor prognosis, would do poorly.

4.2 Electroconvulsive Therapy

Electroconvulsive therapy (ECT) is the oldest of the current somatic treatments, and one for which patterns of use differ somewhat between countries. It still comprises a benchmark against which other therapies for severe depression need to be measured. Six blind comparisons of ECT and simulated ECT have been carried out in the last 15 years in Britain. One (Lambourn and Gill 1978) showed virtually no benefits and in another effects were not very strong (Johnstone et al. 1980a), but the others showed strong treatment effects among severely ill inpatients (Freeman et al. 1978; West 1981; Brandon et al. 1984; Gregory et al. 1985).

Only the Northwick Park study looked at subtype and response (Clinical Research Centre 1984). The superiority of active ECT was found to be mainly in patients with depressive delusions. Other predictor studies also suggest that psychotic depressives show better response (Paykel 1979). In the early Massachusetts collaborative study (Greenblatt et al. 1964) ECT was also markedly superior to placebo in affective psychoses but not neuroses. There have been a number of non-blind randomised comparative trials of ECT and antidepressants with random assignment, mainly among severely ill inpatients, which show ECT to be more effective (Paykel 1979). Among nine comparisons with tricyclic antidepressants, six found ECT better overall, while three studies found equal drug effects. Among comparisons with monoamine oxidase (MAO) inhibitors, the superiority is even more striking, with ECT more effective in all five studies.

4.3 Tricyclic Antidepressants

Tricyclic antidepressants are very well evaluated drugs. Morris and Beck (1974), surveying the limited selection of tricyclic antidepressants then available in the USA, found 93 comparative trials against placebo. Among these, 61 showed drug superior to placebo and 32 failed to do so. There will be more positive studies of additional drugs by now, so the evidence for efficacy is impressive. Some of the negative studies can be attributed to poor trial techniques, such as short treatment periods, low doses and unsatisfactory outcome measures. Some undoubtedly reflect the limited benefit obtained from these drugs.

The view that tricyclics are particularly effective in endogenous depression goes back as early as the initial open studies by Kuhn. However, a critical look at the controlled trials indicates that, although the effect may have been a little better in endogenous depressives, there have been many studies in which a tricyclic was superior to placebo in samples characterised as neurotic or reactive (Ball and Kiloh 1959; Wittenborn et al. 1962; Uhlenhuth and Park 1964; Covi et al. 1974; Friedman 1975; Paykel et al. 1982).

The more recent literature regarding delusional depression also indicates a poor response to tricyclics and better to ECT or neuroleptics (Perry et al. 1982). It would appear that the most severe endogenous or psychotic depressives do not respond very well to tricyclics. There may be a curvilinear relationship in which the best response is shown by patients with the endogenous symptom pattern but moderate severity. This way found in two studies by Coppen and colleagues using the Newcastle Scale (Rao and Coppen 1978; Abou-Saleh and Coppen 1983).

There is increasing evidence that tricyclics have effects outside depression. Marks and O'Sullivan (1988) reviewed a number of studies showing tricyclics superior to placebo in obsessional neurosis and in agoraphobia. Two important studies included a spectrum of anxious and depressed patients. Johnstone et al. (1980b) treated such patients with amitriptyline, diazepam or placebo. Amitriptyline was consistently superior to placebo while diazepam showed only weak effects, even in patients with predominant anxiety. Kahn et al. (1986) carried out a similar study with imipramine, chlordiazepoxide or placebo with similar findings.

We examined effects of tricyclics in mild depression by means of a controlled trial of amitriptyline versus placebo in general practice (Paykel et al. 1988; Hollyman et al. 1988). There were highly significant differences on a wide variety of typical depressive symptoms with amitriptyline impressively superior to placebo. In a series of two-way analyses of covariance incorporating a variety of subclassifications, significant interactions were relatively few, indicating fairly strong and consistent drug effects across most subgroups. Subgroups failing to give rise to interactions included demographic variables, history of chronicity, and endogenous depression. Only in one area, severity, were there interactions. Active drug was clearly superior to placebo in Research Diagnostic Criteria major depressives, but not in minor depressives. When divided on initial Hamilton Score it was only the most mildly ill patients, with Hamilton scores below 13, who showed no benefit from active drug: there were considerable drug–placebo differences in those with initial scores of 13–15 and over 15.

These findings are consistent with a study by Stewart et al. (1985) in which desipramine was superior to placebo in major depression, both with and without melancholia, but not in dysthymic disorder. It was also effective in patients with initial Hamilton scores of 14–18 but not under 14 (Stewart et al. 1983).

The real conclusion about tricyclic antidepressants appears to be that they are truly broad spectrum antidepressants, effective across quite a wide range of depressions, extending to clearly non-endogenous and relatively mild disorders, although with a floor level for severity and also into the spectrum of anxiety disorders. They may have the greatest drug–placebo difference in nonpsychotic depressives showing the endogenous symptom pattern and moderate severity.

4.4 Serotonin Reuptake Inhibitors

There may be more selectivity among the newest recruits to the uptake inhibitors: the specific serotonin reuptake inhibitors. The first of these, zimeldine, was not available long enough for its place to be established firmly. There was a hint from at least one study that it might be effective in anxiety and less so with retardation (Aberg-Wistedt 1982a,b). Since then, among the newer drugs, fluvoxamine has been found superior to maprotiline in panic disorder (Den Boer and Westenberg 1988) and superior to desipramine in obsessional compulsive disorder (Goodman et al. 1990). Both the comparison drugs were chosen as specific noradrenaline uptake inhibitors. The obsessional study is consistent with the suggestions from the earlier literature that clomipramine is particularly effective in obsessionals, including a controlled trial which demonstrated superiority to nortriptyline (Thoren et al. 1980). It may therefore be that there is a particular link between serotonin potentiation and relief of anxiety.

4.5 Dysthymia

Evidence regarding treatment response in dysthymia is sparse so far. The chronicity of the disorder suggests the likelihood of less improvement, irrespective of treatment. Stewart et al. (1985) did not find any evidence that desipramine was superior to placebo in a small dysthymic sample. Guy et al. (1983) found mianserin superior to placebo in patients characterised as chronic dysphorics, a related concept. Kocsis et al. (1988) found imipramine superior to placebo in dysthymics, but almost all had a superimposed major depression, usually chronic. In dysthymic outpatients with additional features of atypical depression, Stewart et al. (1989) found both imipramine and phenelzine superior to placebo. There have recently been some studies employing the 5HT2 antagonist ritanserin but they are not yet conclusive. None of these studies gives strong evidence of specific response to particular types of antidepressant.

4.6 MAO Inhibitors

Although MAO inhibitors (MAOIs) were introduced into therapy before tricyclics, they still have a much more limited place. The clinician who first crystallised a view of a selective clinical place was Sargant. His colleagues, West and Dally (1959), in a retrospective analysis, found patients responding favourably to iproniazid to show absence of self-reproach, morning worsening and early wakening and presence of evening worsening, hysterical symptoms and a history of having been worsened by ECT. Additional features of a syndrome were described, including long illness, phobic anxiety and fatigue.

In the many subsequent papers, three different meanings have really been assigned by different authors to the term atypical depression (Paykel et al. 1983). One is the idea of marked anxiety and phobic symptoms, either accompanied by depression, or assumed to have some relation to an underlying depression as indicated, for instance, by diurnal variation. The second meaning is what would now be described as reversed vegetative symptoms, i.e., depression with a diurnal pattern of evening worsening, insomnia of early rather than late kind or increased sleep, increased appetite and weight, all in the direction opposite to the physiological changes said to characterise endogenous depression. A third meaning, probably closest to the original, was that of non-endogenous depression in general. This usage has gradually dropped out in the last 10 years.

These three meanings in practice identify different groups of patients (Paykel et al. 1983). The concept of atypical depression is somewhat imprecise and it is better to specify which aspect is being emphasised.

The best evidence on the efficacy of MAOIs is for phenelzine. Among 17 controlled trials against placebo in depression (Paykel 1990), there was not a very strong relationship between response and defined subtype, but there was some relationship to treatment setting. Most of the studies showing drug–placebo differences have been in outpatient samples, while studies on inpatients have tended to be negative. Outpatients tend to be less severely ill and more neurotic in symptom pattern. Some re-evaluation may be needed here since most of the inpatient trials were early studies, using doses and treatment periods that were relatively low by modern standards.

Among recent comparisons of MAOIs against tricyclics, we found phenelzine and amitriptyline both superior to placebo in outpatient depressives and mixed anxiety depressives, with surprisingly little difference between them (Rowan et al. 1982; Paykel et al. 1982). On anxiety measures and in more anxious subjects phenelzine was minimally superior to amitriptyline; on depression measures amitriptyline was minimally superior to phenelzine. Similarly, Ravaris et al. (1980) found only weak differences between amitriptyline and phenelzine, with phenelzine having more effect on anxiety measures. Davidson et al. (1986), analysing patients from a number of studies, found weak trends for better effects of MAO inhibitor rather than tricyclic where panic attack and a precipitant were present but where agoraphobia was absent. Georgotas et al. (1987) found only weak differences in elderly depressives, as did Sheehan et al. (1980) in younger subjects with phobic anxiety. Davidson et al. (1988) in a comparative trial of isocarboxazid and placebo found the drug more effective in endogenous depressives but also in patients with reversed vegetative symptoms and in anxious and hostile depressives. Overall these findings favour selectivity for anxiety, but only very weakly and inconsistently.

The New York group have found stronger differences (see Liebowitz et al. 1990; Quitkin et al. 1988, 1989, 1990; Stewart et al. 1989). Selecting patients with reversed vegetative symptoms, they found phenelzine most effective; imipramine was less so although better than placebo. What is most striking in their studies is the limited response of patients with reversed vegetative symptoms to imipramine, although it is superior to placebo.

It remains possible that there is some other variable such as a behavioural one, rather than clinical symptom subtype, which predicts a better response to MAOIs. Some patients appear to respond consistently only to this class of drug. Pare and Mack (1971) found evidence of consistency of response to the same type of antidepressant in successive episodes. The finding of better response in anxiety both for serotonin uptake inhibitors and for MAOIs raises the question as to whether a serotoninergic effect is also involved for the latter.

Taken overall, a general conclusion for MAOIs is that they are weakly selective for anxiety and reversed vegetative symptoms, but the differences from tricyclics are not strong. Clinically, they are used mainly as second choice drugs where tricyclics have failed (Paykel and White 1989). The new generation of MAO-A selective rapidly reversible drugs could very much change this. Little work has been done so far as to whether these drugs effect particular patient subgroups.

5 Recommendations and Conclusions

To move towards conclusions, it is apparent that the differences so far found between different classes of antidepressants in respect of specifically responsive subgroups are small rather than large. There appears to be a common core to all depressions and to the effects of all antidepressants. In favourable cases, most depressions seem to show benefit from most antidepressants. It is only at the extremes that greater selectivity is manifest and even here the selectivity may not so much be in clinical picture but in underlying biochemical factors, not well understood.

Within these limits the broad general findings are that, among the somatic therapies, ECT is the most effective treatment for severe psychotic or retarded depressives; tricyclic antidepressants are broad spectrum antidepressants with effects extending to mild depressives and some anxiety disorders, with probably the best effect where there is moderate severity and possibly where there are endogenous, melancholic or somatic symptoms; serotonin reuptake inhibitors are emerging as having particular effects in anxiety and obsessional disorders. MAOIs show weak specificity towards anxiety or reversed vegetative symptoms. Where does this leave new drug evaluation? It is noteworthy that in practice most pivotal trials of new antidepressants in the last 10 years have made little use of the above evidence, but have tended to test for key efficacy in standard depressions. Initial marketing has usually concentrated on advantages in terms of side effects rather than selective response. It has been left to later studies to extend towards a search for selectivity. This initial evaluation in standard depressed samples has even applied to MAOIs.

This is appropriate, since the selectivity is too weak to warrant undue focus on one particular type during the earlier phases of drug evaluation. There are risks of simply producing more me-too drugs and failing to develop promising drugs of high specificity for specific groups who do not do well at present, but these risks are also inherent in current pharmacological methods of screening for new drugs.

We fall back then on the broader question of the groups which tend to show the largest drug–placebo differences overall. Here the evidence would suggest two guidelines: avoid the most chronic and already unresponsive depressives, and target for the mid-range of severity. Inpatient hospitalised samples are becoming increasingly problematic, although regulatory bodies tend to insist on their use. Most inpatients will have failed to respond to earlier outpatient treatment and will be biased towards nonresponse: the evidence also suggests that drugs are less effective than ECT in such severely ill, deluded or retarded patients.

On the other hand, the most mildly ill subjects do well without drugs and do not show drug–placebo differences. And it is difficult to achieve good study quality control in general practice studies, although, properly selected, such patients do show impressive drug–placebo differences.

The ideal sample for evaluation of a new antidepressant is within the spectrum of the psychiatric outpatient clinic and comprises major depressives, with perhaps a minimum severity of the 17-item Hamilton scale of 18, but without any necessity for selection towards endogenous features. A variety of diagnostic systems should be examined post hoc for influence on response. Later studies should be targeted more on responsive subgroups, depending on clues from the findings of the earlier studies, and any other pointers available and not at all necessarily limited to classical depressives.

References

Aberg-Wistedt A (1982a) A double blind study of zimelidine, a serotonin uptake inhibitor, and desipramine, a noradrenaline uptake inhibitor, in endogenous depression. I. Clinical findings. Acta Psychiatr Scand 66:50–65

Aberg-Wistedt A (1982b) Comparison between zimelidine and desipramine in endogenous depression – a cross-over study. Acta Psychiatr Scand 66:129–138

Abou-Saleh MT, Coppen A (1983) Classification of depression and response to antidepressive therapies. Br J Psychiatry 143:601–603

American Psychiatric Association (1987) Diagnostic and statistical manual of mental disorders, 3rd revised edn. American Psychiatric Association, Washington

Andreasen NC (1982) Concepts, diagnosis and classification. In: Paykel ES (ed) Handbook of affective disorders. Churchill Livingstone, Edinburgh, pp 24–44

Angst J (1966) The aetiology and nosology of endogenous depressive psychoses: a genetic, sociological and clinical study. Springer, Berlin Heidelberg New York

Ball JR, Kiloh LG (1959) A controlled trial of imipramine in treatment of depressive states. Br Med J 2:52–55

Brandon S, Cowley P, McDonald C, Neville P, Palmer R, Wellstood-Eason S (1984) Electroconvulsive therapy: results in depressive illness from the Leicestershire trial. Br Med J 288:22–25

Carroll BJ, Feinberg M, Greden JF et al. (1981) A specific laboratory test for the diagnosis of melancholia: standardisation, validation and clinical utility. Arch Gen Psychiatry 38:15–22

Checkley SA, Glass IB, Thompson C et al. (1984) The GH response to clonidine in endogenous as compared with reactive depression. Psychol Med 14:773–777

Clinical Research Centre, Division of Psychiatry (1984) The Northwick Park ECT trial. Predictors of response to real and simulated ECT. Br J Psychiatry 144:227–237
Coryell W, Winokur G (1992) Course and outcome. In: Paykel ES (ed) Handbook of affective disorders, 2nd edn. Churchill Livingstone, Edinburgh, pp 89–108
Covi L, Lipman RS, Derogatis R, Smith JE, Pattison JH (1974) Drugs and group psychotherapy in neurotic depression. Am J Psychiatry 131:191–198
Davidson JRT, Pelton S, Krishnan RR, Allf B (1986) The Newcastle anxiety depression index in relationship to the effects of MAOI and TCA drugs. J Affect Dis 11:51–61
Davidson JRT, Giller EL, Zisook S, Overall JE (1988) An efficacy study of isocarboxazid and placebo in depression, and its relationship to depressive nosology. Arch Gen Psychiatry 45:120–127
Den Boer JA, Westenberg HGM (1988) Effect of a serotonin and noradrenaline uptake inhibitor in panic disorder; a double-blind comparative study with fluvoxamine and maprotiline. Int Clin Psychopharmacol 3:59–74
Freeman CPL, Basson JV, Creighton A (1978) Double-blind controlled trial of electroconvulsive therapy (ECT) and simulated ECT in depressive illness. Lancet 1:738–740
Friedman AS (1975) Interaction of drug therapy with marital therapy in depressive patients. Arch Gen Psychiatry 32:619–637
Georgotas A, McCue RE, Friedman E, Cooper TB (1987) Response of depressive symptoms to nortriptyline, phenelzine and placebo. Br J Psychiatry 151:102–106
Goodman WK, Price LH, Delgado PL, Palumbo J, Krystal JH, Nagy LM, Rasmussen SA, Heninger GR, Charney DS (1990) Specificity of serotonin reuptake inhibitors in the treatment of obsessive-compulsive disorder. Comparison of fluvoxamine and desipramine. Arch Gen Psychiatry 47:577–585
Greenblatt M, Grosser GH, Wechsler H (1964) Differential response of hospitalised depressed patients to somatic therapy. Am J Psychiatry 120:935–943
Gregory S, Shawcross CR, Gill D (1985) The Nottingham ECT study. A double-blind comparison of bilateral, unilateral and simulated ECT in depressive illness. Br J Psychiatry 146:520–524
Guy W, Ban TA, Schaffer JD (1983) Differential treatment responsiveness among mildly depressed patients. In: Clayton PJ, Barrett JE (eds) Treatment of depression: old controversies and new approaches. Raven, New York, pp 229–250
Hollyman JE, Freeling P, Paykel ES, Bhat A, Sedgwick P (1988) Double-blind placebo-controlled trial of amitriptyline among depressed patients in general practice. J R Coll Gen Pract 109:536–538
Johnstone EC, Deakin JFW, Lawler P, Frith CD, Stevens M, McPherson K, Crow TJ (1980a) The Northwick Park electroconvulsive therapy trial. Lancet 2:1317–1320
Johnstone EC, Cunningham Owens DG, Frith CD, McPherson K, Dowie C, Riley G, Gold A (1980b) Neurotic illness and its response to anxiolytic and antidepressant treatment. Psychol Med 10:321–328
Kahn RJ, McNair DM, Lipman RS, Covi L, Rickels K, Downing R, Fisher S, Frankenthaler LM (1986) Imipramine and chlordiazepoxide in depressive and anxiety disorders. Arch Gen Psychiatry 43:79–85
Kendell RE (1976) The classification of depression: a review of contemporary confusion. Br J Psychiatry 129:15–28
Kocsis JH, Frances AJ, Voss C, Mann JJ, Mason BJ, Sweeney J (1988) Imipramine treatment for chronic depression. Arch Gen Psychiatry 45:253–257
Lambourn J, Gill D (1978) A controlled comparison of simulated and real ECT. Br J Psychiatry 133:514–519
Leff JP (1973) Influence of selection of patients on results of clinical trials. Br Med J 4:156–158
Liebowitz MR, Quitkin FM, Stewart JW, McGrath PJ, Harrison WM, Markowitz JS, Rabkin JG, Tricamo E, Goetz DM, Klein DF (1988) Antidepressant specificity in atypical depression. Arch Gen Psychiatry 45:129–137

Marks I, O'Sullivan G (1988) Drugs and psychological treatments for agoraphobia/panic and obsessive-compulsive disorders: a review. Br J Psychiatry 153:650–658
Morris JB, Beck AT (1974) The efficacy of antidepressant drugs: a review of research (1958–1972). Arch Gen Psychiatry 30:667–674
Pare CMB, Mack JW (1971) Differentiation of two genetically specific types of depression by the response to antidepressant drugs. J Med Genet 8:306–309
Paykel ES (1979) Predictors of treatment response. In: Psychopharmacology of affective disorders. Oxford University Press, Oxford, pp 193–220
Paykel ES (1985) The clinical interview for depression development, reliability and validity. J Affect Dis 9:85–96
Paykel ES (1988) Antidepressants: their efficacy and place in therapy. J Psychopharm 2:105–118
Paykel ES (1990) Monoamine oxidase inhibitors: when should they be used? In: Hawton K, Cowen P (eds) Dilemmas and controversies in the management of psychiatric patients. Oxford University Press, Oxford
Paykel ES, White JL (1989) A European study of views on the use of monoamine oxidase inhibitors. Br J Psychiatry 155(6):9–17
Paykel ES, DiMascio A, Haskell D, Prusoff BA (1975) Effects of maintenance amitriptyline and psychotherapy on symptoms of depression. Psychol Med 5:67–77
Paykel ES, Rowan PR, Parker RR, Bhat AV (1982) Response to phenelzine and amitriptyline in subtypes of neurotic depression. Arch Gen Psychiatry 39:1041–1049
Paykel ES, Parker RR, Rowan RR, Rao BM, Taylor CN (1983) Nosology of atypical depression. Psychol Med 13:131–139
Paykel ES, Rao BM, Taylor CM (1984) Life stress and symptom pattern in outpatient depression. Psychol Med 14:559–568
Paykel ES, Hollyman JA, Freeling P, Sedgwick P (1988) Predictors of therapeutic benefit from amitriptyline in mild depression: a general practice placebo-controlled trial. J Affect Dis 14:83–95
Perris C (1966) A study of bipolar (manic-depressive) and unipolar recurrent affective psychoses. Acta Psychiatr Scand 42 Suppl 194
Perris C (1992) Bipolar and unipolar distinction. In: Paykel ES (ed) Handbook of affective disorders, 2nd edn. Churchill Livingstone, Edinburgh, pp 51–75
Perry PJ, Morgan DE, Smith RE, Tsuang MT (1982) Treatment of unipolar depression accompanied by delusions. ECT versus tricyclic antidepressant-antipsychotic combinations. J Affect Dis 4:195–200
Quitkin FM, Stewart JW, McGrath PJ, Liebowitz MR, Harrison WM, Tricamo E, Klein DF, Rabkin JG, Markowitz JS, Wager SG (1988) Phenelzine versus imipramine in the treatment of probable atypical depression: defining syndrome boundaries of selective MAOI responders. Am J Psychiatry 145:306–311
Quitkin FM, McGrath PJ, Stewart JW, Harrison W, Wager SG, Nunes E, Rabkin JG, Tricamo E, Markowitz J, Klein DF (1989) Phenelzine and imipramine in mood-reactive depressives: further delineation of the syndrome of atypical depression. Arch Gen Psychiatry 46:787–793
Quitkin FM, McGrath PJ, Stewart JW, Harrison W, Tricamo E, Wager SG, Deepek-Welikson K, Nunes E, Rabkin JG, Klein DF (1990) Atypical depressions, panic attacks and response to imipramine and phenelzine. Arch Gen Psychiatry 47:935–941
Rao VA, Coppen A (1978) Classification of depression and response to amitriptyline therapy. Psychol Med 9:3231–3325
Ravaris CL, Robinson DS, Ives JO, Nies A, Bartlett D (1980) Phenelzine and amitriptyline in the treatment of depression. Arch Gen Psychiatry 37:1075–1080
Robinson DS, Nies A, Ravaris CL, Ives JO, Lamborn KR (1974) Treatment response to MAO inhibitors: relation to depressive typology and blood platelet MAO inhibition. In: Angst J (ed) Classification and prediction of outcome of depression. Schattauer, Stuttgart, pp 259–267

Rosenthal SH, Klerman GL (1966) Content and consistency in the endogenous depressive pattern. Br J Psychiatry 112:471–484
Rowan PR, Paykel ES, Parker RR (1982) Phenelzine and amitriptyline: effects on symptoms of neurotic depression. Br J Psychiatry 140:475–483
Sheehan DV, Ballinger J, Jacobsen G (1980) Treatment of endogenous anxiety with phobic, hysterical and hypochondriacal symptoms. Arch Gen Psychiatry 37:51–59
Stewart JW, Quitkin FM, Liebowitz MR, McGrath PJ, Harrison WM, Klein DF (1983) Efficacy of desipramine in depressed outpatients: response according to Research Diagnostic Criteria and severity of illness. Arch Gen Psychiatry 40:202–207
Stewart JW, McGrath PJ, Liebowitz MR, Harrison W, Quitkin F, Rabkin JG (1985) Treatment outcome validation of DSM-III depressive subtypes: clinical usefulness in outpatients with mild to moderate depression. Arch Gen Psychiatry 42:1148–1153
Stewart JW, McGrath PJ, Quitkin FM, Harrison W, Markowitz J, Wager S, Leibowitz MR (1989) Relevance of DSM-III depressive subtype and chronicity of antidepressant efficacy in atypical depression. Arch Gen Psychiatry 46:1080–1087
Thoren P, Asberg M, Cronholm B, Jornestedt L, Traskman L (1980) Clomipramine treatment of obsessive-compulsive disorder. I. A controlled clinical trial. Arch Gen Psychiatry 37:1281–1285
Uhlenhuth EH, Park LC (1964) The influence of medication (imipramine) and doctor in relieving depressed psychoneurotic patients. J Psychiatr Res 2:101
West ED (1981) Electric convulsion therapy in depression: a double-blind controlled trial. Br Med J 282:355–357
West ED, Dally PJ (1959) Effects of iproniazid in depressive syndromes. Br Med J 1:1491–1499
Wittenborn JR, Plante M, Burgess F, Maurer H (1962) A comparison of imipramine, ECT and placebo in the treatment of depression. J Nerv Ment Dis 135:131–137
World Health Organization (1992) The ICD-10 classification of mental and behavioural disorders. Clinical definitions and diagnostic guidelines. WHO, Geneva

Dose–Effect Relationships for Tricyclic Antidepressants: The Basis for Rational Clinical Testing of New Antidepressants

L.F. GRAM

1 Introduction

The dose–effect relationship is a basic element in all research in experimental pharmacology. In clinical pharmacology, the central role of the dose–effect concept has usually been acknowledged, but the actual demonstration of dose–effect relationships in clinical drug research is often extremely difficult. In the early years after the introduction of imipramine and subsequently other tricyclic antidepressants (TCA), the dose–effect problems were not infrequently discussed in the clinical reports, usually on the basis of uncontrolled clinical assessments (Delay and Deniker 1959; Ayd 1959). However, towards the end of the 1960s, the question of appropriate dosing appeared to receive little attention, clinically or in research trials. In a larger review attempting to identify variables important for the therapeutic efficacy of TCA, the *dose* was not even considered (Smith et al. 1969). At that time, the demonstration of pronounced variations in steady state levels in patients on standard TCA (Sjöqvist et al. 1968) gave rise to a series of studies on concentration–effect relationships during the following two decades. For the introduction of new antidepressants, there is an increasing demand for data on the dose–effect relationship. In this situation, it seems awkward that our knowledge about the dose–effect relationship for the usual control therapy, TCA, is rather limited. Also for the clinical use of TCA, the dose–effect issue has been reintroduced by some authors in the 1980s (Quitkin 1985; Roose et al. 1986; Goethe et al. 1988). However, in clinical trials, this problem is seldom even discussed as a source of bias or variability.

2 Dose–Effect Studies of TCA

Several hundred clinical trials with the classical TCA (imipramine, amitriptyline, desipramine, nortriptyline) were reported in the 1960s

Department of Clinical Pharmacology, Odense University, Winsløwparken 19, 5000 Odense C, Denmark

(Bennett 1966; Smith et al. 1969). The vast majority of these studies have either used a flexible dose scheme or a fixed dose scheme with only one dose for each compound studied. In the former case, the dose was selected on the basis of side effects and/or therapeutic effect but usually without operationalized criteria for dose changes. The fixed doses were usually chosen on the basis of earlier uncontrolled dose titration studies, "clinical impression" reports, etc.

Only for imipramine does the literature contain some continuing efforts to clarify the dose–effect problem. This appears partly to be so because of imipramine's status as the classical reference TCA (Quitkin 1985; Goethe et al. 1988). An obvious weakness of the discussion has been that all TCAs apparently have been considered equipotent on a milligram basis (Burt et al. 1962; Bielski and Friedel 1976; Quitkin 1985) although there is no justification for this a priori assumption.

The early controlled studies with imipramine very often employed doses of 200–250 mg/day (Ball and Kiloh 1959; Friedman et al. 1961; Rees et al. 1961, Robin and Langley 1964; Wilson et al. 1962; Waldron and Bates 1965; Paykel et al. 1968; Medical Research Council 1965). In all these studies, imipramine was found to be effective as an antidepressant, whereas studies using desipramine doses of less than 200 mg/day tended to find less convincing effect (Lemere 1959; Hollister et al. 1964; Malitz and Kanzler 1971).

The upper end of the dose range may at least to some extent have been determined by unfavorable experiences with the higher doses. Höhn et al. (1963) thus started out a placebo–imipramine trial with a maximum dose of 400 mg imipraminehydrochloride per day. However, because of several serious toxic reactions early in the study, they reduced the maximum dose to 200 mg imipraminehydrochloride per day.

Wilson et al. (1962) in an ECT–imipramine–placebo comparative study used two doses of imipramine. In the first part of the study, the average imipramine dose was 150 mg/day and in the later part 240 mg/day. Whereas the response on imipramine was poor in the first part of the study, it became good and comparable to electroconvulsive therapy (ECT) in the second part. The uncontrolled conditions and the small number of patients (10–14) limits the power of this study, but later reviews appear to confirm that doses of imipramine less than or equal to 150 mg/day are subtherapeutic in hospitalized, moderately to severely depressed patients (Angst 1970; Quitkin 1985; Roose et al. 1986; Goethe et al. 1988).

The study by Simpson et al. (1976) is the only prospective, double-blind, randomized dose–effect study of TCA. That study compared doses of imipraminehydrochloride 150 mg/day and 300 mg/day, and the main results are shown in Table 1. It seems clear that 300 mg/day was significantly more efficacious than 150 mg/day. The difference in total score reflected corresponding differences in most of the items of the Hamilton scale. Among 12 nonresponding patients, 10 patients received 150 mg/day and two received 300 mg/day.

Table 1. Results of a randomized, double-blind, dose–effect study on imipramine (Simpson et al. 1976)

Type of depression	Imipramine dose					
	150 mg/d			300 mg/d		
	n	Pre[a]	Final[a]	*n*	Pre[a]	Final[a]
Endogenous	21	29.2	14.5	14	30.2	10.7
Neurotic	8	27.0	8.6	8	26.4	3.2
Total	29	28.6	12.9	22	28.8	8.0

[a] Group average total Hamilton rating score (17-item scale) before medication (pre) at last rating (final, usually 4 weeks).

Table 2. Imipramine dose–effect relationship in maintainance therapy of recurrent depression

Study	Imipramine dose (mg/day)	Success rate[a] (%)
Prien et al. (1984)	137 (75–150)	48
Frank et al. (1990)	208 (50–350)[b]	73

[a] 2-year follow-up, placebo success rate about 20% in both studies.
[b] Drug level monitoring, imipramine + desipramine: 308 ± 148 µg/l

Recently published data suggest that these dose–effect relationships for imipramine may also apply to its use in maintenance therapy. A comparison of the study of Prien et al. (1984) and of Frank et al. (1990) (Table 2) indicates that the considerably higher imipramine dose in the latter study markedly influenced the final outcome. In the last study, the dose was determined on the basis of drug level monitoring, and it was required that imipramine + desipramine levels were above 150 µg/l. It remains to be shown whether even more aggressive dosing would have further improved the outcome.

3 Concentration–Effect Studies on TCA

The combination of (1) pronounced interpatient variation in steady state levels when standard doses are given, (2) a narrow therapeutic range, and (3) the lack of reliable clinical effect measurements for dose titration yields unequivocally the classical rationale for drug level monitoring for the TCA (Gram 1977). However, to introduce this principle into clinical patient care or into clinical drug trials requires that the concentration–effect relationships for both therapeutic and toxic effects have been established. Over the past more than two decades, more than 100 papers have been published on this matter (Oliveira et al. 1989). In broad terms, the present status in the field can be summarized as follows:

1. Several studies have reported a correlation between blood concentration (usually plasma or serum) and the antidepressant effect and/or the unintended effects.
2. With one exception (Kragh-Sørensen et al. 1976), these studies have all been *retrospective* in design, and therefore rather hypothesis generating than hypothesis testing.
3. A large number of studies have failed to demonstrate any concentration–effect relationship at all.
4. A number of confounding factors may explain at least some of these discrepancies.

The considerable methodological problems in such studies have been discussed in detail earlier (Gram 1977; Gram et al. 1981, 1982) and are summarized in Table 3. The complex interplay between different methodological factors and the heterogeneity of the studies have made it essentially impossible to make any meaningful meta-analyses. The simple counting of studies with different conclusions is of course not very meaningful. The conclusions made from this literature thus necessarily will have an element of subjectivity. When decisions are to be made as to whether the present literature should have consequences for clinical practice or clinical trial methodology, the balance between the risk of a type 1 error (assuming a nonexisting concentration–effect relationship) and a type 2 error (not taking

Table 3. Concentration–effect relationship studies on tricyclic antidepressants (TCA)

Confounding factors
Study design (retrospective)
Small sample size
Patient heterogeneity
Different effective levels in different diagnostic groups?
Effect measurements
Time factor in response
Low incidence of some toxic reactions
Pharmacokinetics
Stable steady state?
(Standardized dose/sampling schedule)
C_{max}, C_{min} or C_{mean}?
Active metabolites?
Protein binding variable?
Study quality
Drug compliance
Protocol compliance

the consequences of true concentration–effect relationship) is critical and should be weighed against such factors as the possible gain of introducing TCA monitoring or the risk of not introducing this technique in view of the actual costs of the service, etc.

A recent review (Oliveira et al. 1989) concludes in a rather similar manner as done 10–15 years ago (Gram 1977), namely, that a consistent concentration–effect relationship as concerns the antidepressant response has been established for imipramine and nortriptyline, whereas for amitriptyline and clomipramine the picture is less clear in spite of a large number of studies. Furthermore, more recent studies on desipramine appear to permit some conclusions (APA Task Force 1985).

For imipramine, two independent larger studies (n = 60 and 66, respectively, inpatients) carried out simultaneously in New York and Scandinavia (Glassman et al. 1977; Reisby et al. 1977) came to essentially the same conclusion that with steady levels of imipramine + desipramine above 400 nM (~150 µg/l), depressed patients will respond and better so with higher levels until a maximum efficacy appears to be achieved when the combined levels are above 700–800 nM (~250 µg/l).

For *nortriptyline*, a series of studies (Kragh-Sørensen et al. 1973, 1976; Ziegler et al. 1976; Montgomery et al. 1978) including 18–36 patients in each study have confirmed the lack of antidepressant effect at higher steady levels (exceeding 500–600 nM) as first proposed by Åsberg et al. (1971). The data on the lower therapeutically effective nortriptyline concentration are less established but appear to be around 200 nM.

For the other frequently studied TCA, the lower effective concentrations that have been suggested (with considerable uncertainty) are for amitriptyline (+ nortriptyline) ~300 nM, clomipramine (+ desmethylclomipramine) ~500 nM, and for desipramine ~300 nM (Oliveira et al. 1989). For amitriptyline and to less extent the others, there is an inconsistent indication of poor response at high drug levels as for nortriptyline. More recently, Preskorn (1989) on the basis of population studies has drawn attention to the risk of CNS toxicity such as confusion and delirium at high plasma TCA levels. One may speculate whether these effects are related to the absence of antidepressant effect at high nortriptyline plasma levels.

Several sometimes disturbing side effects may occur at subtherapeutic levels. With increasing TCA levels, a sequence of different effects will be seen: anticholinergic effects and orthostatism, moderate sedation, antidepressant effect, confusion – delirium, severe cardiovascular and CNS toxicity.

The latter usually will be seen in cases of overdose (Spiker et al. 1975; Pedersen et al. 1982). Sedation is variable between patients and TCAs. With amitriptyline, the sedation may be pronounced at therapeutic levels.

TCA are therapeutically effective in different conditions and Fig. 1 summarizes our concentration–effect studies with imipramine in nocturnal enuresis (Jørgensen et al. 1980), neuropathy pain (diabetics, Kvinesdal et

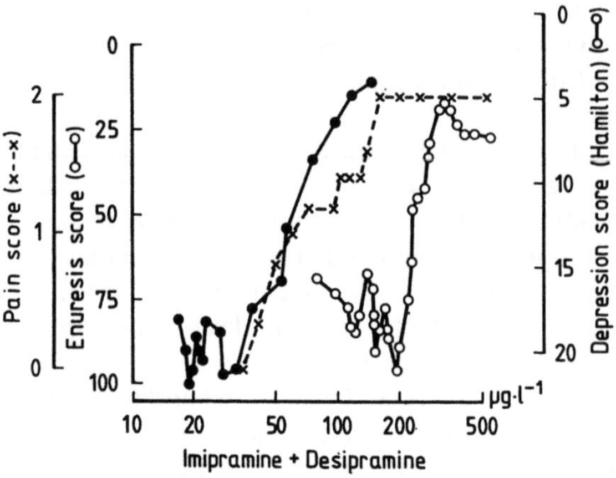

Fig. 1. Concentration–effect relationship in imipramine treatment of three different conditions, endogenous depression (●---●), pain in diabetic neuropathy (X---X), and nocturnal enuresis (O---O). The *curves* were constructed by rank ordering the patients according to steady state concentration and calculation of moving average ($n = 5$) of the corresponding rating score. For depression and enuresis, the values represent residual scores whereas the value for pain represents change in score. (Data from Reisby et al. 1977; Kvinesdal et al. 1984; Jørgensen et al. 1980)

al. 1984) and depression (Reisby et al. 1977). The much lower effective concentrations and the much faster response (maximum within 1 week) in the two former conditions underline that the effect of imipramine in these cases is not related to an antidepressant effect. The arithmetic plot of the concentration–effect curves in pain treatment appears to follow a simple rectangular hyperbola analogous to the Michaelis Menten curve corresponding to a simple E_{max} model. This has been further confirmed in recent studies with both imipramine and paroxetine (Sindrup et al. 1990, 1992). In contrast, for depression treatment, the arithmetic plot is clearly sigmoid with apparently no antidepressant effect at imipramine + desipramine levels below 400–500 nM (~150 μg/l).

To which extent the present evidence of concentration–effect relationships for various TCA can justify drug level monitoring in clinical practice is still being debated. Many clinical centers have introduced this service as a part of their treatment program. Besides, the concrete aid to drug therapy, the psychological effect of such procedures is important and influences both patient and doctor awareness of the importance of proper and stable dosing. Combining the drug level monitoring with a drug information service may further promote good clinical practice in psychotropic drug therapy. In spite of the introduction of TCA monitoring into the routine, prospective studies are still strongly needed. To make such studies prospective and to compare different TCA levels in a controlled, randomized setting requires that predetermined plasma levels can be achieved in the very early phase of the treatment in order not to confuse the effect on response of plasma level and of time. Therefore, it may not be possible to carry out such studies properly unless techniques are available that allow very early dose adjustment. Phenotyping tests, which at least for some TCA seem to be good predictors of steady state levels (Brøsen et al. 1986; Gram and Brøsen 1990), may be a reliable method, one which does not interfere with the pharmacodynamic response.

4 Dose–Effect Problems in Clinical Trials

As discussed above, there is strong evidence that imipramine in doses of 150 mg or less per day is suboptimal for the treatment of major depression. In spite of this, such low doses have been quite customary in clinical trials with new antidepressant drugs for the past 10–20 years.

In early studies comparing imipramine and amitriptyline given in equivalent milligram doses, it seems obvious that the differences observed in favor of amitriptyline could be explained entirely by relative underdosing of imipramine (Hoenig and Visram 1964; Burt et al. 1962). Likewise, genuinely less effective antidepressants may be judged equipotent with TCA if the latter is underdosed (DUAG 1986; DUAG 1990). Dosing problems thus may create both type-1 and type-2 errors.

Low drug doses in clinical trials may be the result of a primarily protocolled low dose and/or the use of a flexible dose schedule. In the latter case, if the patient or the doctor is sensitive to common side effects occurring at subtherapeutic doses, the overall result may be underdosing in a substantial fraction of the patients. A third cause of underdosing may be noncompliance. The magnitude of the problem is difficult to assess since only few publications on clinical trials report on appropriate measures that could document dosing such as pill count or drug level monitoring. Just for this reason, drug level monitoring should be an indispensable standard in clinical trials. Usually the additional costs of including such measures of quality are marginal compared to the total cost of a trial. Indeed drug level monitoring may also allow the identification of patients responding poorly due to low plasma levels because of very fast elimination of the drug.

Recently, a scheme has been developed which allows a quantitative assessment of the consequences of insufficient dosing in relation to sample size and spontaneous recovery in clinical trials (Gram 1990).

For antidepressant treatment, it can be considered justified to analyze the outcome in a dichotomous manner, i.e., as response or nonresponse. An observed therapeutic response may be due to a true effect of the drug or to spontaneous recovery. An observed nonresponse may be due to a true resistance to the drug ("drug resistant depression") or could be the result of insufficient dosing.

The response rate seen when there is no spontaneous recovery and all patients receive a sufficient dose may be termed the *"true" response rate* = X. If the *rate of spontaneous response* = Y and the *rate of insufficient dose* = Z, then it follows:

$$\text{Rate of nonresponse due to insufficient dose} = (1 - Y) \cdot Z \tag{1}$$

$$\text{Drug related response rate} = X(1 - Y)(1 - Z) \tag{2}$$

Observed response rate:

$$R = X(1 - Y)(1 - Z) + Y = X + Y - XY - XZ + XYZ \tag{3}$$

In a trial with two drugs (Nos. 1, 2), there will be two observed response rates (R_1 and R_2) and a *difference in response rate* $D = R_1 - R_2$. In a randomized trial, the rate of spontaneous response (Y) will be the same in the two treatment groups, whereas the rate of insufficient dosing may be different (Z_1 and Z_2) which then yields:

Observed difference in response rates:

$$D = R_1 - R_2 = [X_1 - X_2 - X_1Z_1 + X_2Z_2](1 - Y) \tag{4}$$

As is clear from Eq. 4 and can be seen from Fig. 2, the difference between two treatments will be reduced with increasing rate of placebo response. A high rate of insufficient dosing is particularly critical when it affects the most effective treatment. As an example with a spontaneous response rate (Y) of 15%, the observed difference (D) between treatment X_2 and X_3 (Fig. 2) is 26% when the rate of insufficient dosing is 0 for both treatments, but is reduced to 13% if the rate of insufficient dosing is 30% for treatment X_2. The required number of patients to detect the difference then increases from 2 × 54 to 2 × 246. This example may be representative of what could happen if a TCA on flexible dose in compared with a new, less effective, and less toxic antidepressant.

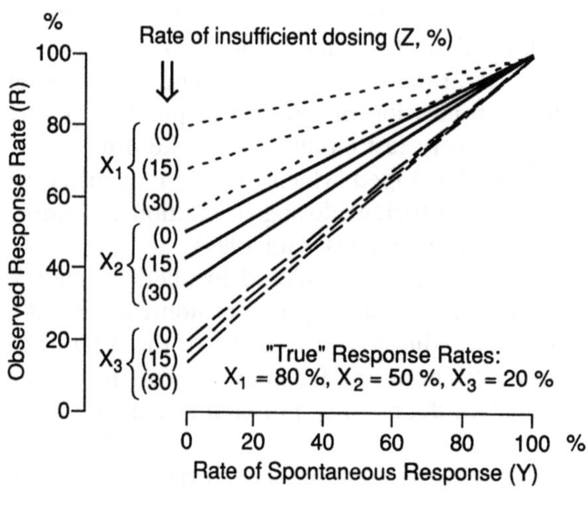

Fig. 2. Observed response rate (R) as a function of the rates of insufficient dosing (Z) and spontaneous response (Y) according to Eq. 3. Examples are shown for three different drugs with true response rates of 80% (X_1), 50% (X_2), and 20% (X_3), respectively

5 Conclusion

The introduction of new antidepressants requires both comparative trials against TCA and documentation on the dose–effect relationships. In this perspective, it is paradoxical that the scientific literature on the dose–effect relationships of TCA is very limited. There is some documentation on concentration–effect relationships for TCA, and it seems logical that this knowledge should be utilized to control that effective TCA doses are given in clinical trials. Insufficient dosing may create the basis for considerable type-1 and type-2 error problems in the evaluation of new antidepressants.

References

Angst J (1970) Klinische Wirkung von Imipramin. In: Angst J, Theobald W, Bleuler M, Kuhn R (eds) Tofranil. Ciba-Geigy, Basel: Stämpfli, Bern, pp 3–82

APA Task Force (1985) Tricyclic antidepressants–blood level measurements and clinical outcome: an APA Task Force report. Am J Psychiatry 142:155–162

Åsberg M, Crönholm B, Sjöqvist F, Tuck D (1971) Relationship between plasma level and therapeutic effect of nortriptyline. Br Med J 3:331–334

Ayd FJ (1959) Antidepressants–1959. Psychosomatics 1:37–41

Ball JRB, Kiloh LG (1959) A controlled trial of imipramine in treatment of depressive states. Br Med J 1052–1055

Bennett IF (1966) Is there a superior antidepressant? In: Garattini S, Dukes MNG (eds) Proceedings of the first international symposium on antidepressant drugs. Excerpta Medica, Amsterdam, pp 375–393

Bielski RJ, Friedel RO (1976) Prediction of tricyclic antidepressant response. Arch Gen Psychiatry 33:1479–1489

Brøsen K, Klysner R, Gram LF, Otton SV, Bech P, Bertilsson L (1986) Steady state concentrations of imipramine and its metabolites in relation to the sparteine/debrisoquine polymorphism. Eur J Clin Pharmacol 30:679–684

Burt CG, Gordon WF, Holt NF, Hordern A (1962) Amitriptyline in depressive states: a controlled trial. J Ment Sci 108:711–730

Danish University Antidepressant Group (DUAG) (1986) Citalopram: clinical effect profile in comparison with clomipramine. A controlled multicenter study. Psychopharmacology (Berl) 90:131–138

Danish University Antidepressant Group (DUAG) (1990) Paroxetine: a selective serotonin reuptake inhibitor showing better tolerance but weaker antidepressant effect than clomipramine in a controlled multicenter study. J Affect Dis 18:289–299

Delay J, Deniker P (1959) Efficacy of tofranil in the treatment of various types of depression: a comparison with other antidepressant drugs. Can Psychiatr Assoc J 4:S100–S112

Frank E, Kupfer DJ, Perel JM, Cornes C, Jarrett DB, Mallinger AG, Thase ME, EcEachran AB, Grochocinski VJ (1990) Three-year outcome for maintenance therapies in recurrent depression. Arch Gen Psychiatry 47:1093–1099

Friedman C, De Mowbray MS, Hamilton V (1961) Imipramine (tofranil) in depressive states. A controlled trial with in-patients. J Ment Sci 107:948–953

Glassman AH, Perel JM, Shostak M, Kantor SJ, Fleiss JL (1977) Clinical implication of imipramine plasma levels for depressive illness. Arch Gen Psychiatry 34:197–204

Goethe JW, Szarek BL, Cook WL (1988) A comparison of adequately vs. inadequately treated depressed patients. J Nerv Ment Dis 176:465–470

Gram LF (1977) Plasma level monitoring of tricyclic antidepressant therapy. Clin Pharmacokinet 2:237–251
Gram LF (1990) Inadequate dosing and pharmacokinetic variability as confounding factors in assessment of efficacy of antidepressants. Clin Neuropharmacol 13 Suppl 1:35–43
Gram LF, Brøsen K (1990) Conditions under which genetic polymorphisms are clinically relevant. In: Alvan G et al. (eds) European consensus conference on pharmacogenetics. Commission of European Communities, Bruxelles, pp 87–96
Gram LF, Bech P, Reisby N, Jørgensen OS (1981) Methodology in plasma level/effect studies on tricyclic antidepressants. In: Usdin E (ed) Clinical pharmacology in psychiatry. Elsevier North-Holland, New York, pp 155–179
Gram LF, Pedersen OL, Kristensen CB, Bjerre M, Kragh-Sørensen P (1982) Drug level monitoring in psychopharmacology: usefulness and clinical problems, with special reference to tricyclic antidepressants. Ther Drug Monit 4:17–25
Hoenig J, Visram S (1964) Amitriptyline versus imipramine in depressive psychoses. Br J Psychiatry 110:840–845
Höhn R, Gross GM, Gross M, Lasagna L (1963) A double-blind comparison of placebo and imipramine in the treatment of depressed patients in a state hospital. J Psychiatr Res 1:76–91
Hollister LE, Overall JE, Johnson M, Pennington V, Katz G, Shelton J (1964) Controlled comparison of amitriptyline, imipramine and placebo in hospitalized depressed patients. J Nerv Ment Dis 139:370–375
Jørgensen OS, Løber M, Christiansen J, Gram LF (1980) Plasma concentrations and clinical effect in imipramine treatment of childhood enuresis. Clin Pharmacokinet 5:386–393
Kragh-Sørensen P, Åsberg M, Eggert-Hansen C (1973) Plasma-nortriptyline levels in endogenous depression. Lancet 2:113–115
Kragh-Sørensen P, Eggert-Hansen C, Baastrup PC, Hvidberg EF (1976) Self-inhibiting action of nortriptylin's antidepressive effect at high plasma levels. A randomized, double-blind study controlled by plasma concentrations in patients with endogenous depression. Psychopharmacologia (Berl) 45:305–312
Kvinesdal B, Molin J, Frøland A, Gram LF (1984) Imipramine treatment of painful diabetic neuropathy. JAMA 251:1727–1730
Lemere F (1959) Negative results in the treatment of depression with imipramine hydrochloride (tofranil). Am J Psychiatry 116:258–259
Malitz S, Kanzler M (1971) Aree antidepressants better than placebo? Am J Psychiatry 127:1605–1611
Medical Research Council (1965) Clinical trial of the treatment of depressive illness. Report to the Medical Research Council by its Clinical Psychiatry Committee. Br Med J 1:881–886
Montgomery S, Braithwaite R, Dawling S, McAuley R (1978) High plasma nortriptyline levels in the treatment of depression. I. Clin Pharmacol Ther 23:309–314
Oliveira IR, Do Prado-Lima PAS, Samuel-Lajeunesse B (1989) Monitoring of tricyclic antidepressant plasma levels and clinical response: a review of the literature. I. Psychiatry Psychobiol 4:43–60
Paykel ES, Price JS, Gillan RU, Palmai G, Chesser ES (1968) A comparative trial of imipramine and chlorpromazine in depressed patients. Br J Psychiatry 114:1281–1287
Pedersen OL, Gram LF, Kristensen CB, Møller M, Thayssen P, Bjerre M, Kragh-Sørensen P, Klitgaard NA, Sindrup E, Hole P, Brinkløv M (1982) Overdosage of antidepressants: clinical and pharmacokinetic aspects. Eur J Clin Pharmacol 239: 513–521
Preskorn SH (1989) Therapeutic drug monitoring of tricyclic antidepressants. A means of avoiding toxicity. In: Dahl SG, Gram LF (eds) Clinical pharmacology in psychiatry: from molecular studies to clinical reality. Springer, Berlin Heidelberg New York, pp 237–243

Prien RF, Kupfer DJ, Mansky PA, Small JG, Tuason VB, Voss CB, Johnson WE (1984) Drug therapy in the prevention of recurrences in unipolar and bipolar affective disorders. Arch Gen Psychiatry 41:1096–1104
Quitkin FM (1985) The importance of dosage in prescribing antidepressants. Br J Psychiatry 147:593–597
Rees L, Brown AC, Benaim S (1961) A controlled trial of imipramine (tofranil) in the treatment of severe depressive states. J Ment Sci 107:552–559
Reisby N, Gram LF, Bech P, Nagy A, Petersen GO, Ortmann J, Ibsen I, Dencker SJ, Jacobsen O, Krautwals O, Søndergaard I, Christiansen J (1977) Imipramine: clinical effects and pharmacokinetic variability. Psychopharmacology (Berl) 54:263–272
Robin AA, Langley GE (1964) A controlled trial of imipramine. Br J Psychiatry 110: 419–422
Roose SP, Glassman AH, Walsh BT, Woodring S (1986) Tricyclic nonresponders: phenomenology and treatment. Am J Psychiatry 143:345–348
Simpson GM, Lee JH, Cuculic Z, Kellner R (1976) Two dosages of imipramine in hospitalized endogenous and neurotic depressives. Arch Gen Psychiatry 33:1093–1102
Sindrup SH, Gram LF, Skjold T, Frøland A, Beck-Nielsen H (1990) Concentration response relationship in imipramine treatment of diabetic neuropathy symptoms. Clin Pharmacol Ther 47:509–515
Sindrup SH, Grodum E, Gram LF, Beck-Nielsen H (1991) Concentration-response relationship in paroxetine treatment of diabetic neuropathy symptoms. Ther Drug Monit 13:408–414
Sjöqvist F, Hammer W, Idestrôm C-M, Lind M, Tuck D, Åsberg M (1968) Plasma level of mono-methylated tricyclic antidepressants and side effects in man. In: Proceedings of the European Society for the study of drug toxicity, Paris 1967. Excerpta Medica, Amsterdam, pp 246–257
Smith A, Traganza E, Harrison G (1969) Studies on the effectiveness of antidepressant drugs. Psychopharmacol Bull [Special Issue] 1–53
Spiker DG, Weiss AN, Chang SS, Ruwitch JF, Biggs JT (1975) Tricyclic antidepressant overdose: clinical presentation and plasma levels. Clin Pharmacol Ther 18:539–546
Waldron J, Bates TJN (1965) The management of depression in hospital. A comparative trial of desipramine and imipramine. Br J Psychiatry 111:511–516
Wilson IC, Vernon JT, Guin T, Sandifer MG (1962) A controlled study of treatments of depression. J Neuropsychiatry 4:331–332
Ziegler VE, Clayton PJ, Taylor JR, Co BT, Biggs JT (1976) Nortriptyline plasma levels and therapeutic response. Clin Pharmacol Ther 20:458–463

Dose–Effect and Concentration–Effect Relationships with New Antidepressants

S.H. PRESKORN

1 Introduction

Depressive disorders are becoming for the psychiatrists what hypertension is for the internists. There exists now a range of medications with different mechanisms and hence different spectra of clinical activity (Table 1). Only a few years ago, tricyclic antidepressants (TCAs) were the main, if not the only, pharmacological option for treating depressed patients. The only choice was which TCA to prescribe and that was mainly based upon side effect profile rather than efficacy considerations. While much was made about whether a given TCA was more effective in "serotoninergic" vs "noradrenergic" depression, there was little empirical data to support such differential effectiveness. Now there are whole classes of drugs with different pharmacological mechanisms both to treat patients and to test for the existence of depressive disorder subtypes having fundamentally different biochemical etiologies (Preskorn 1990).

Against this backdrop, the benefits of establishing reliable dose: effect and concentration: response relationships become clear as do the difficulties inherent in this task. The most elementary principle in pharmacology is establishing a dose: response relationship. Concentration: response relationships are simply a refinement of this concept. From a research standpoint, such relationships establish whether a drug has a putative effect and can aid in determining what is the underlying mechanism. From a clinical standpoint, the establishment of such relationships is necessary to guide the effective and safe use of an agent.

This chapter will consider these issues in terms of the problems encountered during the development of new antidepressant agents and the value of incorporating concentration: response strategies in the development plan. Then, dose: response and concentration: response data from studies of selective serotonin reuptake inhibitors (SSRIs) and the novel agent bupropion will be reviewed as illustrations of the general points.

Psychiatric Research Institute, St. Francis Regional Medical Center and Dept. of Psychiatry, University of Kansas, Wichita, KS 67214, USA

Table 1. Antidepressant chemotherapy

Mixed serotonin and norepinephrine reuptake inhibitors	
Tricyclic antidepressants	
Venlafaxine[a]	
Milnacipran[a]	
Selective serotonin reuptake inhibitors	
Fluoxetine	Fluvoxamine[a]
Sertraline	Citalopram[a]
Paroxetine	Zimelidine
Serotonin-2 antagonists	
Trazodone	
Nefazodone[a]	
Serotonin 1a agonists	
Buspirone	Ipsapirone
Gepirone	Tandospirone
Dopamine reuptake inhibitors	
Bupropion	
Monoamine oxidase inhibitors	
Traditional agents	
Reversible and/or selective agents	
Norepinephrine reuptake inhibitors	
Tomoxetine[a]	
Second messenger system agents[a]	

[a] Investigational in the US.

2 Drug Effects

Most drugs have more than one action and hence more than one effect. Effect may refer to efficacy, nuisance effects (e.g., tolerability), or toxicity. A given drug may have efficacy in more than one condition. These conditions may be as disparate as enuresis, arrhythmias, and depressive disorders, as is the case with TCAs. In such instances, there are likely to be different dose:response and concentration:response relationships (Preskorn 1989). In fact, the demonstration that different dose:response and concentration:response relationships exist for different effects is prima facie evidence that different mechanisms are involved. This perspective must be remembered when considering such relationships.

The purpose of dose:response and concentration:response research is to establish the doses at which a given effect is minimally and maximally present. Since a drug will typically have more than one effect, the issue is the spread between the upper and lower thresholds for these effects. Knowledge of such relationships can allow the clinician to titrate the dose to maximize the desired effect and minimize the other. This issue is most pertinent when considering the therapeutic index for a drug; that is, the difference between the maximally effective dose and the toxic dose.

3 Antidepressant Efficacy: Problems

There are a number of issues which must be managed when testing a drug for antidepressant properties (Table 2). These problems are greater when developing a new class of agents. In fact, experience with a preexisting class may retard rather than facilitate the process.

The reason is that major aspects of antidepressant clinical trials are based upon prior experience. These aspects include inclusion and exclusion criteria, rating scales, timing of assessments, and study duration. The disadvantage for the new agent will be a function of the degree to which it differs from the older agents even though those differences may be desirable.

One goal of developing new agents is to find treatments for patients who do not respond to existing treatments. As many as 30%–50% of depressed patients do not remit when treated with TCAs even when the dose is adjusted to achieve optimal plasma concentrations (Preskorn and Fast 1991). Both SSRIs and bupropion seem to work in a significant percentage of TCA nonresponders and also have some overlap with the population of TCA responders (Aberg-Wisted 1982; Emrich et al. 1987; Lingjaerde et al. 1983; Nystrom et al. 1987; Stern et al. 1983). Conversely, there are TCA responders who do not respond to these agents. To the extent that the inclusion and exclusion criteria inadvertently select for such nonresponders, the new agents will be at a disadvantage.

The problem is that the predictors of responsiveness to a new agent or class will not be known until some experience has accumulated. Unfortunately, clinical trial programs are rarely designed to develop such data even though it would be useful when planning later studies. The other problem is the timetable for drug development and the turnaround time between acquiring clinical data and analyzing it. Both factors work to hamper the efficient use of such information. With SSRIs, there are some

Table 2. Factors affecting antidepressant response studies (from Preskorn and Mac 1984)

Diagnostic heterogeneity
Response assessment
Nonparametric measures
Definition of response
Interrater reliability
Duration of study
Delayed onset of action
Spontaneous remission rate
Study design
Placebo response rate
Nonresponder rate
Sample size
Statistical analysis
Range of plasma drug levels samples

Table 3. Predictor of responsivity to selective serotonin reuptake inhibitors

Clinical	
Late onset[a,b]	
Chronic course[a,b,c]	
TCA nonresponse[a,d]	
Biochemical	
Low CSF 5-HIAA and HVA levels[a,e]	
Low platelet 5-HT uptake[a,f]	

5-HIAA, 5-hydroxyindoleacetic acid; HVA, homovanillic acid; 5-HT, serotonin; TCA, tricyclic antidepressants.
[a] Correlated with low CSF 5-HIAA levels (Cronholm et al. 1977).
[b] Hiramastu et al. (1983).
[c] Nystrom and Hallstrom (1985).
[d] Siwers et al. (1977), Reimherr et al. (1984).
[e] Aberg-Wistedt (1982).
[f] Nystrom et al. (1986).

tentative predictors of responsiveness to these agents which can be incorporated into subsequent clinical trials to test their validity and to increase the ability to demonstrate the efficacy of this class (Table 3).

Another example of the unintentional bias against new agents is the rating scales which exist for antidepressant clinical trials. Scales such as the Hamilton Depression Rating Scale were developed for trials with tertiary amine TCAs. Hence, they give compounds which are sedative and cause weight gain an advantage even though these effects are frequently undesirable. In fact, such scales were not designed to assess response in atypical depressive disorders in which hypersomnia and/or weight gain occur as opposed to insomnia and weight loss. Depending on the severity of the inclusion criteria, the use of such scales may in essence exclude such patients from the trial. Yet, these scales continue to be used because they have been established and because a commitment of necessary resources to develop new scales has not been forthcoming.

Obviously another issue is knowing the optimal dose or concentration of the new agent. Dose ranging studies have built-in biases. They tend to exceed the minimally effective dose and to be mainly limited by side effects. In addition, the dose typically is escalated in nonresponders so that this design has a tendency to produce a curvilinear relationship between dose (or concentration) and response.

4 Toxicity Identification

The number of patients who have been exposed to a novel antidepressant during its clinical trial program generally is in the range of a few thousand. Most of these patients have been exposed to the agent for less than 3 months since the standard length of a clinical trial is 6 weeks and most do not go into an extension protocol. In addition, these patients are carefully screened to be in good physical health and to be on few, if any, concomitant medications, particularly no other psychoactive medications. These facts all reduce the likelihood of detecting rare adverse effects which may become apparent when the drug is marketed.

This problem is compounded when developing a new class of agents. The reasons are the same as given above for efficacy. The researchers and the trial design are sensitive to the toxicity caused by the older class but not necessarily the toxicity of the new one. The fact that most clinical trials are multi-center studies compounds this problem since no single investigator may see enough patients to develop a sense of the problem. In this case, there is a natural tendency to ascribe the adverse event to other factors. Seizures are a good example since a history of a possibly predisposing factor (e.g., a blow to the head) can be found in many patients if aggressively pursued.

These problems are further compounded when dealing with novel psychoactive medication which might cause behavioral toxicity, particularly if that toxicity were an interaction between the drug's effect and an underlying biochemical predisposition. For example, a novel compound might increase impulsivity in a subpopulation of patients. In a multicenter clinical trial, that event might go undetected, even if it occurs at a frequency greater than 1%, unless the loss of impulse control were profound. Otherwise, it might simply be attributed to the underlying illness.

5 Concentration: Response

Concentration: response relationships are simply a refinement of the dose: response concept. Such a refinement may be of only academic and research significance or may be quite valuable clinically depending upon the pharmacology of the specific drug (Table 4). In the case of a drug class such as TCAs, their pharmacokinetic and pharmacodynamic characteristics are such that dose adjustment must be based on concentration: response data rather than upon clinical assessment of the drug's effect (Preskorn and Fast 1991). As discussed later in this chapter, SRIs as a class do not appear to have a profile that makes concentration driven dose adjustment necessary while bupropion does.

Concentration: response data have different implications and uses for drug development (Table 5) compared to clinical practice (Table 6). The latter uses have been addressed elsewhere (Preskorn 1989). The former warrant some elaboration since monitoring drug concentration is not routinely employed during drug development.

Concentration monitoring during the development program can enhance the signal to noise ratio in several ways. First, it can permit detection of

Table 4. Pharmacokinetic and pharmacodynamic factors which determine the usefulness of concentration : response data

Feature	Tricyclic antidepressants	Selective serotonin reuptake inhibitors	Bupropion
Multitude of actions	+	−	?
Small therapeutic index	+	−	+
Large interindividual variability in metabolism	+	+	+
Difficult early detection of toxicity	+	−	+
Long delay in onset of action	+	+	+
Well-defined concentration : response relationships			
Efficacy	+	−	±
Tolerability	−	±	−
Toxicity	+	−	?

Table 5. Drug development reasons to monitor drug plasma levels

Compliance
Detect aberrant metabolizers
- Effect on efficacy
- Effect on toxicity

Detect rare toxicity
Select most optimum dose for future trials
Detect pharmacokinetic problems
- Absorption
- Distribution
- Metabolism
- Elimination

Establish better guidelines for clinical dose titration

Table 6. Clinical reasons to monitor drug plasma levels (Preskorn and Fast 1992)

Check compliance
Increase efficacy
Reduce toxicity
Improve cost effectiveness
Avoid medical-legal problems

patients who fail due to noncompliance. Such patients reduce the power of any study and could jeopardize a development program. Second, such data can complement dose : response data for determining optimum dosing strategies for future studies, particularly if there is substantial interindividual pharmacokinetic variability such that some subjects develop ineffective or toxic concentration on a dose that produces therapeutic concentrations in most patients. Failure to detect and adjust for rapid metabolism may result in an overestimation of the percentage of patients who are truly nonresponsive to the new agent. In contrast, failure to detect a slow metabolizer can lead to failure to identify rare drug toxicity.

An example of the latter is seizures, which might be a rare but concentration dependent event. Since seizures can occur spontaneously and since many individuals can be construed as having predisposing factors (e.g., blow to the head), a drug having a seizure rate of 0.2%–0.3% might well be missed or explained away given the patient database (i.e., numbers and treatment duration) which typically accrues during a clinical trial program. If those seizures were linked to another rare phenomenon, such as unusually slow metabolism or atypical metabolism which results in an unusually high accumulation of an otherwise rare metabolite, then the chances of correctly determining the relationship would be enhanced and could potentially save postmarketing problems.

Examples of rare toxicity being linked to slow or atypical metabolism include the central nervous system (i.e., delirium and seizures) and cardiac (i.e., arrhythmias and cardiac arrests) toxicity of TCAs (Preskorn and Fast 1991). Both result from the gradual accumulation of toxic concentrations in slow metabolizers. The same may be true for bupropion-induced seizures, which will be discussed later (Davidson 1989).

Another drug monitoring issue during drug development is the role metabolites may play in determining the overall effect of the drug. Metabolites may be substantially more or less potent than the parent compound in terms of either a beneficial or adverse effect. This issue is addressed in multiple ways during the drug development process, including pharmacokinetic studies to establish the typical metabolism and elimination of the parent drug and the extent of accumulation of metabolites. The pharmacological effects of metabolites are then tested via in vitro and in vivo preclinical pharmacology studies in the same way as the parent compound.

Often, investigation stops at this point rather than extending into the clinical phase of the drug's development. It could continue by monitoring plasma concentrations of the parent compound and its metabolites during the clinical trials. This data could be examined for unusual metabolizers who either quickly or slowly metabolize the parent drug or who develop unusually high or low levels of one or more metabolites. The concentrations of the parent drug and metabolites can also be examined statistically in terms of their relative contribution to determining a specific beneficial, nuisance, or toxic effect.

In the area of antidepressants, there are multiple examples in which a metabolite had equal or greater effectiveness than did the parent compound. Such examples include tertiary amine TCAs (Preskorn and Fast 1991), fluoxetine (Benfield et al. 1986), and zimelidine (Montgomery et al. 1982). In the case of bupropion, there is reason to suspect that unusual accumulation of one or more of its metabolites is involved in the occurrence of bupropion-induced seizures, as discussed later.

Incorporating concentration monitoring into the drug development process can also permit the detection of pharmacokinetic issues involving drug absorption, metabolism, and elimination which can be valuable when the drug is marketed. Examples include drug: drug interactions such as the effect of concomitantly ingested drugs (e.g., cimetidine). The same would be true for the effects of personal habits such as diet, smoking, or alcohol ingestion. Such interactions may affect the extent of accumulation of either the parent compound or its metabolite(s).

Thus, concentration monitoring can help guide the drug development process. It can also provide important information when the drug is marketed including better guidelines for dose titration and warnings about drug: drug interactions. Such data can also determine whether therapeutic drug monitoring offers any advantage over dose determination based upon clinical response.

6 Application of These Principles

Antidepressant chemotherapy is perhaps the most active area in clinical psychopharmacology (Table 1). The activity is such that a review of all of these classes is beyond the scope of this chapter. Instead, the dose–effect and concentration–effect relationships of SRIs as a class and the novel agent bupropion will next be discussed particularly with regard to how they illustrate the general principles outlined above.

7 Selective Serotonin Reuptake Inhibitors

Members of this class include: fluoxetine, sertraline, fluvoxamine, paroxetine, citalopram, and zimelidine. Fluoxetine, sertraline and paroxetine are marketed now in the United States. Fluvoxamine and citalopram are available in Europe but not in the United States. Fluvoxamine is also in active trial programs in the United States and could be marketed within the next couple of years depending upon the progress of those programs. Zimelidine has been withdrawn from the market due to a toxicity issue which does not appear to generalize to all members of this class.

This class is defined by their selectivity for blocking the serotonin uptake pumps on neurons and platelets. All the members of this class were chosen for development based upon the concept that this mechanism is important in mediating an antidepressant effect in at least a percentage of depressed patients. The candidate agents were also chosen based upon their relative absence of effects on other known neuronal mechanisms such as receptor binding or enzymatic activity.

While all members share a common presumed mechanism of action, this class, in other ways, may be more heterogenous than TCAs. The structure of SSRIs differs from one compound to another to a greater extent than that of TCAs. The metabolism of the compounds is also more variable. For example, fluoxetine has a metabolite, desmethylfluoxetine, which has almost the same pharmacological activity as the parent compound (Fuller et al. 1978) whereas sertraline and paroxetine do not appear to have any metabolites with substantial clinical activity. Fluoxetine and its metabolite also have long half-lives, 2–4 days and 7–15 days, respectively, while sertraline and paroxetine have half-lives of approximately 1 day. Fluvoxamine has a half-life of less than 1 day.

There has been some controversy as to how to position SRIs relative to TCAs. Some have taken the position that they are "weaker" antidepressants relative to TCAs (Bech 1989). This assertion implies a difference in potency which does not seem applicable. Instead, an analogy with antibiotics might be more appropriate. From this vantage, both SRIs and TCAs would be classified as broad-spectrum antidepressants. In 16 double-blind studies containing 2214 patients, SRIs have been found to be superior to the placebo in 13 while placebo was never found to be superior to the SRI (Table 7). In 28 double-blind studies containing 2784 patients, SSRIs were equal in efficacy to TCAs in 24, superior in 3, and inferior in 1 (Table 8).

Yet, the spectra of activity of SRIs and TCAs are not mutually inclusive (Fig. 1). In four crossover studies containing a total of 29 patients, 60%–65% of TCA nonresponders were found to respond to subsequent treatment with a SRI (Aberg-Wistedt 1982; Emrich et al. 1987; Lingjaerde et al. 1983; Nystrom et al. 1987). The converse was also true. While preliminary, these results are intriguing and bear followup.

Thus, clinical trials of these agents could have varying results depending upon whether the population selected for a given study contained more TCA responsive only or SRI responsive only patients. Subjects responsive to both classes would help to distinguish both from placebo but not from each other. In contrast, the remaining two groups (i.e., patients not respon-

Table 7. Summary of placebo-controlled studies (from Aberg-Wistedt 1989)

	Patients (*n*)	Studies (*n*)	Studies showing SSRI > placebo (*n*)	Studies showing SSRI = placebo (*n*)	Studies showing placebo > SSRI (*n*)
Fluoxetine	682	5	5	0	0
Sertraline	623	2	2	0	0
Fluvoxamine	488	4	2	2	0
Citalopram	226	2	1	1	0
Zimeline	195	3	3	0	0
Total	2214	16	13	3	0

Table 8. TCA[a]-controlled studies

	Patients (*n*)	Studies (*n*)	Studies showing SSRI > placebo (*n*)	Studies showing SSRI = placebo (*n*)	Studies showing placebo > SSRI (*n*)
Fluoxetine	792	7	6	1	0
Sertraline	433	2[b]	2	0	0
Fluvoxamine	835	9	7	1	1
Paroxetine	41	1	1	0	0
Femoxetine	162	3	3	0	0
Citalopram	193	2	1	1	0
Zimeline	304	4	4	0	0
Total	2784	28	24	3	1

[a] The comparison TCA in these studies were amitryptyline, AT, in 10 studies; imipramine, IMI, in 13; chlorimipramine, CIMI, in 4.
[b] One study was done in depressive patients aged $\geq$65 years.

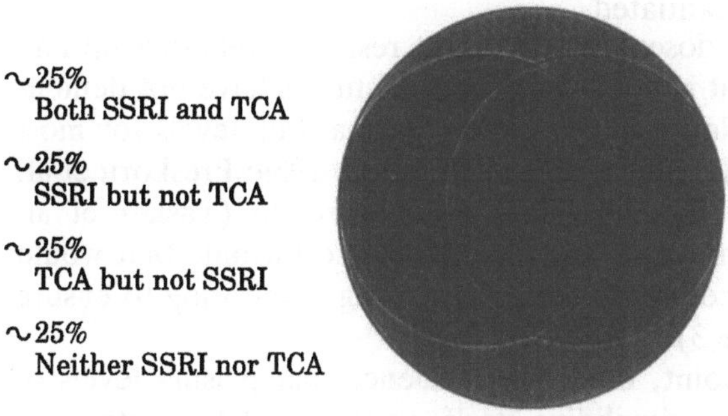

Fig. 1. Percentage of the total population of depressive disorder patients who may be: (a) responsive to both tricyclic antidepressants (TCAs) and serotonin reuptake inhibitors (SSRIs), (b) TCAs but not SSRIs, (c) SSRIs but not TCAs, and (d) neither. The percentages are estimates based upon data from Aberg-Wistedt (1982, 1989), Emrich et al. (1987), Lingjaerde et al. (1983) and Nystrom et al. (1987)

sive to either class and placebo responders) would detract from the ability to separate either class from placebo.

Although there has been extensive research with these compounds, there are only tentative predictors of preferential responsiveness to SRIs (Table 3). It is also not known whether a patient who fails to respond to one SRI will also be unresponsive to others. This lack of information is reflective of the problems discussed above.

As a class, there has generally been difficulty demonstrating dose: antidepressant efficacy relationship with SSRIs. In the case of fluoxetine, there is the suggestion of an inverse relationship between dose and antidepressant response, with daily doses of 40 mg or less being superior to higher doses (Altamura et al. 1988; Schweizer et al. 1990; Wernicke et al. 1988). That finding may be due to the fact that the discontinuation rate due to side effects is dose related with fluoxetine. With sertraline, the dose:

antidepressant response curve is relatively flat over a range of daily doses from 50 to 200 mg (Amin et al. 1989; data on file). However, one study reported a curvilinear relationship with the maximum antidepressant observed at 100 mg per day compared with lower response rates on 50 mg and 200 mg per day (Reimherr et al. 1988). This study has to be interpreted cautiously due to the small numbers in each treatment group (6–11 patients) and the fact that an ascending dose design was used. Citalopram, another SRI, has also failed to show a dose:response relationship (Bjerkenstedt et al. 1985).

The therapeutic index of this class is substantially larger than that of TCAs. Hence, there does not appear to be a clinically relevant upper threshold in terms of dose (or plasma drug concentration) from a safety standpoint. There is an increase in nuisance side effects with dose for this class (Altamura et al. 1988; Schweizer et al. 1990). Nausea, diarrhea, and restlessness all increase in frequency as a function of the daily fluoxetine dose in depressed patients. There has been the suggestion that other patient populations (e.g., obsessive-compulsive disorder and obese patients) might be more resistant to these adverse effects (personal communication) but this assertion remains to be substantiated.

Given the absence of a dose:antidepressant response relationship and the wide therapeutic index, it is not surprising that studies have not demonstrated a clinically useful relationship between plasma drug levels for most members in this class, including fluoxetine (Kelly et al. 1989; Preskorn et al. 1990), sertraline (sertraline data on file), and paroxetine (Tasker et al. 1990). As a class, SRIs do not have the pharmacological profile that would predict the usefulness or necessity of therapeutic drug monitoring to ensure safe and effective use (Table 3).

From a research standpoint, there was evidence that plasma levels of desmethlyzimelidine, but not zimelidine itself, were correlated with antidepressant efficacy (Montgomery et al. 1982; Walinder et al. 1981; Wood et al. 1982). This finding could be interpreted as evidence that the former was the active agent rather than the parent compound. This finding supports the potential value of incorporating concentration monitoring as part of the drug development program.

8 Dopamine Reuptake Inhibitors

A unique antidepressant, bupropion, is the only member in this class. While its mechanism of action is debatable, dopamine reuptake inhibition is its strongest effect on systems thought to be important in treatment of depressive disorders (Preskorn and Othmer 1984).

Like SSRIs, bupropion has a spectrum of antidepressant activity which is not mutually inclusive with TCAs. In double-blind studies, bupropion was found to be more effective in patients who had a history of failing to respond to TCAs than in patients who had a history of TCA responsiveness

(Stern et al. 1983). Like SSRIs, the predictors of which patients will be uniquely responsive to bupropion is not well established. It is also unknown how the spectrum of activity of bupropion compares to SSRIs.

Bupropion is a good example of how the incorporation of concentration monitoring into the drug development program could facilitate that process as well as subsequent clinical use of the compound. First, it meets most of the criteria which predict the usefulness of such monitoring (Table 3). The dose : response curve is truncated, as defined by a lower threshold for antidepressant efficacy and an upper threshold for the occurrence of seizures. This fact coupled with the complicated metabolism of the compound makes it likely that concentration monitoring would be helpful. It also has three metabolites which accumulate such that their concentration under steady-state conditions exceed that of the parent compound by as much as an order of magnitude (Cooper et al. 1984; Laizure et al. 1985; Preskorn and Katz 1989). Moreover, these metabolites are pharmacologically active (Perumal et al. 1986).

There has been a reasonable amount of research done with bupropion examining the relationship between plasma drug levels and antidepressant response. Unfortunately for both this research and the development of the compound, much of the early work was performed with an assay which only measured the parent compound (Butz et al. 1983; Lai and Schroeder 1983). Still, four studies (total $n = 106$ patients) have shown that patients with lower bupropion plasma levels have a better antidepressant response than those with high levels (Fogel et al. 1984; Goodnick and Sandoval 1991; Preskorn 1983; Preskorn et al. 1992). However, all of these studies employed an ascending dose design which would tend to produce this finding (Preskorn 1992a). In the only published study examining antidepressant response in relationship to concentrations of bupropion and three major metabolites, poorer response was associated with higher levels of the three metabolites (Golden et al. 1985). While the bupropion plasma level data did not reach statistical significance in this small study ($n = 10$ with repeat measurements in two patients on different doses), the results were compatible with those from the earlier studies. Taken as a whole, this information suggests that bupropion is effective at low to intermediate concentrations and that higher levels of bupropion and/or its metabolites are associated with a poorer antidepressant response.

This conclusion is complemented by the suspicion that elevated levels of bupropion and/or its metabolites are associated with an elevated seizure risk (Davidson 1989). This suspicion is based upon the following observations. First, the incidence of seizures on bupropion is a function of daily dose. Second, seizures typically occur within a day or a few days of a dose increase and within a few hours of dose administration. Third, individuals with lean body mass (i.e., anoretic-bulimics) have an apparent increased risk.

The only way to confirm this hypothesis is to monitor plasma levels of bupropion and its metabolites and determine whether seizures occur in patients who develop unusually high levels of one or more of the compounds. Unfortunately, this data is lacking despite extensive clinical trials and the fact that it has been marketed in the United States for several years. Had this information been collected during the clinical trial program, it could have increased the likelihood of earlier identification of the seizure risk with bupropion. This information coupled with the antidepressant response data could have indicated that the dose for subsequent clinical trials should have been reduced thus preserving and perhaps augmenting antidepressant efficacy while reducing the risk of seizures. This information would have also supported the use of therapeutic drug monitoring to rationally adjust the dose to increase the safe and effective clinical use of the compound. The latter would have substantially increased the clinical acceptance of the compound. In terms of the drug development process, this information might have also indicated that a change in the delivery system to a more sustained release preparation would have been desirable.

Unfortunately, the absence of such information is problematic since bupropion is not a simple compound to monitor. The fact that the metabolites have substantial different half-lives from the parent compound raises questions as to when to draw a sample and whether more than one time point should be monitored (Preskorn et al. 1990). Also, the sample must be properly treated due to the parent compound's instability at physiological pH (Laizure and DeVane 1985). Although some reference laboratories offer therapeutic drug monitoring of bupropion, clinicians should approach this matter cautiously until more information is available.

9 Conclusions

Antidepressant chemotherapy is becoming more analogous to the treatment of hypertension, with a number of new classes of medications with unique spectra of activity and different pharmacological profiles in terms of nuisance and toxic effects. Recognition of the challenges these developments represent will need to be addressed in clinical trials research. It will be necessary to address the issues of identifying those patients who are most responsive to the new agents and improved strategies to determine optimum dosing guidelines. Incorporation of concentration monitoring into the drug development process can help. The result of this effort will be improved care of patients who do not respond to or do not tolerate existing medications.

References

Aberg-Wistedt A (1982) Comparison between zimelidine and desipramine in endogenous depression: a cross-over study. Acta Psychiatr Scand 66:129–138

Aberg-Wistedt A (1989) The antidepressant effects of 5-HT uptake inhibitors. Br J Psychiatry 155 Suppl 8:32–40
Altamura AC, Montgomery SA, Wernicke JF (1988) The evidence for 20 mg a day of fluoxetine as the optimal in the treatment of depression. Br J Psychiatry 153 Suppl 3:109–112
Amin M, Lehmann H, Mirmiran J (1989) A double-blind, placebo controlled dosefinding study with sertraline. Psychopharmacol Bull 25:164–167
Bech P (1989) Clinical effects of selective serotonin reuptake inhibitors. In: Dahl SG, Graham LF (eds) Clinical Pharmacology in psychiatry. Springer, Berlin Heidelberg New York, pp 81–93
Benfield P, Heel RC, Lewis SP (1986) Fluoxetine: a review of its pharmacodynamic and pharmacokinetic properties and therapeutic efficacy in depressive illness. Drugs 32:481–508
Bjerkenstedt L, Flyckt L, Overo KF et al. (1985) Relationship between clinical effects, serum drug concentration, and serotonin uptake inhibition in depressed patients treated with citalopram: a double-blind comparison of three dose levels. Eur J Clin Pharmacol 28:553–557
Butz RF, Smith PG, Schroeder DH, Findlay JWA (1983) Radio-immunoassay for bupropion in human plasma: comparison of tritiated and iodinated radioligands. Clin Chem 29:462–465
Cooper TB, Suckow RF, Glassman A (1984) Determination of bupropion and its major basic metabolites in plasma by liquid chromatography with dual wave-length u.v. detection. J Pharm Sci 73:1104–1107
Cronholm B, Asberg M, Montgomery S et al. (1977) Suicidal behavior syndrome with low CSF 5-HIAA. Br Med J 60:776
Davidson J (1989) Seizures and bupropion: a review. J Clin Psychiatry 50:256–261
Emrich HM, Berger M, Riemann D et al. (1987) Serotonin reuptake inhibition versus norepinephrine reuptake inhibition: a double-blind differential therapeutic study with fluvoxamine and oxaprotiline in endogenous and neurotic depressives. Pharmacopsychiatrica 20:60–63
Fogel P, Mamer OA, Chouinard G, Farrell PG (1984) Determination of plasma bupropion and its relationship to therapeutic effect. Biomed Mass Spectrom 11:629–632
Fuller RW, Snoddy HD, Perry KW et al. (1978) Importance of duration of action in the antagonism of p-chloroamphetamine depletion of brain serotonin: comparison of fluoxetine and chlorimipramine. Biochem Pharmacol 27:193–198
Golden RN, DeVane CL, Laizure SC, Rudorfer MD, Sherer MA, Potter WZ (1985) Bupropion in depression: the role of metabolites in clinical outcome. Arch Gen Psychiatry 45:145–149
Goodnick PJ, Sandoval R (1991) Wellbutrin blood levels and clinical response. 144th Annual Meeting of the American Psychiatric Association, New Orleans
Hiramatsu KI, Takahashi R, Mori A et al. (1983) A multicenter, double-blind comparative trial of zimelidine and imipramine in primary major depressive disorders. Act Psychiatr Scand 68 Suppl 308:31–54
Kelly MW, Perry PJ, Holstead SG, Garvey JM (1989) Serum fluoxetine and norfluoxetine concentrations and antidepressant response. Ther Drug Monit 11:165–170
Lai AA, Schroeder DH (1983) Clinical pharmacokinetics of bupropion: a review. J Clin Psychiatry 44:82–84
Laizure SC, DeVane CL (1985) Stability of bupropion and its major metabolites in human plasma. Ther Drug Monit 7:447–450
Laizure SC, DeVane CL, Stewart JT, Dommisse CS, Lai AA (1985) Pharmacokinetics of bupropion and its major basic metabolites in normal subjects after a single dose. Clin Pharmacol Ther 38:586–589
Lingjaerde O, Bratfos O, Bratlid T et al. (1983) A double-blind comparison of zimelidine and desipramine in endogenous depression. Acta Psychiatr Scand 68:22–30

Montgomery SA, Montgomery DB, McAule R et al. (1982) Profile of antidepressant action of zimelidine and norzimelidine compared with amitriptyline. In: Costa E, Racagni G (eds) Atypical antidepressants: clinical practices. Raven, New York

Nystrom C, Hallstrom T (1985) Double-blind comparison between serotonin and norepinephrine reuptake blocker in the treatment of depressed patients: clinical aspects. Acta Psychiatr Scand 72:6–15

Nystrom C, Ross SB, Hallstrom T et al. (1986) Comparison between serotonin and norepinephrine reuptake blocker in the treatment of depressed outpatients: biochemical aspects. Acta Psychiatr Scand 73:133–138

Nystrom C, Ross SB, Hallstrom T et al. (1987) Comparison between serotonin and norepinephrine reuptake blocker in the treatment of depressed outpatients: a cross-over study. Acta Psychiatr Scand 75:377–382

Perumal AS, Smith TM, Suckow RF, Cooper TB (1986) Effect of plasma from patients containing bupropion and its metabolites on the uptake of norepinephrine. Neuropharmacology 25:199–202

Preskorn SH (1983) Antidepressant response and plasma concentrations of bupropion. J Clin Psychiatry 44:137–139

Preskorn S (1989) Tricyclic antidepressants: whys and hows of therapeutic drug monitoring. J Clin Psychiatry 50 Suppl:34–42

Preskorn SH (1990) The future of psychopharmacology: needs and potentials. Psychiatr Annu 20(11):625–633

Preskorn SH (1992a) Should bupropoin doseage be adjusted based upon therapeutic drug monitoring? Psychopharmacol Bull 27:637–643

Preskorn SH, Fast G (1992b) Therapeutic drug monitoring of tricyclic antidepressants: efficacy, safety, and cost effectiveness. J Clin Psychiatry 52, 6 [Suppl]:23–33

Preskorn SH, Katz SE (1989) Bupropion plasma levels: intraindividual and interindividual variability. Ann Clin Psychiatry 1:59–61

Preskorn SH, Mac D (1984) The implication of concentration-response studies of tricyclic antidepressants for psychiatric research and practice. Psychiatr Dev 3:201–222

Preskorn S, Othmer S (1984a) Bupropion: a monocyclic antidepressant. J Clin Psychiatry Monogr Ser 2(5):23–26

Preskorn S, Othmer S (1984) Evaluation of bupropion hydrochloride: the first of a new class of atypical antidepressants Pharmacotherapy 4:20–34

Preskorn SH, Fleck RJ, Schroeder DH (1990) Therapeutic drug monitoring of bupropion. Am J Psychiatry 147(12):1690

Preskorn SH, Silkey B, Beber J, Dorey C (1991) Antidepressant response and plasma concentration of fluoxetine. Ann Clin Psychiatry 3:147–153

Preskorn SH, Hughes CW, Othmer SC, Othmer E, Kumar R (1992) Bupropion: concentration-response relationship. Ann Clin Psychiatry (in press)

Reimherr FW, Wood DR, Byerley B et al. (1984) Characteristics of responders to fluoxetine. Psychopharmacol Bull 20:70–72

Reimherr FW, Byerley WF, Ward MF, Lebegue BJ, Wender PH (1988) Sertraline, a selective inhibitor of serotonin uptake, for the treatment of outpatients with major depressive disorder. Psychopharmacol Bull 24:200–205

Schweizer E, Rickels K, Amsterdam JD, Fox I, Puzzuoli G, Weise C (1990) What constitutes an adequate antidepressant trial for fluoxetine. J Clin Psychiatry 51:8–11

Siwers B, Ringberg VA, Tuck JR (1977) Initial clinical trial based on biochemical methodology of zimelidine (a serotonin uptake inhibitor) in depressed patients. Clin Pharmacol Ther 21:194–200

Stern WC, Harto-Truax N, Bauer N (1983) Efficacy of bupropion in tricyclic-resistant or intolerant patients J Clin Psychiatry 44(52):148–152

Tasker TCG, Kaye CM, Zussman DB, Link CGG (1990) Paroxetine plasma levels: lack of correlation with efficacy or adverse events. Acta Psychiatr Scand 80 Suppl 350:152–155

Walinder J, Skott A, Carlsson A, Persson R (1981) 5-HT reuptake inhibitors plus tryptophan in endogenous depression. Acta Psychiatr Scand 69 Suppl 290:179–190

Wernicke J, Dunlop SR, Dorniseif BE et al. (1988) Low-dose fluoxetine therapy for depression. Psychopharmacol Bull 24:183–188

Wood KM, Swade CC, Coppen AJ (1982) Zimelidine: a pharmacokinetic and pharmacodynamic study in depressive illness. Br J Clin Pract 19 Suppl:42–47

Therapeutic Potentials of Recently Introduced Antidepressants

P. Vestergaard, L.F. Gram, P. Kragh-Sørensen,
P. Bech, N. Reisby, T.G. Bolwig,
and the Danish University Antidepressant Group

1 Introduction

Antidepressant drugs have not been classified very systematically and no commonly accepted nomenclature has been developed. Classification has been based upon criteria as different as the time of development of the drugs, their chemical structure, their biochemical properties, and their behavioral effects.

Table 1 shows as an example different groups of antidepressant drugs currently available in the United States and Denmark classified according to the time of their development. The division between traditional and recent drugs can be broadly defined as the 1970s. Subgrouping is based upon the chemical structure of the drugs (cyclic), biochemical properties (enzyme and transmitter reuptake inhibition), or whether they are typical compared with the other subgroups. Stimulant drugs such as bupropion, an antidepressant currently not available in the two countries, could also be added to the group of atypical antidepressants. Alprazolam, a benzodiazepine analogue, may also belong to this group when used as an antidepressant. The most striking difference between the two countries is that in Denmark as in most other European countries larger numbers of the recently developed antidepressants have been registered.

Only for traditional tricyclic antidepressants has the clinical efficacy been firmly established for severely (endogenously) depressed patients (Baldessarini 1989; Davis 1985; Morris and Beck 1974). As regards monoamine oxidase (MAO) inhibitors, although clinically effective, it is still uncertain which types of depressed patients benefit the most from treatment with these drugs (Baldessarini 1989; Davis 1985; Morris and Beck 1975). For other cyclic and recently introduced antidepressant drugs it is fair to state that although the antidepressant effect of these drugs has been more or less convincingly established through placebo-controlled studies, two issues remain to be settled: whether the effect of these drugs is specifically antidepressant or rather an unspecific sedative or anxiolytic effect, and whether the antidepressant effect of the recently introduced drugs reaches the same

Psychiatric Hospital in Aarhus, 8240 Risskov, Denmark

Table 1. Antidepressant drugs currently available in the United States and Denmark

	US	Denmark
Traditional		
Tricyclic		
Amitriptyline	X	X
Clomipramine		X
Desipramine	X	X
Dosulepin		X
Doxepin	X	X
Imipramine	X	X
Lofepramine		X
Nortriptyline	X	X
Protriptyline	X	X
Trimipramine	X	X
Opipramol		X
MAO inhibitors		
Isocarboxazid	X	X
Phenelzine	X	
Tranylcypramine	X	
Other cyclic		
Amoxapine	X	X
Maprotiline	X	X
Mianserin		X
Recent		
Serotonin reuptake inhibitors		
Citalopram		X
Fluvoxamine		X
Fluoxetine	X	X
Reversible MAO inhibitors		
Moclobemide		X
Atypical		
Trazodone	X	

level of efficacy as has been obtained with the traditional tricyclic antidepressants, which, roughly estimated, is a substantial improvement in 60%–80% of the patients treated. The answer to the last question has been the objective of the Danish University Antidepressant Group (DUAG) through a series of multisite randomized clinical trials.

2 Danish University Antidepressant Group Trials

Table 2 shows the list of trials carried out by DUAG in which the efficacy of recent antidepressant drugs has been compared with that of clomipramine, a traditional tricyclic antidepressant. With the exception of some minor modifications in principle all trials have been performed according to the same protocol. The most important features of the trials are listed in Table

Table 2. Antidepressant drug trials carried out by the Danish University Antidepressant Group (DUAG)

Time period	Phase	Drugs
1980–1983	DUAG-1	Clomipramine vs citalopram
1985–1987	DUAG-2	Clomipramine vs paroxetine
1987–1990	DUAG-3	Clomipramine vs moclobemide
1990 on	DUAG-4	Clomipramine dose–response

Table 3. Characteristics of the DUAG multicenter randomized antidepressant drug trials

Large, homogeneous patient groups
Fixed dose regimens
6 Weeks' duration
High interrater reliability
Predefined outcome measures
Rules for drop-out and withdrawal
Control of compliance with drug monitoring

3. They include the recruitment of a homogeneous group of hospitalized, moderately to severely depressed patients sufficiently large for the detection of a clinically relevant difference in efficacy with a sufficient degree of certainty, the use of a fixed dose regimen throughout the entire treatment period, the constant surveillance of interrater reliability within and between participating centers, the establishment of predefined principles for data analysis which include the definition of response categories and rules for drop-out and early termination and, finally, the control of patient compliance through drug monitoring. All patients who completed more than 2 weeks of active treatment were included in the final analysis. Nonparametric methods were applied in the statistical analyses. The diagnostic assessments of patients allowed classification according to DSM-III and separation into groups of endogeneous and non-endogeneous depression following scoring on the Newcastle inventory. For quantitative assessments the Hamilton Depression Scale (HDS) was used.

The DUAG centers are coordinated by a steering committee, a permanent secretariat, and a company-independent laboratory service and data analysis facility. Monthly rating sessions are performed throughout the entire trial periods between participating centers and weekly or biweekly within individual centers. For each new trial satellite centers are invited to join the four permanent university based centers if requirements for training of participating clinicians and a sufficient number of patients to be included are met.

3 Results of DUAG Trials

So far three recently introduced antidepressant drugs have been evaluated in DUAG trials. Two of these drugs, citalopram and paroxetine, belong to the class of selective serotonin reuptake inhibitors (SSRI), one of them, moclobemide, to the selective and reversible MAO inhibitors. Results from the SSRI studies have been published in detail (DUAG 1986, 1990). The moclobemide results have not yet been fully analyzed. A survey of the results is presented in Table 4. This table shows for all three studies an average reduction in the HDS score of approximately 10 points for the test drugs as compared with approximately 15 points for the reference drug, clomipramine, after 4–6 weeks of treatment. In all three studies the differences in score reduction between the test drugs and clomipramine were statistically significant for the last weeks of treatment. Statistically significant differences were found when analyses were performed for response categories as shown in Table 5. Complete recovery, defined as HDS score below 7 points, was obtained for clomipramine in 34%–60% of patients in the three trials. For the three test drugs the comparative figures were 21%–28% (Table 5). Complete plus partial recovery (HDS $\leq$ 15 points) was obtained in 73%–87% of patients treated with clomipramine compared

Table 4. Outcome of DUAG trials: reduction on Hamilton Depression Scale (HDS)

	Test drug	Clomipramine
Citalopram, 1980–1983	10	15
Paroxetine, 1985–1987	10	15
Moclobemide, 1987–1990	9	13

Table 5. Outcome of DUAG trials

	Test drug (%)	Clomipramine (%)	*p* value
Citalopram, 1980–1983			
CR	28	60	0.002
NR	30	25	0.7
Paroxetine, 1985–1987			
CR	22	57	0.001
NR	48	13	0.001
Moclobemide, 1987–1990			
CR	22	34	0.01
NR	53	27	0.01

CR, complete response = HDS $\leq$ 7; NR, non response = HDS $\geq$ 16.

Table 6. Drop-out due to adverse drug reactions in DUAG trials

Drug and reaction	Drop-out (*n*)
Clomipramine (*n* = 173)	
Mania	3
Grand mal	1
Orthostatic hypotension	12
Other	10
Citalopram (*n* = 57)	
None	0
Paroxetine (*n* = 62)	
Anxiety	1
Moclobemide (*n* = 57)	
Mania	1
Hypertension	1
Other	4

Numbers in parentheses indicate total number of patients.

with 47%–70% treated with the test drugs (Table 5). Only for citalopram was the difference between test drug and clomipramine not statistically significant when the category complete plus partial response was analyzed. The analysis of unwanted effects showed the occurrence of well-known anticholinergic side effects from treatment with clomipramine. In the groups of patients receiving SSRI drugs side effects were less pronounced and headache and nausea were the dominating ones. No cardiovascular toxicity was recorded for either clomipramine or test drugs.

Drop-out due to adverse drug reactions is summarized in Table 6. For clomipramine drop-out rates were high, with an average of nine patients or approximately 15% in each trial. The development of mania and orthostatic hypotenstion dominated the list. These drop-out rates, however, were more than outweighed by rates of approximately 20% due to deterioration in the clinical condition of the patients who received the test drugs. In spite of the many patients who experienced adverse drug reactions or unpleasant side effects due to clomipramine more than 75% of the "intention to treat" group of patients on clomipramine obtained a satisfactory antidepressant response.

This brief summary demonstrates that in the DUAG multisite trials all three test drugs statistically significantly failed to reach the same degree of antidepressant efficacy as that of the traditional tricyclic antidepressant clomipramine. These results are at variance with most of those published of the same and of other recently introduced antidepressant drugs. In general, other studies have shown the new drugs to be more efficacious than placebo and to possess the same degree of efficacy as the tricyclic antidepressants, which were used as reference drugs (Dechant and Clissold 1991; Stabl et al. 1989; Benfield et al. 1986; Boyer and Feighner 1991).

4 Reasons for Discrepancies Between DUAG and Other Studies

There are at least two possible explanations for the differences in outcome between the DUAG studies and the vast majority of other studies of recent antidepressant drugs. One explanation may be that the DUAG studies were performed on predominantly endogeneously depressed hospitalized patients whereas almost all other studies of recent antidepressant drugs have been carried out on groups of outpatients who are likely to suffer from milder depressions of a less homogeneous character. The drugs under study may well exert different effects on different subgroups of depressed patients.

The other possibility for an explanation of the differences in outcome lies in an examination of the different types of bias which may distort the conclusions of drug trials (Kraemer and Pruyn 1990; Gøtzsche 1990). Important sources of bias in studies of antidepressant drugs can be extracted from the list of characteristics of the DUAG trials (Table 3). In the DUAG studies much effort was invested in minimizing the influence of bias from these sources. Large groups of diagnostically homogeneous patients were recruited after power calculations in order that valid clinical conclusions could be drawn from the statistical analyses with a sufficient degree of certainty. Fixed dose regimens were used in order to ensure that patients treated with reference tricyclic antidepressants (clomipramine) obtained sufficient doses and plasma concentration levels; multisite problems with regard to size and composition of individual patient groups were analyzed and reported and a high level of interrater reliability was secured through frequent co-rating sessions between participating centers. In the analysis of data emphasis was placed upon differences between predefined response categories. The definition of the DUAG response categories carried the advantage of underlining the total number of patients who actually became well during the treatment period. Also reporting and analysis of patient withdrawal and drop-out was carried out according to predefined rules in order to ensure that all patients who entered the trials were accounted for. The final analysis in the DUAG studies was performed on the "intention to treat" sample of patients who completed at least 2 weeks of active treatment. Finally in the DUAG studies much effort was invested in controlling compliance through monitoring of serum drug concentrations. This measure is important since noncompliance is responsible for a high proportion of the variance in patients' response to drugs (Harter and Peck 1991).

The majority of studies of recent antidepressant drugs differ from the DUAG studies in most or all of the above-mentioned factors. As mentioned, almost every one of the other studies was made up of outpatients often with liberally defined major depressive episodes and the majority of studies operated with groups of 15 to 30 patients, too small to avoid a considerable risk of committing statistical errors of the second kind. Therefore many of the studies erroneously may have concluded that a recent antidepressant test drug was as effective as the reference drug when no statistically significant difference was found in the analysis of outcome. In most studies with reference drugs flexible dose regimens were employed. This procedure often led to reference drug doses too small to offer fair comparison with the test drug. Doses ranging from 75 to 150 mg per day of tricyclic antidepressants were the rule. Interestingly, in one of the very few other studies (Peselow et al. 1989) in which a reference drug, imipramine, was also found to be superior to a recent drug, paroxetine, the maximum imipramine dose was 210 mg, far higher than the doses used in most other studies, but comparable with the 150 mg of clomipramine used in the DUAG studies. The interrater reliability in other multisite trials hardly ever received a comment; neither did the possible differences in the composition of individual patient groups regarding age, sex, and diagnosis. In most studies the reasons for drop-out and withdrawal were not reported and consequently not analyzed. Differences in outcome were generally reported as group average reductions on the HDS scores. Such average values may obscure the possibility that the majority of the patients treated in one or both drug groups remained moderately ill and that possibly only a small fraction of patients recovered completely.

Apart from the differences in trial design and data analysis which may introduce bias when conclusions about differences or similarities between various drugs are drawn, the qualities of a new drug may be obscured through publication bias. Many results from antidepressant drug studies were never published in detail but appeared in abstracts from company-sponsered symposia or in summary reports in symposia publications printed as a supplement to international journals. Also, data may exist "on file with the drug company," a reference not seldomly seen in the information material passed out by the companies (Smith Kline Beecham 1990). Finally, data may only exist as part of metaanalytical studies based upon unpublished smaller trials. Partial or indirect data from these sources may not necessarily be incorrect but their validity is difficult to assess. Counting paroxetine studies as an example, 21 trials seem to have been performed. Only 11 of these were published, the majority in a summarized form, and only four of them appeared in reviewed journals.

5 Summary and Conclusion

The DUAG studies showed that in well-designed and rigorously executed multisite drug trials three representatives (citalopram, paroxetine, and moclobemide) from two classes of recent antidepressant drugs were less effective than the standard reference drug, clomipramine. The most important reasons for the superiority of clomipramine was probably that clomipramine was given in a high and fixed dose of 150 mg per day throughout the entire treatment period and that patient compliance was ensured through drug monitoring. When the DUAG studies are compared with "no difference" studies, the difference between DUAG and others lies not so much in a different efficacy of the test drugs but in the efficacy of the reference drugs, where clomipramine in the DUAG studies was more effective than reference tricyclics in most other studies with flexible dose regimens. A relatively high rate of adverse drug reactions with clomipramine administered in high and fixed doses was probably due to a considerable interindividual variability in the pharmacokinetic properties (Gram 1990), and the development of side effects may be predicted and prevented when better knowledge of plasma concentration and dose–response relations for classical tricyclic antidepressants allow individual dose adjustments. Such studies are under way with in the DUAG. The results of such studies may reduce the need for new antidepressants which, although less toxic than the classical tricyclics, may prove to be also less potent.

The DUAG studies were performed in hospitalized, moderately to severely, endogeneously depressed adult patients and conclusions from the DUAG studies about the superiority of clomipramine over three recent antidepressants cannot readily be generalized to cover less homogeneous groups of outpatients with milder depression. Neither are the conclusions from the DUAG studies necessarily valid for other recent antidepressants or other drug doses than the ones applied. For outpatients with milder depression recent antidepressant drugs, by virtue of their milder side effects, may be alternatives to traditional antidepressants and to psychotherapy.

References

Baldessarini RJ (1989) Current status of antidepressants: clinical pharmacology and therapy. J Clin Psychiatry 50:117–126

Benfield P, Heel RC, Lewis SP (1986) Fluoxetine. A review of its pharmacodynamic and pharmacokinetic properties, and therapeutic efficacy in depressive illness. Drugs 32:481–508

Boyer WF, Feighner JP (1991) The efficacy of selective serotonin re-uptake inhibitors in depression. In: Feighner JP, Boyer WF (eds) Selective serotonin re-uptake inhibitors. Wiley, Chichester, pp 89–108

Danish University Antidepressant Group (DUAG) (1986) Citalopram: clinical effect profile in comparison with clomipramine. A controlled multicenter study. Psychopharmacology (Berl) 90:131–138

Danish University Antidepressant Group (DUAG) (1990) Paroxetine: a selective serotonin reuptake inhibitor showing better tolerance, but weaker antidepressant effect than clomipramine in a controlled multicenter study. J Affect Dis 18:289–299

Davis JN (1985) Antidepressant drugs. In: Kapland HI, Saddock BJ (eds) Comprehensive textbook of psychiatry, vol 4, 4th edn. Williams and Wilkins, Baltimore, pp 1513–1537

Dechant KL, Clissold SP (1991) Paroxetine. A review of its pharmacodynamic and pharmacokinetic properties, and therapeutical potential in depressive illness. Drugs 41:225–253

Gøtzsche PC (1990) Bias in double-blind trials. Dan Med Bull 37:329–336

Gram LF (1990) Inadequate dosing and pharmacokinetic variability as confounding factors in assessment of efficacy of antidepressants. Clin Neuropharmacol 13 Suppl 1:S35–S44

Harter JG, Peck CC (1991) Chronobiology: suggestions for integrating it into drug development. Ann NY Acad Sci 618:563–571

Kraemer HC, Pruyn JP (1990) The evaluation of different approaches to randomized clinical trials. Arch Gen Psychiatry 47:1163–1169

Morris JB, Beck AT (1974) The efficacy of antidepressant drugs. Arch Gen Psychiatry 30:667–674

Peselow ED, Filippi A-M, Goodnick P, Barouche F, Fieve RR (1989) The short- and long-term efficacy of paroxetine HCI. A. Data from a 6-week double-blind parallel design trial vs imipramine and placebo. Psychopharmacol Bull 25:267–271

Smith Kline Beecham (1990) Paroxetine. A review of preclinical and clinical studies. Franklin Scientific Projects, London

Stabl M, Bizière K, Schmid-Burgk W, Amrein R (1989) Review of comparative clinical trials. Moclobemide vs tricyclic antidepressants and vs placebo in depressive states. J Neural Transm 28:77–89

Role of Genetic Polymorphism in Psychopharmacology – An Update

K. Brøsen, S.H. Sindrup, E. Skjelbo, K.K. Nielsen, and L.F. Gram

1 Introduction

Pharmacogenetics is concerned with the genetic basis for interindividual differences in the clinical reponse to drugs. The study of genetic polymorphism in drug metabolism has been an area of particular interest. A genetic polymorphism is a monogenic or mendelian trait that exists in the population in at least two phenotypes (and presumably in at least two genotypes), the rarest of whom exists in at least 1%–2% (Vogel and Motulsky 1982). Thus, two phenotypes are discernible in the case of genetic polymorphism in drug metabolism: a slowly metabolizing phenotype who may develop toxic plasma (tissue) concentrations when a standard dose regimen is employed and a rapidly metabolizing phenotype who may develop subtherapeutic concentrations.

Oxidation is the most important primary step in the metabolism and hence elimination of most psychotropic drugs. Drug oxidations are catalyzed by a group of related heme proteins, socalled isozymes, which are designated cytochrome P450. The P450s are located to the membranes of the smooth endoplasmic reticulum of a number of tissues, in particular in liver tissue. It is estimated that there are between 20 and 200 drug-metabolizing P450s in humans, and each is encoded by a separate gene. At the biochemical level, P450 isozymes differ from each other by their amino acid composition. P450 genes are classified into families (designated by an Arabic numeral) and subfamilies (designated by a capital letter) according to the degree of amino acid homology of the encoded isozymes (Nebert et al. 1991). At the functional level most drug-metabolizing P450s display a marked regio- and stereoselectivity and have a wide substrate specificity.

Two independent genetic polymorphisms of drug oxidation, each related to a distinct P450, have been extensively studied during the last 10–15 years: the mephenytoin oxidation polymorphism which is related to a P450 in the 2C subfamily and the sparteine/debrisoquine oxidation polymorphism the source of which is the CYP2D6.

Department of Clinical Pharmacology, Odense University, Winsløwparken 19, 5000 Odense C, Denmark

2 The Mephenytoin Oxidation Polymorphism

The mephenytoin oxidation polymorphism was revealed by the demonstration of a bimodal distribution of the ability to perform the aromatic 4-hydroxylation of *S*-mephenytoin in the Swiss population (Küpfer and Preisig 1984). Thus, in white Caucasian populations about 3% are poor metabolizers (PM) of *S*-mephenytoin, and the remainder more than 90% are extensive metabolizers (EM). Family studies showed that PM are homozygous for an autosomal recessive allele and that EM comprise both the heterozygotes and the homozygous dominants (reviewed in Drøhse et al. 1989).

The mephenytoin oxidation polymorphism displays marked interethnic differences. Thus, the PM frequency is about 10% in East Greenlanders (Clasen et al. 1991) and 15%–20% in Japanese and Chinese (reviewed in Wilkinson et al. 1989).

The defect in mephenytoin hydroxylation has not yet been characterized at the DNA/RNA level. The source of the mephenytoin oxidation polymorphism is an enzyme in the CYP2C subfamily, tentatively designated CYP2C9 (Nebert et al. 1991). The CYP2C is one of a group of closely regulated and almost identical isozymes, and it is presently not known which one of these is defective in the PM (Ged et al. 1988).

The metabolism of the antimalarial prodrug proguanil to its active metabolite cycloguanil heavily depends on the mephenytoin oxidation polymorphism (Ward et al. 1991). The mephenytoin oxidation polymorphism is partially responsible for the *N*-demethylation of diazepam, of *N*-desmethyldiazepam (Bertilsson et al. 1989), of imipramine (Skjelbo et al. 1991) of clomipramine (K.K. Nielsen, personal communication), and of citalopram (Sindrup et al. 1993). For the psychotropic drugs mentioned the ratio between the average clearance in EM is about twice the value in PM, and there is some overlapping in the clearance values between the two phenotypes. This suggests that the *N*-demethylations are catalyzed only in part by the CYP2C9. Alternatively, it may be hypothesized that the oxidation of *S*-mephenytoin and the *N*-demethylation of the psychotropic drugs are catalyzed by distinct but closely regulated P450s in the 2C subfamily.

3 The Sparteine/Debrisoquine Oxidation Polymorphism

3.1 Background

The sparteine/debrisoquine oxidation polymorphism was discovered nearly 15 years ago (Evans et al. 1980; Eichelbaum et al. 1979). In white Caucasians about 7% of the population are PM of sparteine and debrisoquine and the remainder more than 90% are EM. Family studies showed that PM are homozygous for an autosomal recessive allele and that EM are either heterozygotes or homozygous dominants (Evans et al. 1980). Studies in Blacks, Orientals and Eskimos have shown that the PM frequency in these populations is only about 1%–3% (reviewed in Steiner et al. 1989).

A distinct P450, now referred to as the CYP2D6 (Nebert et al. 1991), is the source of the sparteine/debrisoquine oxidation polymorphism. The CYP2D6 is absent from the livers of PM (Zanger et al. 1988), and in this phenotype substrates of the isozyme are predominantly eliminated by alternative low-affinity P450s, by other enzymes, or by renal excretion.

Different types of point mutations, gene deletions, and gene duplications in the CYP2D6 gene explain why the CYP2D6 is not expressed in the livers of the PM (Kagimoto et al. 1990; Gaedigk et al. 1991). Moreover, the characterization of the most common gene anomalies of the CYP2D6 has provided the basis for the development of an allele-specific polymerase chain reaction (PCR) amplification genotype test (Heim and Meyer 1990).

The sparteine/debrisoquine oxidation polymorphism is a major determinant of interindividual differences in the elimination of tricyclic antidepressants (Brøsen and Gram 1989; Sjöqvist 1989; Brøsen 1990), some neuroleptics (Bertilsson et al., this volume, p. 230), 5HT-reuptake inhibitors (Sindrup et al. 1992a,b), beta-blockers, and antiarrhythmics (Eichelbaum and Gross 1990) (Table 1).

3.2 The Clinical Pharmacokinetics of Drug Metabolism via the CYP2D6

The major functional characteristics of the CYP2D6 are genetic polymorphism (sparteine/debrisoquine type), inhibition by many drugs, saturation kinetics for many substrates, and stereoselective metabolism (Brøsen 1990). In EM, drug elimination proceeds in parallel by the CYP2D6 (major route) and by alternative low-affinity P450s, by other enzymes, or by renal excretion (minor routes) (Brøsen 1990).

The study of the sparteine/debrisoquine oxidation polymorphism has targeted the CYP2D6 as the site for inter- as well as intraindividual differences in the metabolism of several groups of clinically important drugs. The intraindividual differences in drug metabolism are due to intraindividual differences in the relative importance of the CYP2D6 for the overall drug elimination (Table 2). The CYP2D6 becomes more important by selective induction, by renal dysfunction, or by selective inhibition or saturation of alternative P450s (Table 2). Conversely, CYP2D6 becomes less important by saturation or by selective inhibition of the isozyme or by induction of alternative P450s (Table 2).

Studies with human liver microsome preparations have shown that many commonly used drugs, notably some antiarrhythmics, some neuroleptics and some serotonin (5HT)-reuptake inhibitors are very potent, selective inhibitors of CYP2D6, having apparent inhibitor constant (K_i) values of

Table 1. Psychotropic drugs in relation to CYP2D6, the source of the sparteine/debrisoquine oxidation polymorphism

Drug	K_i[a] μM	Model drug[b]	Reference	Cl_{EM}/CL_{PM}[c]	Reference
Tricyclic antidepressants					
Amitriptyline	50	Sparteine	Otton et al. (1983)	~2	Mellström et al. (1983)
Nortriptyline	15	Sparteine	Otton et al. (1983)	~5	Bertilsson et al. (1980)
Imipramine	40	Sparteine	Otton et al. (1983)	~2	Brøsen et al. (1986)
Desipramine	6	Sparteine	Otton et al. (1983)	~6	Brøsen et al. (1986)
Clomipramine	16	Imipramine	Skjelbo and Brøsen (1992)	~2.5	Kramer Nielsen et al. (1992)
N-desmethylclomipramine	8	Imipramine	Skjelbo and Brøsen (1992)	~3.0	Kramer Nielsen et al. (1992)
Neuroleptics					
Clorpromazine	7	Sparteine	Otton et al. (1983)	?	–
Clozapine	4	Dextrometorphan	Fischer et al. (1992)	?	–
Fluphenazine	1	Bufuralol	Fonné-Fister and Meyer (1988)	?	–
Haloperidol	1	Sparteine	Inaba et al. (1985)	~2	Llerena et al. (1992)
Levomepromazine	1	Imipramine	Brøsen et al. (1991b)	?	–
Perphenazine	0.16	Imipramine	Brøsen and Brøsen (1992)	~4	Dahl-Puustinen et al. (1989)
Pipamperone	No inhibition	Imipramine	Brøsen and Brøsen (1992)	?	–
Remoxipride	?	–	–	~2	Steiner et al. (1988)
Thioridazine	0.75	Desipramine	von Bahr et al. (1985)	~3	von Bahr et al. (1991)
Trifluperidol	0.7	Bufuralol	Fonné-Fister and Meyer (1988)	?	
Zuclopentixol	Apparently no inhibition	Imipramine	Skjelbo and Brøsen (1992)	~2.5	Dahl et al. (1991)

5-HT reuptake inhibitors					
Citalopram	19	Imipramine	Skjelbo and Brøsen (1992)	~1	Sindrup et al. (in press)
N-desmethylcitalopram	1.3	Imipramine	Skjelbo and Brøsen (1992)	~1.5	Sindrup et al. (in press)
Fluvoxamine	4	Imipramine	Skjelbo and Brøsen (1992)	?	
Fluoxetine	0.5	Imipramine	Brøsen and Skjelbo (1991)	?	–
Norfluoxetine	0.6	Imipramine	Brøsen and Skjelbo (1991)	?	–
Paroxetine	0.8	Bufuralol	Brøsen et al. (1991a)	~7 and	Sindrup et al. (1992a)
	0.4	Imipramine	Skjelbo and Brøsen (1992)	~2[d]	Sindrup et al. (1992a)
Sertraline	0.7	Sparteine	Crewe et al. (1991)	?	–
Miscellaneous					
Diazepam	No inhibition	Sparteine	Inaba et al. (1985)	~1	Bertilsson et al. (1989)
N-desmethyldiazepam	162	Sparteine	Inaba et al. (1985)	~1	Bertilsson et al. (1989)
Mianserin	7	Imipramine	Skjelbo and Brøsen (1992)	?	–
Moclobemide	140	Imipramine	Skjelbo and Brøsen (1992)	?	–

[a] Apparent inhibitor constant in human liver microsomes.
[b] Inhibition experiments carried out with human liver microsome preparations.
[c] Ratio between average clearance in extensive and poor metabolizers.
[d] See Table 3.

Table 2. Factors and mechanisms which are responsible for *intra*individual differences in the relative importance of CYP2D6[a] for the overall elimination of drugs

	Consequence for total plasma clearance EM	PM	Comment
Increased importance of CYP2D6			
Selective induction of CYP2D6	Increase	No change	Probably not important
Inhibition of alternative P450s	Decrease	Decrease	Decrease in clearance is relatively more pronounced in PM
Saturation of alternative P450s	Decrease	Decrease	Decrease in clearance is relatively more pronounced in PM
Impairment of renal function	Decrease	Decrease	Decrease in clearance is relatively more pronounced in PM (e.g., flecainide)
Decreased importance of CYP2D6			
Saturation of CYP2D6	Decrease	No change	The difference in total clearance between EM and PM will diminish, but not disappear (see tex)
Selective inhibition of CYP2D6	Decrease	No change	The difference between EM and PM with regard to clearance may be completely abolished with an appropriate dose of a potent inhibitor
Selective induction of alternative P450s	Increase	Increase	The relative increase in total clearance is larger in PM than in EM, but the phenotype difference will not disappear

EM, extensive metabolizers; PM, poor metabolizers.
[a] The target of the sparteine/debrisoquine oxidation polymorphism.

about 1 μM or less (Table 1). Thus the pharmacogenetic difference in drug metabolism between EM and PM is practically abolished during concomitant intake of a potent inhibitor (Brinn et al. 1986).

As a consequence of saturation of CYP2D6, the difference between EM and PM with regard to drug clearance will be reduced as the dose is increased or repeated. However, the phenotype difference will never disappear completely because there will always be a contribution from the CYP2D6 to the overall drug elimination in EM but not in PM. A recent panel study of the single and repeated oral dose kinetics of paroxetine illustrates this concept (Table 3).

Table 3. The single dose and steady-state kinetics of paroxetine in nine extensive metabolizers and eight poor metabolizers of sparteine (median and range; data from Sindrup et al. 1992a)

	AUC_{sd}[a] ($nmol\,h^{-1}l^{-1}$)	AUC_{ss}[b]
EM	550 (240–1230)	2550 (1360–3890)
Wilcoxon test (ss vs sd)	**	
PM	3910 (1710–7510)	4410 (2230–7770)
Wilcoxon test (ss vs sd)	NS	
Mann-Whitney test (EM vs PM)	***	*

AUC, area under curve; sd, single dose; ss, steady state; EM, extensive metabolizers; PM, poor metabolizers; NS, not significant.
$^*p < 0.05$; $^{**}p < 0.01$; $^{***}p < 0.001$.
[a] After a single oral dose of 30 mg paroxetine.
[b] Plasma AUC from 0–24 h after 2 weeks of repeated paroxetine dosing (30 mg/day).

4 Clinical Significance of Genetic Polymorphism in Drug Metabolism

Phenotyping before treatment would be of value for drugs where the parent compound and/or active metabolite are eliminated almost exclusively via the polymorphic pathway (Figs. 1, 2) and for which plasma level monitoring is considered necessary (Brøsen and Gram 1989; Brøsen 1990). Thus, in psychopharmacology mephenytoin testing cannot at present be recommended as a routine test. However, sparteine or debrisoquine testing would certainly be of value in relation to therapeutic drug monitoring of tricyclic antidepressants and neuroleptics (Brøsen and Gram 1989; Brøsen 1990; Bertilsson et al. 1991).

The selective 5-HT reuptake inhibitor paroxetine is partially metabolized via CYP2D6 (Table 3) (Sindrup et al. 1992a,b). However a therapeutic plasma concentration range for the use of paroxetine as an antidepressant has not been established (DUAG 1989). At plasma levels above 200 n*M*, paroxetine is also useful against the symptoms of painful diabetic neuropathy (Sindrup et al. 1990a), but clinical dose titration is readily performed (Sindrup et al. 1991) and phenotyping is probably not required.

The utility of sparteine and debrisoquine testing in psychopharmacology is hampered by the frequent coadministration of drugs which are potent inhibitors of CYP2D6 (Table 1) (Syvälathi et al. 1986). This problem may be overcome by the use of genotyping for the CYP2D6 gene by means of allele-specific PCR amplification (Heim and Meyer 1990). The disadvantage of the PCR genotyping test is that about 10% of the PM are misclassified as EM (Nørremark Nielsen et al., in preparation) and, further, that the test is

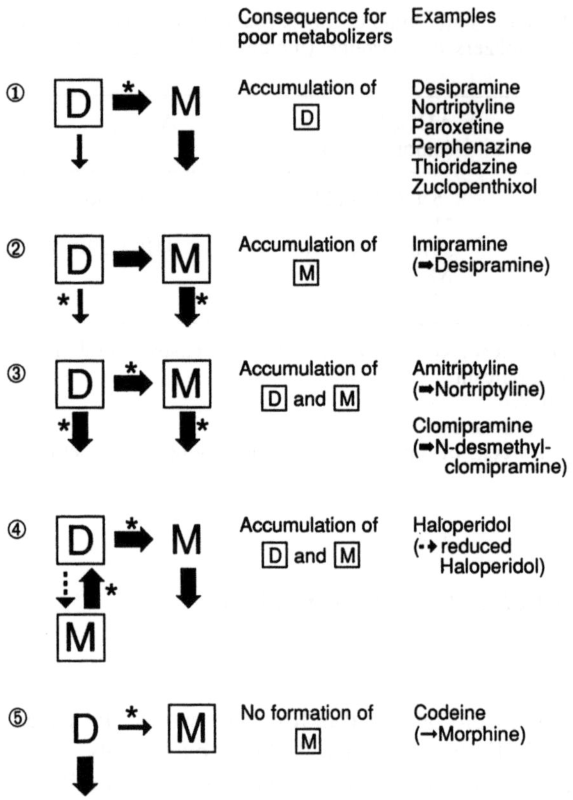

Fig. 1. Five consequences of the sparteine/debrisoquine oxidation polymorphism for the pharmacokinetics of psychotropic drugs. □, Active; *, via the sparteine/debrisoquine oxidation polymorphism; *D*, parent compound; *M*, metabolite; ➧, major oxidative route; →, minor oxidative route; ---▶, nonoxidative route. (Data on haloperidol according to Tyndale et al. 1991a)

a poor predictor of the CYP2D6 function in the EM group, which comprises more than 90% of the patients.

There are a number of clinically important exceptions to the general rule that the sparteine/debrisoquine oxidation polymorphism is important only if the overall metabolism of the drug is catalyzed by the CYP2D6. The best documented example hereof is the prodrug codeine, of which 10% or less of the dose is *O*-demethylated via CYP2D6 to the active metabolite morphine (Yue et al. 1989). Thus, very little morphine is formed in the PM, and it has recently been shown that pain thresholds are elevated in EM but not in PM after codeine intake (Sindrup et al. 1990b).

Remoxipride appears to be another example. On average, the total plasma clearance of remoxipride is about two times higher in EM as compared to the value in PM (Steiner et al. 1988), which suggests that remoxipride is only metabolized in part by the CYP2D6. However, in a recent clinical study, 16 EM subjects were treated with remoxipride 100 mg twice daily for 3 days and no adverse effects were observed except for light acathesia in a few subjects. However, at the same dose four out of four PM subjects dropped out of the study, three due to acute dystonia and one due to severe

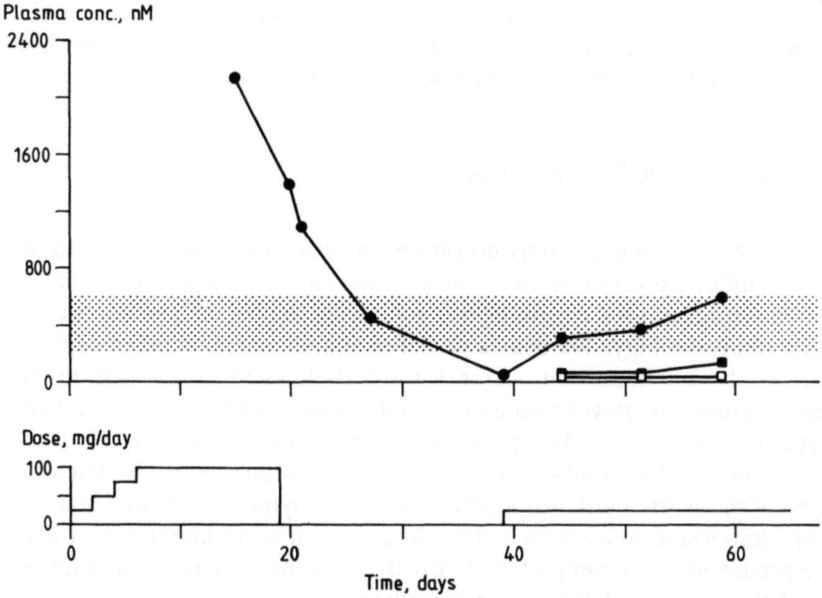

Fig. 2. Serum concentrations of nortriptyline (●), 10-E-OH-nortriptyline (□), 10-Z-OH-nortriptyline (■) during treatment of a 42-year-old female poor metabolizer of sparteine with nortriptyline 25–100 mg per day. After about 2 weeks of treatment the patient complained over severe constipation, accommodation disturbance, urinary retention, and a feeling of tightness in the chest. There was a moderate prolongation of the PQ interval and a widening of the QRS complex on the ECG. Later, the patient recovered during treatment with 25 mg nortriptyline/day. □, Therapeutic plasma concentration range. (From Petersen and Brøsen 1991)

acathesia (L.F. Gram, personal communication). The discrepancy between the moderate pharmacokinetic difference between EM and PM and the dramatic pharmacodynamic difference is difficult to explain. It is possible, however, that the CYP2D6 is expressed in the brain in EM but not in PM (Niznik et al. 1990; Tyndale et al. 1991b) and that here it may contribute to the local removal and, hence, modification of the clinical effects of remoxipride (Britto and Wedlund 1992).

5 Interactions Due to Inhibition of CYP2D6

When a substrate and an inhibitor of the CYP2D6 are coadministered there is the possibility of a drug–drug interaction. This will be a particular problem when a potent inhibitor is given in combination with a drug which is extensively metabolized by CYP2D6 and for which plasma level monitoring is considered useful. The potent inhibition of neuroleptics on the metabolism of tricyclic antidepressants (Gram and Overø 1972) and of fluoxetine and paroxetine on the metabolism of tricyclic antidepressants and of haloperidol (Bell and Cole 1988; Goff et al. 1991; Brøsen et al. 1993) represent the best documented and clinically the most relevant examples hereof.

6 Conclusion and Perspectives

The discovery of genetic polymorphism in drug oxidation has had an enormous influence on drug metabolism research. The mephenytoin oxidation polymorphism still seems to be of a somewhat limited clinical importance in psychopharmacology. The sparteine/debrisoquine oxidation polymorphism appears to be an important factor for interindividual differences in the clinical response to tricyclic antidepressants, some neuroleptics, and some 5HT-reuptake inhibitors. The possibility of a rational prediction of drug–drug interactions due to inhibition of CYP2D6 is emphasized. The intensive studying of the sparteine/debrisoquine oxidation polymorphism has generated the very important concept that the clinical elimination kinetics of a drug can be predicted if the metabolism of the drug can be assigned to a functionally well characterized P450 or another enzyme.

References

Bell IR, Cole JO (1988) Fluoxetine induces elevation of desipramine level and exacerbation of geriatric non psychotic depression. J Clin Psychopharmacol 8:447–448

Bertilsson L, Eichelbaum M, Mellström B, Säwe J, Schulz H-U, Sjöqvist F (1980) Nortriptyline and amitriptyline clearance in relation to debrisoquine hydroxylation in man. Life Sci 27:1673–1677

Bertilsson L, Henthorn TK, Sanch E, Tybring G, Säwe J et al. (1989) Importance of genetic factors in the regulation of diazepam metabolism: relationship to S-mephenytoin, but not debrisoquin hydroxylation phenotype. Clin Pharmacol Ther 45:348–355

Brinn R, Brøsen K, Gram LF, Haghfelt T, Otton SV (1986) Sparteine oxidation is practically abolished in quinidine-treated patients. Br J Clin Pharmacol 22:194–197

Britto MR, Wedlund PJ (1992) Cytochrome P-450 in the brain-potential evolutionary and therapeutic relevance of localization of drug metabolizing enzymes. Drug Metab Dispos 20:446–450

Brøsen K (1990) Recent developments in hepatic drug oxidation – implications for clinical pharmacokinetics. Clin Pharmacokinet 18:220–239

Brøsen K, Gram LF (1989) Clinical significance of the sparteine/debrisoquine oxidation polymorphism. Eur J Clin Pharmacol 36:537–547

Brøsen K, Skjelbo E (1991) Fluoxetine and norfluoxetine are potent inhibitors of P450IID6 – the source of the sparteine/debrisoquine oxidation polymorphism. Br J Clin Pharmacol 32:136–137

Brøsen K, Otton SV, Gram LF (1986) Imipramine demethylation and hydroxylation: impact of the sparteine oxidation phenotype. Clin Pharmacol Ther 40:543–549

Brøsen K, Gram LF, Kragh-Sørensen P (1991a) Extremely slow metabolism of amitriptyline but normal metabolism of imipramine and desipramine in an extensive metabolizer of sparteine, debrisoquine and mephenytoin. Ther Drug Monit 13:177–182

Brøsen K, Zeugin T, Meyer UA (1991b) Role of P450IID6, the target of the sparteine/debrisoquin oxidation polymorphism in the metabolism of imipramine. Clin Pharmacol Ther 49:609–617

Brøsen K, Hansen MGJ, Nielsen KK, Sindrup SH, Gram LF (1993) Inhibition by paroxetine of desipramine in extensive but not in poor metabolizers of sparteine. Eur J Clin Pharmacol (in press)

Clasen K, Madsen L, Brøsen K, Albøge K, Husfeldt S, Gram LF (1991) Sparteine and mephenytoin oxidation: genetic polymorphisms in East- and West Greenland. Clin Pharmacol Ther 49:624–631

Crewe HK, Lennard MS, Tucker GT, Woods FR, Haddock RE (1992) The effect of selective serotonin re-uptake inhibitors on cytochrome P4502D6 (CYP2D6) activity in human liver microsomes. Br J Clin Pharmacol 34:262–265

Dahl ML, Ekqvist B, Widen J, Bertilsson L (1991) Disposition of the neuroleptic zuclopenthixol co-segregates with the polymorphic hydroxylation of debrisoquine. Acta Psychiatr Scand 84:99–102

Dahl-Puustinen ML, Liden A, Alm C, Nordin C, Bertilsson L (1989) Disposition of perphenazine is related to polymorphic debrisoquine hydroxylation in human beings. Clin Pharmacol Ther 46:78–81

Danish University Antidepressant Group (DUAG) (1990) Paroxetine: a selective serotonin reuptake inhibitor showing better tolerance but weaker antidepressant effect than clomipramine in a controlled multicenter study. J Affect Dis 18:289–299

Drøhse A, Bathum L, Brøsen K, Gram LF (1989) Mephenytoin and sparteine oxidation: genetic polymorphisms in Denmark. Br J Clin Pharmacol 27:620–625

Eichelbaum M, Gross A (1990) The genetic polymorphism of debrisoquine/sparteine metabolism – clinical aspects. Pharmacol Ther 46:377–394

Eichelbaum M, Spannbrucker N, Steincke B, Dengler HJ (1979) Defective N-oxidation of sparteine in man: a new pharmacogenetic defect. Eur J Clin Pharmacol 16:183–187

Evans DAP, Mahgroup A, Sloan TP, Idle JR, Smith RL (1980) A family and population study of genetic polymorphism of debrisoquine oxidation in a white British population. Med Genet 17:102–105

Fischer V, Vogels B, Maurer G, Tynes R (1992) The antipsychotic clozapine is metabolized by the polymorphic human microsomal and recombinant cytochrome 2D6. J Pharmacol Exp Ther (in press)

Fonné-Fister R, Meyer UA (1988) Xenobiotic and endobiotic inhibitors of cytochrome P450db1 function, the target of the debrisoquine/sparteine type polymorphism. Biochem Pharmacol 37:3829–3835

Gaedigk A, Blum M, Gaedigk R, Eichelbaum M, Meyer UA (1991) Deletion of the entire cytochrome P450 CYP2D6 gene as a cause of impaired drug metabolism in poor metabolizers of the debrisoquine/sparteine polymorphism. Am J Hum Genet 48:943–950

Ged C, Umbenhauer DR, Bellew TM, Bork RW, Srivastava PK et al. (1988) Characterization of cDNAs, mRNAs and proteins related to human liver microsomal cytochrome P-450 (S)-mephenytoin 4′-hydroxylation. Biochemistry 27:6929–6940

Goff DC, Midha KK, Brotman AW, Waites M, Baldessarini RJ (1991) Elevation of plasma concentrations of haloperiodol after the addition of fluoxetine. Am J Psychiatry 148:790–792

Gram LF, Overø KF (1972) Drug interaction: inhibitory effect of neuroleptics on the metabolism of tricyclic antidepressants in man. Br Med J 163:463–465

Heim M, Meyer UA (1990) Genotyping of poor metabolisers of debrisoquine by allele-specific PCR amplification. Lancet 2:529–532

Inaba T, Jurima M, Mahon WA, Kalow W (1988) In vitro studies of two isozymes of human liver cytochrome P450. Mephenytoin p-hydroxylase and sparteine monooxygenase. Drug Metab Dispos 13:443–448

Kagimoto M, Heim M, Kagimoto K, Zeugin T, Meyer UA (1990) Multiple mutations of the human cytochrome P450IID6 gene (CYP2D6) in poor metabolizers of debrisoquine. J Biol Chem 265:17209–17214

Kramer Nielsen K, Brøsen K, Gram LF, Danish University Antidepressant Group (1992) The steady-state plasma levels of clomirpamine and its metabolites: impact of the sparteine/debrisoquine oxidation polymorphism. Eur J Clin Pharmacol (in press)

Küpfer A, Preisig R (1984) Pharmacogenetics of mephenytoin: a new drug hydroxylation polymorphism in man. Eur J Clin Pharmacol 26:753–759

Llerena A, Alm C, Dahl M-L, Ekqvist B, Bertilsson L (1992) Haloperidol disposition is dependent on the debrisoquine hydroxylation phenotype. Ther Drug Monit 14:92–97

Mellström B, Bertilsson L, Lou Y-C, Säwe J, Sjöqvist F (1983) Amitriptyline metabolism: relationship to polymorphic debrisoquine hydroxylation. Clin Pharmacol Ther 34: 516–520

Nebert DW, Nelson DR, Coon MJ, Estabrook RW, Feyereisen R et al. (1991) The P450 superfamily: update on new sequences, gene mapping and recommended nomenclature. DNA Cell Biol 10:1–14

Niznik HB, Tyndale RF, Sallee FR, Conzalez FJ, Hardwick JP, Inaba T, Kalow W (1990) The dopamine transporter and cytochrome P450IID1 (debrisoquine hydroxylase) in brain: resolution and identification of two distinct [^{3}H] GBR-12935 binding proteins. Arch Biochem Biophys 276:424–432

Otton SV, Inaba T, Kalow W (1983) Inhibition of sparteine oxidation in human liver by tricyclic antidepressants and other drugs. Life Sci 32:795–800

Petersen P, Brøsen K (1991) Severe nortriptyline poisoning in poor metabolizers of sparteine type. Ugeskr Læger 153:443–444

Sindrup SH, Gram LF, Brøsen K, Eshøj O, Mogensen EF (1990a) The selective serotonin reuptake inhibitor paroxetine is effective in the treatment of diabetic neuropathy symptoms. Pain 42:135–144

Sindrup SH, Brøsen K, Bjerring P, Arendt-Nielsen L, Larsen U, Angelo HR, Gram LF (1990b) Codeine increases pain thresholds to copper vapor laser stimuli in extensive but not poor metabolizers of sparteine. Clin Pharmacol Ther 48:686–693

Sindrup SH, Grodum E, Gram LF, Beck-Nielsen H (1991) Concentration-response relationship in paroxetine treatment of diabetic neuropathy symptoms. A patient-blinded dose-escalation study. Ther Drug Monit 13:408–414

Sindrup SH, Brøsen K, Gram LF, Hallas J, Skjelbo E et al. (1992a) The relationship between paroxetine and the sparteine oxidation polymorphism. Clin Pharmacol Ther 51:278–287

Sindrup SH, Brøsen K, Gram LF (1992b) Pharmacokinetics of the selective serotonin reuptake inhibitor paroxetine – nonlinearity and relation to the sparteine oxidation polymorphism. Clin Pharmacol Ther 51:288–295

Sindrup SH, Brøsen K, Hansen MGJ, Aaes-Jørgensen T, Overø K, Gram LF (1993) The pharmacokinetics of citalopram in relation to the sparteine and mephenytoin oxidation polymorphisms. Ther D Monit (in press)

Sjöqvist F (1989) Pharmacogenetics of antidepressants. In: Dahl SG, Gram LF (eds) Clinical pharmacology in psychiatry – from molecular studies to clinical reality. Springer, Berlin Heidelberg New York, pp 181–191

Skjelbo E, Brøsen K (1992) Inhibitors of imipramine metabolism by human liver microsomes. Br J Clin Pharmacol 34 (in press)

Skjelbo E, Brøsen K, Hallas J, Gram LF (1991) The mephenytoin oxidation polymorphism is partially responsible for the N-demethylation of imipramine. Clin Pharmacol Ther 49:18–23

Steiner E, Movin G, Wahlen A, Nilsson L, Lindberg A (1988) Pharmacokinetics of the potential antipsychotic drug remoxipride in rapid and slow hydroxylators of debrisoquine. Internal report. ASTRA Alab, Clinical Research, Södertälje

Steiner E, Bertilsson L, Säwe J, Bethling I, Sjöqvist F (1989) Polymorphic debrisoquine hydroxylation in 757 Swedish subjects. Clin Pharmacol Ther 44:431–435

Syvälahti E, Lindberg R, Kallio J, de Vocht M (1986) Inhibitory effects of neuroleptics on debrisoquine oxidation in man. Br J Clin Pharmacol 22:89–92

Tyndale RF, Kalow W, Inaba T (1991a) Oxidation of reduced haloperidol to haloperidol: involvement of human P450IID6 (sparteine/debrisoquine monooxygenase). Br J Clin Pharmacol 31:655–660

Tyndale RF, Sunahara R, Inaba T, Kalow W, Gonzalez FJ, Niznik HB (1991b) Neuronal cytochrome P450IID1 (debrisoquine/sparteine-type): potent inhibition of activity by (-)-cocaine and nucleotide sequence identity to human hepatic P450 gene CYP2D6. Mol Pharmacol 40:63–68

Vogel F, Motulsky AD (1982) Human genetics, problems and approaches. Springer, Berlin Heidelberg New York

Von Bahr C, Spina E, Birgersson C (1985) Inhibition of desmethylimipramine 2-hydroxylation by drugs in human liver microsomes. Biochem Pharmacol 14: 2501–2505

Von Bahr C, Movin G, Nordin C, Liden A, Odenaes MH, Hedberg A, Ring H, Sjöqvist F (1991) Plasma levels of thioridazine and metabolites are influenced by the debrisoquin hydroxylation phenotype. Clin Pharmacol Ther 49:234–240

Ward SA, Helsby NA, Skjelbo E, Brøsen K, Gram LF, Breckenridge AM (1991) The activation of the biguanide antimalarial proguanil co-segregates with the mephenytoin oxidation polymorphism – a panel study. Br J Clin Pharmacol 31:689–692

Wilkinson GR, Guengerich FP, Branch RA (1989) Genetic polymorphism of S-mephenytoin hydroxylation. Pharmacol Ther 43:53–76

Yue QY, Svensson JO, Alm C, Sjöqvist F, Säwe J (1989) Codeine O-demethylation co-segregates with polymorphic debrisoquine hydroxylation. Br J Clin Pharmacol 28: 639–645

Zanger UM, Vilbois F, Hardwick J, Meyer UA (1988) Absence of hepatic cytochrome P450bufI causes genetically deficient debrisoquine oxidation in man. Biochemistry 27:5447–5454

Psychotropic Drug Metabolism and Clinical Monitoring

A.E. Balant-Gorgia[1] and L.P. Balant[2]

1 Introduction

The major causes of variability in blood concentrations of psychoactive substances are presystemic and systemic hepatic clearances, with a few exceptions such as lithium or sulpiride. The main reason for this variability is to be found in the lipophilic nature of most psychotropes which favors elimination by metabolism rather than by renal excretion of the unchanged drug. The nature of this variability is, in part, of defined genetic origin (see Brøsen et al., this volume) and, in part, of undefined genetic or poorly controlled environment factors, which interfere with aging, or pathological conditions. Analysis of the interplay of drug metabolism and therapeutic monitoring would thus imply a review of all the aspects of biotransformation which may induce intra- and interindividual variability. Confronted with this (almost) insuperable task, we have decided to concentrate on selected aspects of metabolism. The criteria behind these choices are summarized by three questions: (1) which substances (parent drug and/or metabolite) should be mentioned? (2) how should they be determined? and (3) which approach should be adopted for the interpretation of the concentration data? For each area of interest, we have tried to summarize current knowledge and to express an opinion, which is not necessarily the result of a general consensus.

2 Active Metabolites of Phenothiazines

2.1 Pharmacological and Pharmacokinetic Properties

Phenothiazines are metabolized in humans to numerous metabolites, and a number of them have been shown to possess pharmacological activity (Jørgensen 1986). As postulated by Dahl (1981), it may be assumed that, in

[1] Therapeutic Drug Monitoring Unit, Institutions Universitaires de Psychiatrie, 1225 Chêne-Bourg, Switzerland
[2] Clinical Research Unit, Institutions Universitaires de Psychiatrie, 47 rue du XXXI Décembre, 1207 Geneva, Switzerland

order to contribute significantly to the clinical effect or to the possible side effects of a drug, a metabolite should fulfill the following criteria: (a) possess a certain intrinsic pharmacological or toxicological activity; (b) be formed in sufficient amounts after therapeutic doses of the drug; and (c) have pharmacokinetic properties such that it reaches sufficiently high concentrations at the site of action.

Even today, after years of research, little is known about the exact "profile" of all phenothiazine metabolites. There are numerous reasons for this lack of information. One of them is that the number of phenothiazine metabolites which are formed in such amounts that they may be expected to contribute to the effects of the drug in humans is usually much lower than the total number of identified or postulated metabolites (Dahl et al. 1983). As a consequence, it is often difficult to determine a priori from urinary excretion data which metabolites should be synthesized in order to test their in vitro and (if possible) in vivo behavior and effects. Another complicating factor is that metabolites may be inactive (Dahl et al. 1981) or may show different pharmacological effects. As an example, it has been suggested that 3-hydroxy-levomepromazine may contribute to the neuroleptic effects of levomepromazine in humans, while *N*-monodesmethyl-levomepromazine may contribute significantly to the sedative effect of this drug (Dahl et al. 1983). It is thus probable that the different routes of metabolism lead to compounds with quite different physicochemical properties and pharmacological profiles (and not only potencies) than those of the parent molecule (Dahl 1982)

2.2 Interindividual Variability in Metabolic Patterns

It is well demonstrated that there are important interindividual differences in the "metabolic spectrum" formed in patients. These differences might, in part, be the consequence of polymorphic metabolism, as demonstrated recently in healthy volunteers for thioridazine (von Bahr et al. 1991). As an example from the clinical setting, Midha et al. (1987b) found that, in patients treated with fluphenazine decanoate, the concentrations of fluphenazine sulfoxide were nearly as high as those of the parent drug. Since there was a considerable amount of variation in sulfoxide levels among patients, it is conceivable that differences among patients in metabolism may be clinically important although the precise pharmacological activity of this metabolite and its binding capacity to receptor sites is still unclear (Marder et al. 1989a).

2.3 Present Situation

The relevance of including measurement of pharmacologically active metabolites has, for example, been investigated and discussed for chlorpromazine (Mackay et al. 1974; Wode-Helgodt and Alfredsson 1981), thioridazine (Axelsson and Mårtensson 1983; Mårtensson and Nyberg 1989), and levomepromazine (Loennechen et al. 1990). Extensive reviews have been published on this subject (Dahl 1981, 1982, 1986). It is usually hypothesized that some of these metabolites contribute to the therapeutic and/or toxic effects of the phenothiazine neuroleptics. However, today no definitive information exists on this matter.

Presently there is no consensus on the utility of monitoring plasma concentrations of these phenothiazines, with or without active metabolites. Some investigators consider that such an approach is not useful when administering these compounds (Balant-Gorgia and Balant 1987; Dahl 1986), whereas others have found measurement of the parent compound alone useful for therapeutic drug monitoring. There is, however, better agreement on the usefulness of monitoring plasma concentrations of haloperidol, fluphenazine, perphenazine, thiothixene, flupentixol, and zuclopenthixol. This position is, however, susceptible to modification as new information becomes available.

3 Demethylated Metabolites of Tricyclic Antidepressants

3.1 Routine Plasma Concentration Monitoring

When monitoring concentrations of amitriptyline, imipramine, or clomipramine, it is now usual to measure also the demethylated metabolites and to relate the clinical and unwanted effects to the sum of the parent compound and its active metabolite. This procedure could be criticized on the ground that their physicochemical properties (important for blood/brain partitioning) and their pharmacological profiles are different and, as a consequence, that they contribute to the antidepressive effect in a way that is not simply related to the sum of their plasma concentrations. Presently the answer to this question is based on the rather pragmatic observation that such an approach is probably more appropriate than neglecting one of the two "partners." As discussed below for clomipramine, the respective concentrations of the two active moieties greatly differ among individuals and their sum represents probably the most reliable parameter to estimate the amount of "pharmacological activity" present in the blood of patients. It could thus be advocated that nonspecific methods based, for example, on immunological techniques could be a valid alternative to the use of specific chemical methods. In our opinion this is not correct since the relative importance of parent drug and demethylated metabolite are indicative of potential pharmacokinetic anomalies.

3.2 Prediction of Steady-State Concentrations

At the end of the 1970s considerable interest was raised by the possibility of predicting steady-state concentrations of tricyclic antidepressants from a single test dose. The rationale of this approach was that the gradual increase in daily dose could delay response (Brunswick et al. 1979) and that the search for a reliable kinetic predictor for clinical response which could be easily adapted for routine use in inpatients and outpatients would contribute to maximize the antidepressant effect and reduce the risk of toxicity (Montgomery et al. 1979). Among the parameters crucial for accurate prediction are the time between administration of the "spot dose" and sampling, the elimination half-life, and linearity of disposition kinetics (Slattery et al. 1980). The methods proposed for maintenance-dose prediction may work for nortriptyline and desipramine (Nelson et al. 1987). For clomipramine, the fact that the apparent elimination half-life of clomipramine is about 24 h and that of desmethyl-clomipramine about 96 h renders this approach quite difficult to apply. In addition, it has been shown that the pharmacokinetics of imipramine show considerable nonlinearity (Brøsen et al. 1986; Sindrup et al. 1990); this is probably a serious drawback for any method designed to predict steady-state concentrations using a single-dose/single-point approach. Recently it has also been shown that desipramine exhibits substancial nonlinear kinetics in about 30% of patients (Nelson and Jatlow 1987) and the linearity of the kinetics of amitriptyline and nortriptyline has been questioned (Vandel et al. 1989, 1990). An additional factor which might complicate this matter is the well known fact that hydroxylation of tricyclic antidepressants is under the control of a polymorphic enzymatic system (see Brøsen, this volume).

3.3 Concentration–Effects Relationships

The existence of linear or curvilinear concentration–effect relationships for tricyclic antidepressants has been extensively investigated. The situation found for clomipramine is representative of the difficulty inherent to this type of exercise. Both a linear (Faravelli et al. 1984) and a curvilinear (Broadhurst et al. 1977; Della Corte et al. 1979; Vandel et al. 1982) relationship between clinical effect and concentrations of clomipramine (CLO) and/or desmethyl-clomipramine (DECLO) have been described. Vandel et al. (1982) noted a relationship between clinical response and plasma concentrations of CLO, DECLO, and the sum of the two compounds, whereas Della Corte et al. (1979) found a relationship only with the metabolite. Reisby et al. (1979) observed a relationship between clinical outcome and concentration only for the parent compound in one group of patients and no relationship at all in another: in the first group of patients, the relation was apparently curvilinear if total Hamilton scores were used, but linear if a subset of items was utilized. Finally, some investigators have failed to detect any relationship (Jones and Luscombe 1976; Montgomery et al. 1980; Moyes et al. 1980).

3.4 Metabolic Ratios

Despite the complicated interchange between concentrations of dimethylated parent compound and demethylated metabolite, involving demethylation and hydroxylation, clinically relevant information can be obtained from the analysis of the ratio of parent compound to metabolite under steady-state conditions.

As an example, the following rules can be derived for clomipramine: (1) Under normal conditions, the ratio CLO/DECLO is about 0.4, indicating that DECLO concentrations are about 2.5 times higher than those of CLO. (2) In patients showing poor hydroxylation capacities of the debrisoquine/sparteine phenotype the ratio may be decreased to 0.2 with a marked relative increase of DECLO levels (Balant-Gorgia et al. 1989). (3) Concomitant phenothiazine administration may transform an extensive hydroxylator into a poor hydroxylator with the same consequences as for the debrisoquine/sparteine polymorphism. (4) Liver insufficiency or chronic alcohol abuse may lead to an "inversion" of the ratio with values higher than 1, indicating low demethylation and relatively normal hydroxylation (Balant-Gorgia, unpublished observations). (5) Noncompliance or partial compliance is often associated with ratios close to 1, since CLO ($t_{1/2}$ = about 24 h) steady-state concentrations are reached faster than DECLO concentrations ($t_{1/2}$ = about 96 h).

Similar findings have been published for imipramine (IMI)/desipramine (DMI) with normal values for IMI/DMI around 0.85 and poor metabolizers showing decreased ratios of about 0.085. It has been advocated that the ratio IMI/DMI might be useful as an indicator of the effectiveness of a treatment with IMI (Rigal et al. 1987). It is, however, presently not clear whether a ratio within the "normal" range is an indicator of an optimum proportion of the two "therapeutic ingredients" or if ratios outside this range are indicative of pharmacokinetic problems which may interfere with the therapeutic effect, due to too low or too high concentrations of the active moieties.

3.5 Present Situations

Normal practice for starting tricyclic therapy is a progressive increase of the daily dose over about 1 week. This procedure is applied whether or not drug level monitoring facilities are available. The single-dose/single point method requires that the clinical laboratory be equipped with appropriate methods to assay samples at low concentration and to provide rapid turnabout time for results (Nelson et al. 1989). This is certainly technically feasible, however, despite more than 10 years of investigations this procedure has not been clearly validated as far as faster clinical response is considered. This is probably due to the fact that many factors other than drug concentration play a decisive role in this process; among those the "therapeutic alliance" between physician and patient probably are just as important in achieving rapid relief of the symptoms of depression.

As far as data interpretation is concerned, it is probable that no clear-cut and univocal "correlation" (in the statistical sense) will ever be found between concentrations of tricyclic drugs and/or their desmethylated derivatives since, in our opinion, the clinical endpoints cannot be reduced to a "percentual decrease of a depression score after 4 weeks." Accordingly, the concept of a therapeutic concentration range in which the greatest proportion of patients have a good probability to respond to therapy without suffering life threatening side effects remains the most robust concept for data interpretation in therapeutic drug monitoring of antidepressant medication.

Drug to metabolite ratios represent, despite their shortcomings, an elegant way to detect metabolic anomalies or compliance problems. Analytical methods allowing separate quantification of the two types of species should be used for drug monitoring.

4 Hydroxylated Metabolites of Tricyclic Antidepressants

4.1 Historical Perspective

The role of active metabolites of tricyclic antidepressants was discussed 10 years ago by Potter (1981), who stated that "the boundaries of moving from in vitro potency to a clinical situation have not been defined" and that "it is unlikely that comparison of sums, ratios, or weighted proportions of tertiary and secondary amines plus hydroxylated metabolites with effect(s) will provide the precise demonstrations that are needed." It must be realized that 10 years later our understanding of the role of hydroxylated metabolites of tricyclic antidepressants has not progressed much, despite a considerable number of investigations. One of the problems, already mentioned by Potter, is that most hydroxylated metabolites of these drugs are not approved for administration to humans. Accordingly, our knowledge about their kinetics and the variables susceptible to modify their behavior stems only from indirect observations.

The difficulties encountered in such investigations is well demonstrated by two studies performed by Nelson et al. (1983, 1988a). In the first study (1983), a fixed dose of DMI was administered, and the results suggested that 2-hydroxy-desipramine (2-OH-DMI) concentrations contributed little to the drug's effect. In the second study (1988a), DMI concentration variability was controlled with a flexible dose regimen, and a contribution of 2-OH-

DMI to the correlation between drug levels and antidepressant response was observed. Although response was correlated more strongly with DMI levels alone, the strongest correlation for each measure of response was with total DMI + 2-OH-DMI. Finally, the authors reported that in their study DMI threshold concentrations were just as useful as total drug levels in discriminating between responders and nonresponders. One of the reasons for this finding may be that, contrary to the situation observed with nortriptyline, the concentrations of 2-OH-DMI are usually much lower than those of the parent compound (Potter et al. 1982; Sutfin et al. 1988). In addition it was found that the concentrations of hydroxydesipramine were higher in patients over 60 years than in younger patients, but that the differences were not clinically relevant (Nelson et al. 1988b). The same applies for the hydroxylated metabolites of CLO and DECLO (Balant-Gorgia et al. 1986; Gex-Fabry et al. 1990; Linnoila et al. 1982).

In view of the numerous methodological problems encountered with hydroxylated metabolites of tricyclic antidepressants and in order to limit the present discussion, only one example will be presented (i.e., hydroxy-nortriptyline) because in recent years one of these compounds has been available for administration to healthy volunteers (Bertilsson et al. 1986).

4.2 Stereospecific Metabolism

Due to the double bond linking of the side chain to the ring system of amitriptyline and nortriptyline, 10-hydroxylation may be stereospecific (Mellström et al. 1981; Bock et al. 1982). The disposition of nortriptyline has been particularly well investigated and studies in patients at steady-state have been performed, during which hydroxy-nortriptylines were measured (Nordin et al. 1987). *Trans*(E)-10-hydroxy-nortriptyline (E-10-OH-NT) is the major metabolite in humans, whereas *cis*(Z)-10-hydroxy-nortriptyline is pharmacokinetically of minor importance. By measuring the excretion of nortriptyline metabolites in urine, it was shown that the metabolic clearance of nortriptyline by hydroxylation in the E-position, but not in the Z-position, correlated even better with the debrisoquine metabolic ratio than the total clearance of nortriptyline (Mellström et al. 1981). E-10-OH-NT itself has a chiral center that gives rise to two enantiomers. This compound is about 50% as potent as nortriptyline as an inhibitor of the neuronal uptake of noradrenaline in vitro. However, it has much less affinity to muscarinic receptors in vitro and also fewer anticholinergic side effects (Bertilsson et al. 1989). In addition, compared with the parent compound, the disposition of E-10-OH-NT exhibits less variation between individuals per se, because it is eliminated by glucuroconjugation and as the unchanged substance in urine and not by polymorphic hydroxylation, as is the case for nortriptyline. Due to its pharmacodynamic and pharmacokinetic properties, it has been advocated to develop this compound as a novel antidepressant with particular usefulness in elderly patients (Bertilsson et al. 1989). However, other authors have linked cardiotoxicity to elevated concentrations of 10-OH-NT in elderly patients (Schneider et al. 1988; Young et al. 1988). Accordingly, this matter is far from being fully clarified (Pollock and Perel 1989). With the objective to develop E-10-OH-NT as a novel antidepressant, the disposition of racemic E-10-OH-NT has been studied in healthy volunteers (Dahl-Puustinen et al. 1989). Results indicate that first-pass glucuronidation and tubular secretion of this substance are enantioselective, but that the debrisoquine hydroxylation status was not associated with the investigated kinetic processes.

The series of investigations related here are a good illustration of the complexity of tricyclic antidepressant metabolism in relation to the search for possible relationships between plasma concentrations and effects.

4.3 Present Situation

It has been shown that the plasma concentrations of 10-OH-nortriptylines often exceed those of the parent drug during nortriptyline treatment and that CSF concentrations are comparable, showing that 10-OH-NTs pass into the central nervous system (Bertilsson et al. 1983). In view of the possible clinical and/or toxic effects of these metabolites, the question is thus raised as to the potential usefulness of measuring these metabolites for routine nortriptyline concentration monitoring. Presently this seems not to be the case in the great majority of laboratories although it may be particularly useful in elderly patients or patients with renal insufficiency (Schneider et al. 1990).

For the other tricyclic antidepressants, routine plasma or full blood concentration monitoring can be performed ignoring the concentrations of the hydroxylated compounds. It is, however, strongly suggested that for research purposes these metabolites should always be measured. Neglecting their presence may lead to artifactual conclusions, in particular in patients with pharmacokinetic anomalies. This has recently been suggested by Stern et al. (1991) for 2-hydroxy-DMI.

5 Reduced Haloperidol

5.1 Pharmacokinetics

Haloperidol (HAL) is metabolized in humans by cleavage of the molecule by oxidative dealkylation. HAL is also metabolized via reversible reduction transforming a ketone function to its alcohol. In recent years numerous investigators have studied interconversion between HAL and its reduced metabolite (REHAL), first in animals and later in humans (Froemming et al. 1989). It is interesting to note that the human studies in healthy volunteers needed the development of sensitive and specific analytical methods since, for obvious reasons, they have to be performed using very low doses of the drug or its metabolite (Midha et al. 1988). It appears in Caucasians that the overall interconversion favors reduction of HAL to its metabolite in most of the subjects (Chang et al. 1991), although there may be exceptions (Chakraborty et al. 1989). When analyzing pharmacokinetic data and calculating REHAL/HAL ratios great care must be taken not to reach conclusions based on artifacts. The first problem is encountered with the determination of the half-life of the two compounds. If, for practical reasons and clinical purposes, one may assume that the elimination of HAL is about 24 h, this is not true from a strict pharmacokinetic point of view since the "apparent elimination half-life" tends to increase with time, probably reflecting the interconversion of the two compounds. The second problem arises when comparing areas under the curves (AUCs) measured after the administration of a single dose or steady-state concentrations. As an example, Midha et al. (1989) could detect REHAL in only 6 out of 28 subjects after a single dose of HAL, whereas Shostak et al. (1987) and Ko et al. (1989) measured REHAL in all of their 17 and 15 patients, respectively. They observed REHAL/HAL ratios ranging from 0.25 to 4.75. In contrast Altamura et al. (1989) found 5 out of 30 patients with no detectable metabolite concentrations.

5.2 Interethnic Differences?

Steady-state concentrations have been measured in a variety of patients and the ratio of REHAL/HAL shows high interindividual variability. If an arbitrary cut-off point of one is taken, 3 out of 17, 12 out of 15, or 19 out of 30 patients had a ratio lower than one in the studies of Shostak, Ko, and Altamura, respectively. The numbers of patients included in these studies are clearly too low to permit extrapolations about the distribution of this ratio in the general population. Accordingly, it is difficult to compare this type of results to those of Chang et al. (1987), reporting that all of their 12 Chinese patients had a ratio below 0.5, or those of Someya et al. (1990), reporting that 37 out of 45 Japanese patients had relatively low ratios (mean 0.42) and that the distribution was bimodal. This problem is certainly worth further investigation since it appears that in Chinese patients (Potkin et al. 1984) HAL concentrations are more elevated and that Asians in general need lower doses of antipsychotic drugs than non-Asians (Lin and Finder 1983). In contrast, there seems to be no difference in kinetics of HAL between black and white healthy subjects (Midha et al. 1989).

5.3 Clinical Relevance

In different pharmacological models REHAL has been found to be considerably less active than its parent compound. Thus, the apparent activity of the metabolite is, at least in part, attributable to its conversion into HAL. As a consequence, it is very difficult to separate the intrinsic activity of the two compounds. At the present time there is still controversy about the shape of the dose-response curve of HAL and its therapeutic and toxic plasma level ranges. It is thus possible that REHAL contributes to the difficulty in establishing these parameters. The available information on the possible role of REHAL is still preliminary since, as stated by Dahl (1990), certain conditions should have been fulfilled in order to obtain clinically useful results from studies investigating plasma drug concentrations vs effect relationships, and the number of patients investigated has been limited.

5.4 Present Situation

The therapeutic range for HAL seems reasonably well established on the basis of the concentrations of the parent compound alone. For normal "routine" monitoring there is probaly no need to include measurements of the reduced metabolite. However, if the simultaneous measurement is feasible, it should be performed in well defined patient subgroups in order to try to better assess the clinical relevance of high, medium, or low concentrations of the metabolite or the potential importance of the metabolic ratio.

6 Miscellaneous Questions

6.1 Clozapine

Until recently, clozapine concentration monitoring has received little attention due to its relatively confined use. However, in a recent paper Lovdahl et al. (1991) have described a method for the measurement of clozapine and its active metabolite *N*-desmethyl-clozapine. Since blood samples are obligatorily taken for cell counts, it would be interesting to measure the parent compound and metabolite in order to gain more insight into possible concentration-effect relationships.

6.2 Fluoxetine

The half-life of the desmethyl metabolite of fluoxetine (norfluoxetine) is long (approximately 6–14 days), but steady-state levels were, interestingly, observed at 3 weeks. Plasma concentrations of parent compound and metabolite have been found to be of the same order of magnitude. Exploration of relationships between clinical effect and plasma concentrations suggest that fluoxetine may contribute very little to the response and that the active pharmacological agent is norfluoxetine (Montgomery et al. 1990). In this case, fluoxetine would be an (inactive?) prodrug. Clearly, as with other psychotropic agents, more information is needed before this information can be fully validated.

6.3 Depot Neuroleptics

From a pharmacokinetic point of view, depot neuroleptics are inactive prodrugs which have to be bioconverted to their active moiety. It seems that the ester bond used for this class of drugs is labile in the plasma and/or liver, showing no detectable interindividual variability. There are two practical consequences of the slow release from the depot and the rapid hydrolysis of these prodrugs. The first is the well known "flip-flop" kinetics of depot neuroleptics and the second is the lack of first-pass metabolism. The potential differences in "metabolite spectrum" after oral and depot administration have not been thoroughly investigated and results have often been conflicting (Marder et al. 1989b). In a recent study performed with fluphenazine it was found that sulfoxidation of the parent compound is likely to be a much more important factor for patients treated with oral as opposed to a depot phenothiazine (Marder et al. 1989a). However, as stated by these authors, determining the clinical importance of such findings will be a difficult challenge.

6.4 Stereospecific Metabolism of Flupentixol

Flupentixol represents a rare case in pharmaceutical chemistry. The oral form is a 1:1 mixture of *cis*(Z)-flupentixol (the active isomer) and *trans*(E)-flupentixol which is inactive, whereas the depot formulation contains only the active form. The two isomers are not biotransformed at the same rate and these rates vary in individual patients (Balant-Gorgia et al. 1987). As a consequence, steady-state ratios of *trans*(E)/*cis*(Z) concentrations are not constant around one, but the inactive isomer is usually present at higher concentrations than the active compound. The "isomeric ratio" varies from 0.75 to 6.0 with about 60% of the patients showing values between 1.5 and 2.5. As a consequence, total concentrations of flupentixol are a poor reflection of the concentration of the active moiety. An additional problem is raised when comparisons between oral and depot administrations are based, respectively, on total concentrations (i.e., *cis*+*trans*) and on *cis*(Z)-flupentixol concentrations only. It is thus recommended to use a stereospecific capillary column GC method for therapeutic drug monitoring of this neuroleptic.

7 Implication for the Choice of Analytical Methods

7.1 Receptor Assays

As discussed by Jørgensen in 1986, an increasing number of investigators are trying to avoid the problems raised by active metabolites of neuroleptics by measuring "activity" in plasma using a radioreceptor assay based on dopamine receptors from the corpus striatum and regarding this activity as a measure of therapeutic moiety concentration. This approach will, of course, give the combined activity of the parent drug and its metabolites in plasma, but since the ratio of parent drug to metabolites is most certainly very different in the plasma and in the brain, because of differences in lipophilicity, this activity cannot be used as a measure of the drug concentration in the brain. In addition, radioreceptor assays presently lack the sensitivity and the reproducibility that are required for therapeutic monitoring. As a conclusion, Jørgensen stated that the radioreceptor assay is no alternative to separate measurement of all active compounds in plasma by specific analytical methods. The same conclusions were reached by Guthrie et al. (1987).

7.2 Immunoassays

Immunoassays have good sensitivity and are usually easy to perform. HAL and its reduced metabolite illustrate the problem encountered with immunoassays since the antibody does not distinguish between the two compounds. The method thus depends on an elaborate scheme for the extraction, derivatization, and separation of the two substances (Browning et al. 1985). In addition, immunoassays may be expensive if they are used for daily monitoring, which may require a full calibration curve for one or two samples.

7.3 Chemical Methods

Usually, drug monitoring is based on plasma concentrations. We have introduced whole blood measurements for tricyclic antidepressants in order to overcome any problem related to ex vivo plasma-erythrocyte "repartitioning," although plasma and whole blood concentrations seem to be very close. This is, however, not necessarily always the case, as illustrated for REHAL which seems to accumulate significantly in red blood cells (Ko et al. 1989). It has also been advocated to measure neuroleptics in CSF or in plasma water. The first approach, although theoretically interesting, is clearly not possible for routine measurements. The use of free concentrations in plasma has received little attention up to now (Garver 1989) and it is thus difficult to predict if the potential added value for clinical monitoring would outweigh the added time and expense required to prepare the sample and perform the assay.

As far as the relative values of gas chromatography (GC) and high pressure liquid chromatography (HPLC) are concerned, GC methods are usually faster, but they often do not allow the possibility to measure all metabolites. However, caution is also necessary with HPLC methods as demonstrated by Midha et al. (1987a) for the simultaneous measurement of chlorpromazine and six of its presumably active metabolites.

7.4 Present Situation

As pointed out by Jørgensen (1986), we believe that the use of specific chemical methods is still preferable for drug monitoring of extensively metabolized psychoactive substances. In addition to providing reliable estimates of the concentrations of the different molecular species, they also allow the detection of other, potentially interfering, lipophilic xenobiotics which may be indicative of parallel medication intake. GC is a reliable method for routine clinical measurements of tricyclic antidepressants and neuroleptics such as HAL, flupentixol, or zuclopenthixol. For research purposes, or for drugs showing many metabolites, HPLC might be preferable. In our opinion, the value of immunological identification and quantification remains to be demonstrated.

8 Conclusions

Tricyclic antidepressants and neuroleptics have been available for about 30 years, but many questions related to their metabolites remain unanswered as far as therapeutic monitoring is concerned. One of the issues that has found no general consensus is the potential utility of drug concentration monitoring, despite the fact that in centers where this approach is available there seems to be an agreement among physicians that the method is useful for many patients. One of the key issues to be solved before agreement can be reached is the role of active metabolites and the best way to use this information when it becomes available. As a consequence, more efforts should be undertaken to measure active metabolites in plasma of patients for which therapeutic monitoring is performed in order to increase the basic knowledge on the interplay between parent drug and active metabolites, their pharmacokinetic and pharmacodynamic properties, and their respective impacts on therapeutic and unwanted effects. When developing new psychotropic drugs, great care should be taken not to neglect these aspects and to perform, as early as possible, ad hoc studies during phase I, II, and III clinical trials.

References

Altamura AC, Mauri M, Cavallaro R, Regazzetti MG, Bareggi SR (1989) Hydroxyhaloperidol and clinical outcome in schizophrenia. In: Dahl SG, Gram LF (eds) Clinical pharmacology in psychiatry. Springer Berlin Heidelberg New York, pp 263–268 (Psychopharmacology series 7)

Axelsson R, Mårtensson E (1983) Clinical effects related to the serum concentrations of thioridazine and its metabolites. In: Gram LF, Usdin E, Dahl SG, Krag-Sørensen P, Sjöqvist F, Morselli PL (eds) Clinical pharmacology in psychiatry. Macmillan, London, pp 165–174

Balant-Gorgia AE, Balant LP (1987) Antipsychotic drugs: Clinical pharmacokinetics of potential candidates for plasma concentration monitoring. Clin Pharmacokinet 13:65–90

Balant-Gorgia AE, Balant LP, Genet C, Dayer P, Aeschlimann JM, Garrone G (1986) Importance of oxidative polymorphism and levomepromazine treatment on the steady-state blood concentrations of clomipramine and its major metabolites. Eur J Clin Pharmacol 31:449–455

Balant-Gorgia AE, Balant LP, Gex-Fabry M, Genet C (1987) Stereoselective disposition of flupentixol: influence on steady-state plasma concentrations in schizophrenic patients. Eur J Drug Metab Pharmacokinet 12:123–128

Balant-Gorgia AE, Balant LP, Garrone G (1989) High blood concentrations of imipramine or clomipramine and therapeutic failure: a case report study using drug monitoring data. Ther Drug Monit 11:415–420

Bertilsson L, Mellström B, Nordin C, Siwers B, Sjöqvist F (1983) Stereospecific 10-hydroxylation of nortriptyline: genetic aspects and importance for biochemical and clinical effects. In: Gram LF, Usdin E, Dahl SG, Krag-Sørensen P, Sjöqvist F, Morselli PL (eds) Clinical pharmacology in psychiatry. Macmillan, London, pp 217–226

Bertilsson L, Nordin C, Otani K, Resul B, Scheinin M, Siwers B, Sjöqvist F (1986) Disposition of single oral doses of E-10-hydroxynortriptyline in healthy subjects, with some observations on pharmacodynamic effects. Clin Pharmacol Ther 40:261–267

Bertilsson L, Dahl-Puustinen ML, Nordin C (1989) E-10-hydroxynortriptyline: effects and disposition of a potential novel antidepressant. In: Dahl SG, Gram LF (eds) Clinical pharmacology in psychiatry. Springer, Berlin Heidelberg New York, pp 52–59 (Psychopharmacology series 7)

Bock JL, Giller E, Gray S, Jatlow P (1982) Steady-state plasma concentrations of cis- and trans-10-OH-amitriptyline metabolites. Clin Pharmacol Ther 31:609–616

Broadhurst AD, James HD, Della Corte L, Heeley AF (1977) Clomipramine plasma level and clinical response. Postgrad Med J 53 Suppl 4:139–145

Brøsen K, Gram LF, Klysner R, Bech P (1986) Steady-state levels of imipramine and its metabolites: significance of dose-dependent kinetics. Eur J Clin Pharmacol 30:43–49

Browning JL, Harrington CA, Davis CM (1985) Quantification of reduced haloperidol and haloperidol by radioimmunoassay. J Immunoassay 6:45–66

Brunswick DJ, Amsterdam JD, Mendels J, Stern SL (1979) Prediction of steady-state imipramine and desmethylimipramine plasma concentrations from single-dose data. Clin Pharmacol Ther 25:605–610

Chakraborty BS, Hubbard JW, Hawes EM, McKay G, Cooper JK, Gurnsey T, Korchinsky ED, Midha KK (1989) Interconversion between haloperidol and reduced haloperidol in healthy volunteers. Eur J Clin Pharmacol 37:45–48

Chang WH, Chen TY, Lee CF, Hu WH, Yeh EK (1987) Low plasma reduced haloperido/haloperidol ratios in Chinese patients. Biol Psychiatry 22:1406–1408

Chang WH, Lin SK, Jann MW (1991) Interconversion between haloperidol and reduced haloperidol in schizophrenic patients and guinea pigs: a steady-state study. J Clin Psychopharmacol 11:99–105

Dahl SG (1981) Active metabolites of phenothiazine drugs. In: Usdin E, Dahl SG, Gram LF, Lingjaerde O (eds) Clinical pharmacology in psychiatry. Macmillan, London, pp 125–137

Dahl SG (1982) Actives metabolites of neuroleptic drugs: possible contribution to therapeutic and toxic effects. In: Raven, New York 4:33–40

Dahl SG (1986) Plasma level monitoring of antipsychotic drugs clinical utility. Clin Pharmacol 11:36–61

Dahl SG (1990) Conditions for meaningful plasma level monitoring of neuroleptics. In: Stefanis CN, Rabavilas AD, Soldatos CR (eds) Psychiatry: a world perspective, vol 3. Excerpta Medica, Amsterdam

Dahl SG, Hjorth M, Hough E (1981) Chlorpromazine, metrotrimeprazine, and metabolites. Structural changes accompanying the loss of neuroleptic potency by ring sulfoxidation. Mol Pharmacol 21:409–414

Dahl SG, Hals PA, Johnsen H, Morel E, Lloyd KG (1982) Possible role of hydroxymetabolites in the action of neuroleptics. In: Gram LF, Usdin E, Dahl SG Krag-Sørensen P, Sjöqvist F, Morselli PL (eds) Clinical pharmacology in psychiatry. Macmillan, London, pp 136–149

Dahl-Puustinen ML, Perry TL, Dumont E, von Bahr C, Nordin C, Bertilsson L (1989) Stereoselective disposition of racemin E-10-hydroxynortriptyline in human beings. Clin Pharmacol Ther 45:650–656

Della Corte L, Broadhurst AD, Sgaragli GP, Filippini S, Heeley AF, Faravelli C, Pazzagli A (1979) Clinical response and tricyclic plasma levels during treatment with clomipramine. Br J Psychiatry 134:390–400

Faravelli C, Ballerini A, Ambonetti A, Broadhurst AD, Das M (1984) Plasma levels and clinical response during treatment with clomipramine. J Affect Dis 6:95–107

Froemming JS, Francis Lam YW, Jann MW, Davis CM (1989) Pharmacokinetics of haloperidol. Clin Pharmacokinet 17:396–423

Garver DL (1989) Neuroleptic drug levels and antipsychotic effects: a difficult correlation; potential advantage of free (or derivative) versus total plasma levels. J Clin Psychopharmacol 9:277–281

Gex-Fabry M, Balant-Gorgia A, Balant LP, Garrone G (1990) Clomipramine metabolism: model-based analysis of variability factors from drug monitoring data. Clin Pharmacokinet 19:241–255

Guthrie S, Lane EA, Linnoila M (1987) Monitoring of plasma drug concentrations in clinical psychopharmacology. In: Mellzer HY (ed) Psychopharmacology: the third generation of progress. Raven, New York, pp 1323–1338

Jones RB, Luscombe DK (1976) Plasma levels of clomipramine and its N-desmethyl metabolite following oral administration of clomipramine in man. Br J Pharmacol 57:430P

Jørgensen A (1986) Metabolism and pharmacokinetics of antipsychotic drugs. Prog Drug Metab 9:111–174

Ko GN, Korpi ER, Kirch DG (1989) Haloperidol and reduced haloperidol concentrations in plasma and red blood cells from chronic schizophrenic patients. J Clin Psychopharmacol 9:186–190

Lin KM, Finder E (1983) Neuroleptic dosage for Asians. Am J Psychiatry 140:490–491

Linnoila M, Insel T, Kilts C, Potter WZ, Murphy DL (1982) Plasma steady-state concentrations of hydroxylated metabolites of clomipramine. Clin Pharmacol Ther 32:208–211

Loennechen T, Andersen A, Hals PA, Dahl SG (1990) High-performance liquid chromatographic determination of levomepromazine (metrotrimeprazine) and its mains metabolites in serum and urine. Ther Drug Monit 12:574–581

Lovdahl MJ, Perry PJ, Miller DD (1991) The assay of clozapine and N-Desmethylclozapine in human plasma by high-performance liquid chromatography. Ther Drug Monit 13:69–72

Mackay AVP, Heeley AF, Baker J (1974) The relationship of plasma chlorpromazine to its 7-hydroxy and sulphoxide metabolites in a large population of chronic schizophrenics. Br J Clin Pharmacol 1:425–430

Marder SR, Van Putten T, Aravagiri M (1989a) Plasma level monitoring for maintenance neuroleptic therapy. In: Dahl SG, Gram LF (eds) Clinical pharmacology in psychiatry. Springer, Berlin Heidelberg New York, pp 269–279 (Psychopharmacology series 7)

Marder SR, Hubbard JW, Van Putten T, Midha KK (1989b) Pharmacokinetics of long-acting injectable neuroleptic drugs: Clinical implications. Psychopharmacology (Berl) 98:433–439

Mårtensson E, Nyberg G (1989) Active metabolites of neuroleptics in plasma and CSF: Implications for therapeutic drug monitoring. In: Dahl SG, Gram LF (eds) Clinical pharmacology in psychiatry. Springer Berlin Heidelberg New York, pp 257–262 (Psychopharmacology series 7)

Mellström B, Bertilsson L, Säwe J, Schulz HU, Sjöqvist F (1981) E- and Z-10-hydroxylation of nortriptyline: relationship to polymorphic debrisoquine hydroxylation. Clin Pharmacol Ther 30:189–193

Midha KK, Hubbard JW, Cooper JK, Gurnsey T, Hawes EM, McKay G, Chakraborty BS, Yeung PKF (1987a) Therapeutic monitoring of chlorpromazine IV: comparison of a new high-performance liquid chromatographic method with radioimmunoassays for parent drug and some of its major metabolites. Ther Drug Monit 9:358–365

Midha KK, Hubbard JW, Marder SR, Hawes EM, Van Putten T, McKay G, May PRA (1987b) The sulfoxidation of fluphenazine in schizophrenic patients maintained on fluphenazine decanoate. Psychopharmacology (Berl) 93:369–373

Midha KK, Cooper JK, Hawes EM, Hubbard JW, Korchinski ED, McKay G (1988) An ultrasensitive method for measurement of haloperidol and reduced haloperidol in plasma by high-performance liquid chromatography with coulometric detection. Ther Drug Monit 10:177–183

Midha KK, Chakraborty BS, Ganes DA, Hawes EM, Hubbard JW, Keegan DL, Korchinski ED, McKay G (1989) Intersubject variation in the pharmacokinetics of haloperidol and reduced haloperidol. J Clin Psychopharmacol 9:98–104

Montgomery SA, McAuley R, Montgomery DB, Braithwaite RA, Dawling S (1979) Dosage adjustment from simple nortriptyline spot level predictor tests in depressed patients. Clin Pharmacokinet 4:129–136

Montgomery SA, McAuley R, Montgomery DB, Dawling S, Braithwaite RA (1980) Plasma concentration of clomipramine and desmethylclomipramine and clinical response in depressed patients. Postgrad Med J 56 Suppl 1:130–133

Montgomery SA, Baldwin D, Shah A, Fineberg N, Montgomery D (1990) Plasma-level response with fluoxetine and zimelidine. Clin Neuropharmacol 13 Suppl 1:S71–S75

Moyes ICA, Ray RL, Moyes RB (1980) Plasma levels and clinical improvement: a comparative study of clomipramine and amitriptyline in depression. Postgrad Med J 56 Suppl 1:127–129

Nelson JC, Jatlow PI (1987) Nonlinear desipramine kinetics: prevalence and importance. Clin Pharmacol Ther 6:666–670

Nelson JC, Bock JL, Jatlow PI (1983) Clinical implications of 2-hydroxydesipramine plasma concentrations. Clin Pharmacol Ther 33:183–189

Nelson JC, Jatlow PI, Mazure C (1987) Rapid desipramine dose adjustment using 24-hour levels. Clin Psychopharmacol 7:72–77

Nelson JC, Mazure C, Jatlow PI (1988a) Antidepressant activity of 2-hydroxydesipramine. Clin Pharmacol Ther 44:283–288

Nelson JC, Atillasoy E, Mazure C, Jatlow PI (1988b) Hydroxydesipramine in the elderly. J Clin Psychopharmacol 8:428–433

Nelson JC, Mazure C, Jatlow PI (1989) Clinical implications of the pharmacokinetics of tricyclic antidepressants. In: Dahl SG, Gram LF (eds) Clinical pharmacology in

psychiatry. Springer, Berlin Heidelberg New York, pp 219–227 (Psychopharmacology series 7)
Nordin C, Bertilsson L, Siwers B (1987) Clinical and biochemical effects during treatment of depression with nortriptyline: the role of 10-hydroxynortriptyline. Clin Pharmacol Ther 42:10–19
Pollock BG, Perel JM (1989) Hydroxy metabolites of tricyclic antidepressants: evaluation of relative cardiotoxicity. In: Dahl SG, Gram LF (eds) Clinical pharmacology in psychiatry. Springer, Berlin Heidelberg New York, pp 232–236 (Psychopharmacology series 7)
Potkin DG, Shen YC, Pardes H, Phelps BH, Zhou DF, Shu L, Korpi ER, Wyatt RJ (1984) Haloperidol concentration elevated in Chinese patients. Psychiatry Res 12:167–172
Potter WZ (1981) Active metabolites of tricyclic antidepressants. In: Usdin E, Dahl SG, Gram LF, Lingjaerde O (eds) Clinical pharmacology in psychiatry. Macmillan, London, pp 139–153
Potter WZ, Calil HM, Sutfin TA, Zavadil AP, Jusko WJ, Rapoport J, Goodwin FK (1982) Active metabolites of imipramine and desipramine. Clin Pharmacol Ther 31:393–401
Reisby N, Gram LF, Bech P, Sihm F, Krautwald O, Elley J, Christiansen J (1979) Clomipramine: plasma levels and clinical effects. Commun Psychopharmacol 3:341–351
Rigal JG, Albin HC, Duchier AR, D'Aulnay JM, Fenelon JH, Vincon GA, Demotes-Mainard FM (1987) Imipramine blood levels and clinical outcome. J Clin Psychopharmacol 7:222–229
Schneider LS, Cooper TB, Severson JA, Zemplenyi T, Sloane RB (1988) Electrocardiographic changes with nortriptyline and 10-hydroxynortriptyline in elderly depressed outpatients. J Clin Psychopharmacol 8:402–408
Schneider LS, Cooper TB, Suckow RF, Lyness SA, Haugen C, Palmer R, Sloane RB (1990) Relationship of hydroxynortriptyline to nortriptyline concentration and creatinine clearance in depressed elderly outpatients. J Clin Psychopharmacol 10:333–337
Shostak M, Perel JM, Stiller RL, Wyman W, Curran S (1987) Plasma haloperidol and clinical response. A role for reduced haloperidol in antipsychotic activity? J Clin Psychopharmacol 7:394–400
Sindrup SH, Brøsen K, Gram LF (1990) Nonlinear kinetics of imipramine in low and medium plasma level ranges. Ther Drug Monit 12:445–449
Slattery JT, Gibaldi M, Koup JR (1980) Prediction of maintenance dose required to attain a desired drug concentration at steady-state from a single determination of concentration after an initial dose. Clin Pharmacokinet 5:377–385
Someya T, Takahashi S, Shibasaki M, Inaba T, Cheung SW, Tang SW (1990) Reduced haloperidol/haloperidol ratios in plasma: polymorphism in Japanese psychiatric patients. Psychiatry Res 31:111–120
Stern SL, Ribner HS, Cooper TB, Nelson LD, Johnson MH, Suckow RF (1991) 2-Hydroxydesipramine and desipramine plasma levels and electrocardiographic effects in depressed younger adults. J Clin Psychopharmacol 11:93–98
Sutfin TA, Perini GI, Molnar G, Jusko WJ (1988) Multiple-dose pharmacokinetics of imipramine and its major active and conjugated metabolites in depressed patients. J Clin Psychopharmacol 8:48–53
Vandel B, Vandel S, Jounet JM, Allers G, Volmat R (1982) Relationship between the plasma concentration of clomipramine and desmethylclomipramine in depressive patients and the clinical response. Eur J Clin Pharmacol 22:15–20
Vandel S, Bertschy G, Vandel B, Allers G, Volmat R (1989) Amitriptyline: linear or nonlinear kinetics in every day practice? Eur J Pharmacol 37:595–598
Vandel S, Bertschy G, Allers G, Volmat R (1990) Nonlinear Kinetics of nortriptyline in every day practice. Eur J Clin Pharmacol 39:97–98

Von Bahr C, Movin G, Nordin C, Lidén A, Hammarlund-Udenaes M, Hedberg A, Ring H, Sjöqvist F (1991) Plasma levels of thioridazine and metabolites are influenced by the debrisoquin hydroxylation phenotype. Clin Pharmacol Ther 49:234–240

Wode-Helgodt B, Alfredsson G (1981) Concentrations of chlorpromazine and two of its active metabolites in plasma and cerebrospinal fluid of psychotic patients treated with fixed drug doses. Psychopharmacology (Berl) 73:55–62

Young RC, Dhar AK, Kutt H, Alexopoulos GS (1988) Isomers of 10-hydroxynortriptyline in geriatric depression. Ther Drug Monit 10:164–167

Disposition of the Neuroleptics Perphenazine, Zuclopenthixol, and Haloperidol Cosegregates with Polymorphic Debrisoquine Hydroxylation

L. BERTILSSON, M.L. DAHL, B. EKQVIST, and A. LLERENA

1 Introduction

Dosage requirements and the therapeutic response vary widely between patients treated with neuroleptic drugs. There are large interindividual differences in the elimination kinetics and in the steady state plasma levels achieved during treatment with a fixed dose of a neuroleptic (Dahl 1986). Thus, pharmacokinetic factors contribute to the variability in drug response. One of the major aims in optimizing neuroleptic treatment has been to search for concentration–effect rather than dose–effect relationships as discussed by Baldessarini et al. (1988). Knowledge of the factors contributing to the pharmacokinetic variability is thus of importance for individualization of drug therapy.

Neuroleptic drugs are metabolized in the liver by the cytochrome P450 enzyme system. Activity of one of the hepatic P450 isoenzymes, CYP2D6 or "debrisoquine hydroxylase," is polymorphic in Caucasian populations. Some 5%–10% of Caucasians lack this isoenzyme and are classified as poor metabolizers (PM) of debrisoquine, while the rest are extensive metabolizers (EM) (Evans et al. 1980; Steiner et al. 1988). The debrisoquine/4-hydroxydebrisoquine metabolic ratio (MR), measured in 8-h urine after the intake of a single oral dose of debrisoquine, is a measure of this enzyme activity and shows bimodal distribution, dividing Caucasian populations into PM and EM (Fig. 1).

The metabolism of a number of important drugs, including tricyclic antidepressants, some antiarrythmic drugs, and beta-blockers, cosegregates with the capacity to hydroxylate debrisoquine (Brøsen and Gram 1989). In vitro, the neuroleptics thioridazine and chlorpromazine inhibit the metabolism of sparteine and desipramine which covary with the 4-hydroxylation of debrisoquine (Otton et al. 1983; von Bahr et al. 1985). Moreover, Syvälahti et al. (1986) have shown that patients treated with the neuroleptics thioridazine and levomepromazine had significantly higher urinary MRs of debrisoquine than patients not treated with neuroleptics. These studies show that neuro-

Department of Clinical Pharmacology, Karolinska Institute, Huddinge Hospital, 141 86 Huddinge, Sweden

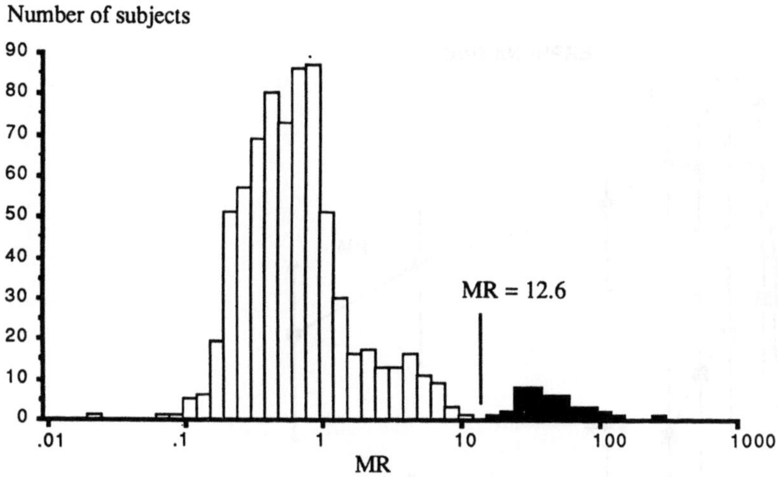

Fig. 1. Distibution of the debrisoquine/4-hydroxydebrisoquine metabolic ratio (*MR*) in 757 healthy Swedish subjects given an oral dose of 10 mg debrisoquine. The antimode at MR 12.6 between extensive and poor metabolizers is indicated. (From Steiner et al. 1988)

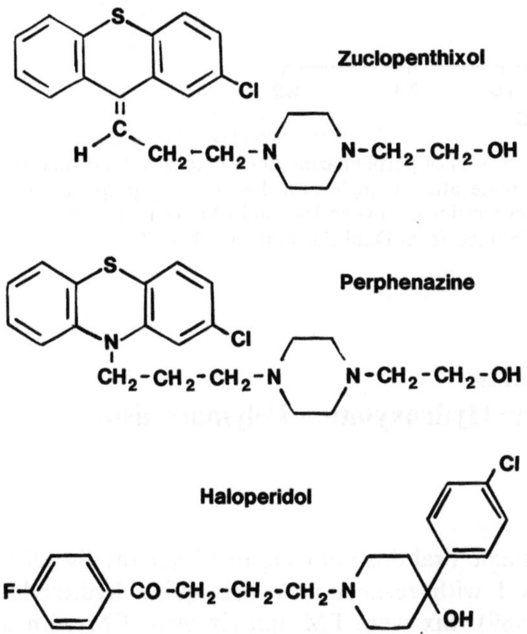

Fig. 2. Chemical structures of zuclopenthixol, perphenazine, and haloperidol

leptics are inhibitors of CYP2D6 and they might therefore also be substrates for this enzyme. In this review we present data showing that the disposition of the neuroleptics perphenazine, zuclopenthixol, and haloperidol (Fig. 2) is genetically regulated and related to the polymorphic hydroxylation of debrisoquine.

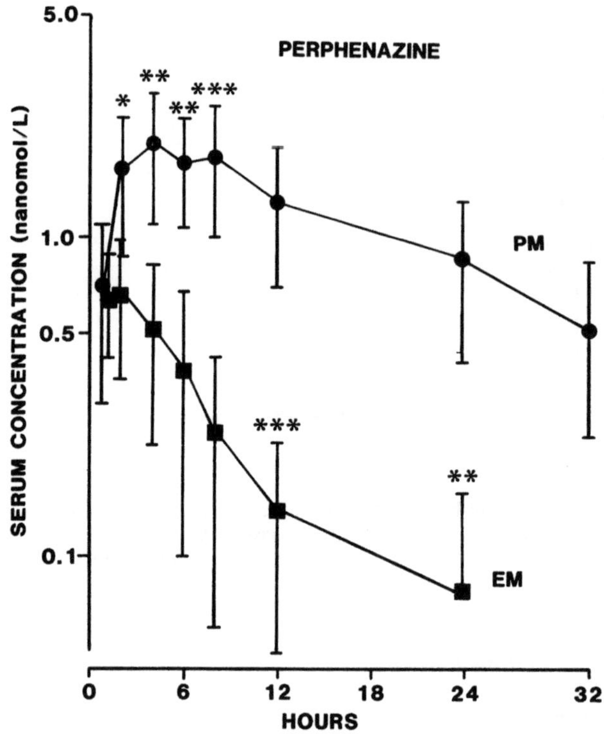

Fig. 3. Serum concentrations (mean ± SD) of perphenazine in six extensive (*EM*) and six poor metabolizers (*PM*) of debrisoquine after a single oral dose of 6 mg perphenazine. Significant differences in serum concentrations between EM and PM are indicated: $^{*}p < 0.05$; $^{**}p < 0.01$; $^{***}p < 0.001$. (Modified from Dahl-Puustinen et al. 1989)

2 Disposition of Neuroleptics in Relation to Debrisoquine Hydroxylation Polymorphism

2.1 Perphenazine

Perphenazine was given as a single oral dose of 6 mg to 12 healthy Swedish subjects previously phenotyped with respect to debrisoquine hydroxylation (Dahl-Puustinen et al. 1989). Six were PM and six were EM with a debrisoquine MR of less than 1. As shown in Fig. 3, the peak serum concentrations were higher in PM than in EM (2.4 ± 0.6 versus 0.7 ± 0.3 nmol/l; $p < 0.001$), indicating involvement of the debrisoquine hydroxylase in the first pass metabolism of the drug. A similar difference between the two phenotypes was also seen in the systemic elimination of the drug. The serum concentrations were 10 times higher in PM than in EM 24 h after drug intake. The study shows that the elimination of perphenazine is to a great extent dependent on the activity of the debrisoquine hydroxylase.

2.2 Zuclopenthixol

Zuclopenthixol is a neuroleptic drug with a chemical structure very similar to that of perphenazine (Fig. 2). Single oral doses of 10 or 6 mg of zuclopenthixol were given to six EM and six PM of debrisoquine (Dahl et al. 1991). The peak plasma levels of zuclopenthixol did not differ between the phenotypes, whereas the plasma elimination half-life was significantly longer in PM than in EM (29.9 ± 6.6 versus 17.6 ± 6.9 h; $p < 0.05$; Fig. 4). Accordingly, the total oral plasma clearance was lower in PM than in EM (0.78 ± 0.27 versus 2.12 ± 0.651 $h^{-1} kg^{-1}$; $p < 0.001$). Thus, the disposition of zuclopenthixol as well as that of perphenazine is related to the debrisoquine hydroxylation phenotype.

Ten of the subjects who received zuclopenthixol had previously participated in the perphenazine study. The oral clearances of these two drugs correlated significantly ($r_s = 0.83$; $p < 0.01$; Fig. 5). The variation in the oral clearance of perphenazine was about 40-fold among these selected subjects of PM and EM phenotype, whereas that of zuclopenthixol was only six fold (Fig. 5). This is in accordance with data from patients showing large interindividual differences in the steady state plasma levels of perphenazine (Bolvig Hansen and Larsen 1977; Bolvig Hansen et al. 1981). The disposition of zuclopenthixol, on the other hand, has been reported to show relatively little variation between individuals (Aes-Jørgensen et al. 1981).

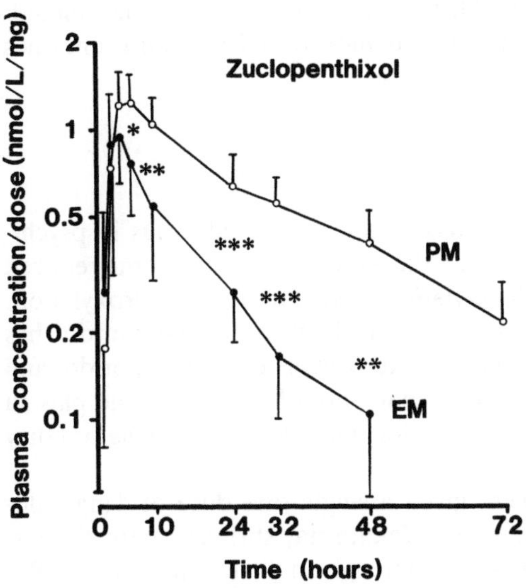

Fig. 4. Plasma concentrations of zuclopenthixol per dose unit (nmol $l^{-1} mg^{-1}$; mean ± SD) in six extensive (*EM*; ●) and six poor metabolizers (*PM*; ○) who received an oral dose of either 10 or 6 mg zuclopenthixol. $^{*}p < 0.05$; $^{**}p < 0.01$; $^{***}p < 0.001$ (from Dahl et al. 1991)

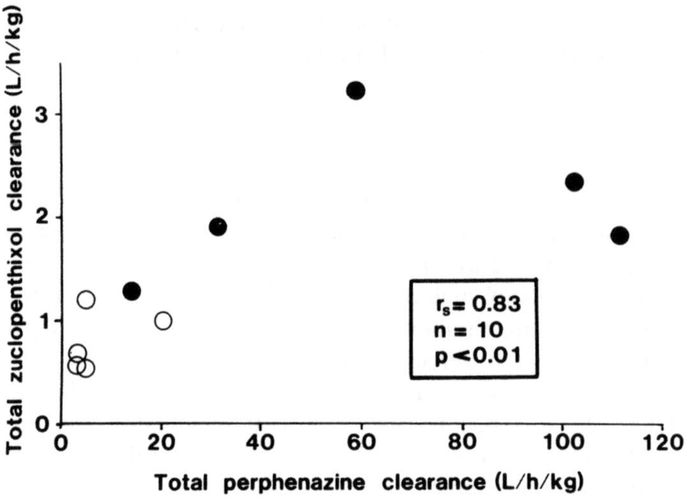

Fig. 5. Correlation between the total oral clearance of perphenazine and that of zuclopenthixol in five extensive (●) and five poor metabolizers (○) who received both drugs on separate occasions

The debrisoquine hydroxylase activity thus seems to be more important for the elimination of perphenazine than for that of zuclopenthixol.

Among the five EM given both perphenazine and zuclopenthixol one subject had a low clearance of both neuroleptics similar to the group of five PM. This subject was an EM of debrisoquine, but a PM of *S*-mephenytoin. It can therefore not be excluded that the polymorphic *S*-mephenytoin hydroxylase, in addition to the debrisoquine hydroxylase, is involved in the metabolism of these neuroleptics. This remains, however, to be studied. Brøsen et al. (this volume) have recently demonstrated that both enzymes are involved in the metabolism of imipramine.

2.3 Haloperidol

Haloperidol is worldwide one of the most commonly used drugs in psychiatry. It is metabolized by reduction of the ketone group to form reduced haloperidol as well as by *N*-dealkylation and aromatic hydroxylation. The role of reduced haloperidol in the clinical effects of haloperidol has been discussed (Froemming et al. 1989). Interconversion of haloperidol and reduced haloperidol is known to occur as haloperidol is found in the plasma after administration of reduced haloperidol and vice versa (Chakraborty et al. 1989).

Three PM of debrisoquine were given a single oral dose of 4 mg haloperidol. All three developed side effects (akathisia, stiffness, paresthesias, restlessness) and a 2-mg dose was therefore given to the next three PM

Table 1. Plasma pharmacokinetics of an oral dose of haloperidol to five EM[a] and six PM[b] of debrisoquine (from LLerena et al. 1992a)

	EM	PM	*p* value
C_{max}/dose ($nmol\,l^{-1}\,mg^{-1}$)	0.93 ± 0.34	1.10 ± 0.46	NS
Half-life (h)	16.3 ± 6.4	29.4 ± 4.2	<0.01
Clearance ($l\,h^{-1}\,kg^{-1}$)	2.49 ± 1.31	1.16 ± 0.36	<0.05

EM, extensive metabolizers; PM, poor metabolizers.
[a] Six EM were given 4 mg of haloperidol, but in one subject the elimination was so rapid that accurate kinetics could not be calculated.
[b] The dose of haloperidol was 4 mg in three PM and 2 mg in three PM.

(LLerena et al. 1992a). All six EM received a 4-mg dose without side effects. As shown in Table 1, the elimination of haloperidol was faster in EM than in PM. Peak plasma concentrations, calculated per dose unit, did not differ between the phenotypes. The PM also had significantly ($p < 0.05$) higher concentrations of reduced haloperidol in plasma compared to EM at 10, 48 and 72 h after haloperidol intake (LLerena et al. 1992b). Thus, the levels of both haloperidol and reduced haloperidol were higher in PM than in EM subjects. Interestingly, Tyndale et al. (1991) recently reported evidence suggesting that the debrisoquine hydroxylase is involved in the oxidation of reduced haloperidol to haloperidol in vitro in human liver microsomes.

3 Conclusions

The disposition of the neuroleptic drugs perphenazine, zuclopenthixol, and haloperidol is related to the genetically determined capacity to hydroxylate debrisoquine. Von Bahr et al. (1991) have shown that this is true also for thioridazine. Higher steady state plasma levels due to slower elimination in PM than in EM might expose PM to an increased risk of side effects if treated with the same doses of these drugs as EM. On the other hand, extremely rapid EM might need higher doses than usual. This has previously been pointed out for the use of tricyclic antidepressants in extremely rapid EM of debrisoquine (Bertilsson et al. 1985). The contribution of this genetically determined variability in relation to other sources of variation remains to be studied in patients during long-term treatment with neuroleptics.

Acknowledgements. These studies were supported by Swedish Medical Research Council (3902) and were carried out in coordination with COST B1. Dr. LLerena was a postdoctoral fellow from Department of Pharmacology and Psychiatry, University of Extremadura, Badajoz, Spain, supported by the Spanish Ministry of Education and Science. We thank Ms. Christina Alm, RN, and Ms. Jolanta Widén for skillful assistance.

References

Aaes-Jørgensen T, Gravem A, Jørgensen A (1981) Serum levels of the isomers of clopenthixol in patients given cis (Z)-clopenthixol or cis(Z)/trans(E)-clopenthixol. Acta Psychiatr Scand 64 Suppl 294:70–77

Baldessarini RJ, Cohen BM, Teicher MH (1988) Significance of neuroleptic dose and plasma level in the pharmacological treatment of psychoses. Arch Gen Psychiatry 45:79–91

Bertilsson L, Åberg-Wistedt A, Gustafsson LL, Nordin C (1985) Extremely rapid hydroxylation of debrisoquine – a case report with implication for treatment with nortriptyline and other tricyclic antidepressants. Ther Drug Monit 7:478–480

Bolvig Hansen L, Larsen NE (1977) Plasma concentrations of perhenazine and its sulphoxide metabolite during continuous oral treatment. Psychopharmacology (Berl) 53:127–130

Bolvig Hansen L, Larsen NE, Vestergård P (1981) Plasma levels of perphenazine (Trilafon) related to development of extrapyramidal side effects. Psychopharmacology (Berl) 74:306–309

Brøsen K, Gram LF (1989) Clinical significance of the sparteine/debrisoquine oxidation polymorphism. Eur J Clin Pharmacol 36:537–547

Chakraborty BS, Hubbard JW, Hawes EM, McKay G, Cooper JK, Gurnsey T, Korchinski ED, Midha KK (1989) Interconversion between haloperidol and reduced haloperidol in healthy volunteers. Eur J Clin Pharmacol 37:45–48

Dahl SG (1986) Plasma level monitoring of antipsychotic drugs. Clinical utility. Clin Pharmacokinet 11:36–61

Dahl M-L, Ekqvist B, Widen J, Bertilsson L (1991) Disposition of the neuroleptic zuclopenthixol cosegregates with the polymorphic hydroxylation of debrisoquine in humans. Acta Psychiatr Scand 84:99–102

Dahl-Puustinen M-L, Lidén A, Alm C, Nordin C, Bertilsson L (1989) Disposition of perphenazine is related to polymorphic debrisoquine hydroxylation in human beings. Clin Pharmacol Ther 46:78–81

Evans DAP, Mahgoub A, Sloan TP, Idle JR, Smith RL (1980) A family and population study of the genetic polymorphism of debrisoquine oxidation in a white British population. J Med Genet 17:102–105

Froemming JS, Francis Lam YW, Jann MW, Davis CM (1989) Pharmacokinetics of haloperidol. Clin Pharmacokinet 17:396–423

LLerena A, Alm C, Dahl M-L, Ekqvist B, Bertilsson L (1992a) Haloperidol disposition is dependent on debrisoquine hydroxylation phenotype. Ther Drug Monit 14:92–97

LLerena A, Dahl M-L, Ekqvist B, Bertilsson L (1992b) Haloperidol disposition is dependent on the debrisoquine hydroxylation phenotype: Increased plasma levels of the reduced metabolite in poor metabolizers. Ther Drug Monit 14:261–264

Otton SV, Inaba T, Kalow W (1983) Inhibition of sparteine oxidation in human liver by tricyclic antidepressants and other drugs. Life Sci 32:795–800

Steiner E, Bertilsson L, Säwe J, Bertling I, Sjöqvist F (1988) Polymorphic debrisoquine hydroxylation in 757 Swedish subjects. Clin Pharmacol Ther 44:431–435

Syvälahti EKG, Lindberg R, Kallio J, de Vocht M (1986) Inhibitory effects of neuroleptics on debrisoquine oxidation in man. Br J Clin Pharmacol 22:89–92

Tyndale RF, Kalow W, Inaba T (1991) Oxidation of reduced haloperidol to haloperidol: involvement of human P450IID6 (sparteine/debrisoquine monooxygenase). Br J Clin Pharmacol 31:655–660

Von Bahr C, Spina E, Birgersson C, Ericsson Ö, Göransson M, Henthorn T, Sjöqvist F (1985) Inhibition of desmethylimipramine 2-hydroxylation by drugs in human liver microsomes. Biochem Pharmacol 34:2501–2505

Von Bahr C, Movin G, Nordin C, Lidén A, Hammarlund-Udenaes M, Hedberg A, Ring H, Sjöqvist F (1991) Plasma levels of thioridazine and metabolites are influenced by the debrisoquine hydroxylation phenotype. Clin Pharmacol Ther 49:234–240

Phenotypes for Psychotropic Drug Metabolism in the Elderly

B.G. Pollock and J.M. Perel

1 Psychotropic Use and Adverse Effects in the Elderly

In elderly people, illness caused by medications may be the most significant treatable health problem (Beers and Ouslander 1989). One-sixth of all U.S. hospital admissions of patients over 70 years of age, compared with 1 in 35 admissions in the rest of the population, have been attributed to adverse drug reactions (National Council on Patient Information 1988). In Britain, 10% of all hospital admissions to geriatric medicine departments were found to be due to medication toxicity. A total of 25.4% of patients admitted under these circumstances were taking four to six drugs and 12% were taking psychotropics (Williamson and Chopin 1980).

Psychotropic drugs, because of their extensive use and narrow therapeutic indices, rank with cardiovascular medications as the most common cause of serious adverse reactions in the elderly. Depression is the most prevalent psychiatric disorder in old age and such patients are prone to serious adverse effects from antidepressant medication, which has been related to the particular drug, its concentration, the presence of other drugs, and the preexisting state of the patient (Glassman et al. 1984). Preskorn and Jerkovich (1990), in an extensive meta-analysis, found that 6% of 976 tricyclic-treated patients developed CNS toxicity involving psychotic, cognitive, or affective symptoms evolving into delirium. Elevated antidepressant plasma levels and age were the most important risk factors for the development of delirium.

Neuroleptic-induced side effects are common in older patients and parkinsonian effects are particularly troubling; 50% of all patients between 60 and 80 develop at least some extrapyramidal effects even with the lower potency antipsychotic drugs (Mason and Granacher 1980). The prevalence of tardive dyskinesia has been consistently positively correlated with increasing age (Casey 1991).

The use of benzodiazepines, phenothiazines, and antidepressants by the elderly living in the community was found to be the single greatest risk

Department of Psychiatry, Clinical Pharmacology Program, University of Pittsburgh School of Medicine, Western Psychiatric Institute and Clinic, 3811 O'Hara St., Pittsburgh, PA 15213, USA factor associated with falls and was much greater than the risk associated with cognitive impairment and depression (Tinetti et al. 1988). There was no association found between falling and the use of diuretics, antihypertensive agents, and cardiovascular medications in this study. Tricyclic antidepressants and antipsychotics have been found to increase the risk of hip fractures by twofold in a dose-dependent manner (Ray et al. 1987). Elderly patients prescribed long half-life, compared with short half-life, benzodiazepines also appear to be at increased risk for hip fractures (Ray et al. 1989).

2 Relevance of Drug Metabolism

The cytochrome P450 isozyme CYP2D6 or debrisoquine (DBQ) hydroxylase is involved in the metabolism of at least 25 drugs including antihypertensives, antiarrhythmics, antidepressants, and major tranquilizers (Brosen and Gram 1989), all of which are commonly prescribed to older patients. Mephenytoin (MPH) has exhibited a new and different polymorphic oxidation (CYP2C) independent of the DBQ type. The deficiency of hydroxylation is confined to the 4-hydroxylation of *S*-MPH. The incidence of the poor metabolizer phenotype in a young Caucasian population is approximately 3%–5% (Wedlund et al. 1984) but rises to 18%–23% in a Japanese sample (Nakamura et al. 1985). There is evidence (Bertilsson et al. 1989) that the metabolism of diazepam and desmethyldiazepam and citalopram and the demethylation of imipramine (Skjelbo et al. 1991) cosegregate with the oxidation of MPH. Interestingly, the first demonstration of an age-related preferential decline in stereoselective metabolism has been with a medication utilizing *S*-MPH hydroxylase, hexobarbital (Chandler et al. 1988).

For drugs with a narrow therapeutic range, it would seem appropriate to avoid standard doses in slow metabolizers. It may be particularly important to recognize the slow metabolizer phenotype among the elderly, who may have exaggerated drug responses due to physiological or pharmacodynamic reasons (Pollock et al. 1990). Not only do poor metabolizers have difficulty eliminating specific drugs, but patients taking a variety of concurrent medications will have significantly elevated metabolic ratios. It is of equal importance, however, to recognize that those older patients found to be extensive metabolizers, may be undertreated with medication, because dosages are inappropriately lowered due to the patient's age alone.

Although experiments with senescent rodents have suggested an age associated decline in drug metabolizing enzyme activity (Kato et al. 1964; Rikans 1989), recent human in vito data argues strongly against this (Schmucker et al. 1990). Antipyrine has been widely used as a model substrate for studying the influence of disease and environment on hepatic metabolism. It has also been used in geriatric subjects, in whom only 3% of variance in metabolic clearance could be explained by age alone (Vestal et al. 1975). Although antipyrine, as a low-clearance drug, reflects oxidative metabolism in a general way, polymorphism in its metabolism and clearance has never been shown, nor has it been assigned to a specific P450.

3 Current Studies

We have assessed the feasibility of simultaneously determining DBQ and MPH phenotypes in an elderly population. A total of 171 subjects of mean age 75 years (range 59–96 years) were studied. All subjects had liver function tests within normal ranges, and all were medication-free for minimally 2 weeks (5 weeks after fluoxetine). The procedure using single doses of 10 mg of DBQ plus 100 mg of MPH and an 8 h urine collection was well tolerated. Even in frail subjects, no adverse effects were observed. DBQ/4-hydroxy-DBQ was analyzed by reverse phase high performance liquid chromatography (HPLC) (Harrison et al. 1986). *S*- and *R*- mephenytoin (MPH) were quantified by capillary gas chromatogrophy (GC) with a chiral column (Wedlund et al. 1984). All those with elevated S:R ratios underwent confirmation by HPLC assay for the 4-OH-metabolite. Precautions to minimize the decomposition of an acid labile metabolite (Zhang et al. 1991) included adding preservative, refrigerating the container at all times, rapid freezing of specimens at −80°c, and assay for S:R ratios within 6 weeks.

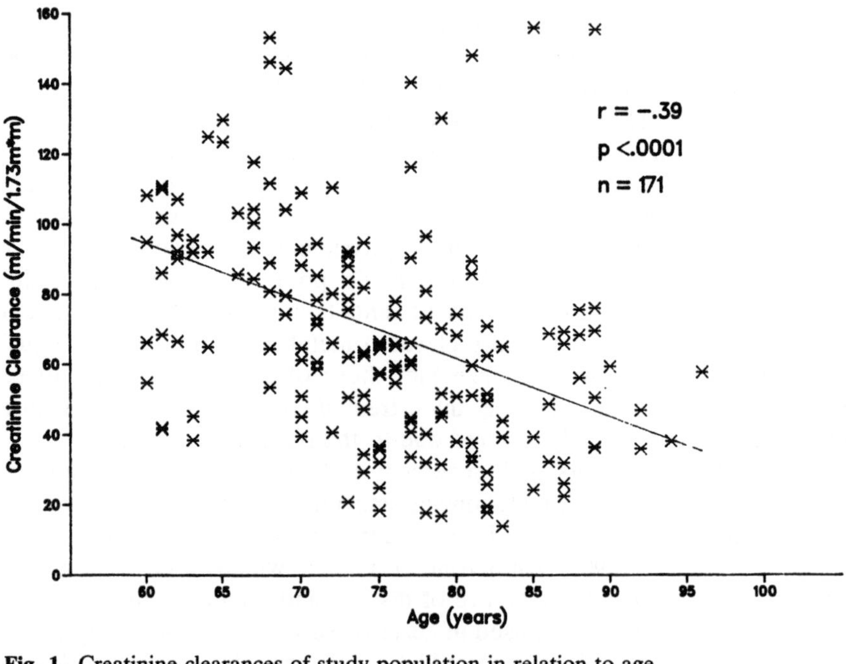

Fig. 1. Creatinine clearances of study population in relation to age

While the expected correlation of increasing age and decline in creatinine clearance was found ($r = -0.40$) (Fig. 1), there was no correlation of age or creatinine clearance with either metabolic ratio (Figs. 2 and 3). There were no significant differences in proportions of slow metabolizers between males and females or controls vs dementia or depression. Kernel density analysis was used to examine population discontinuities (Silverman 1981; Herman and Laverty 1989). This procedure determined an antimode of 11.6 for the bimodal DBQ distribution. The incidence of categorically slow DBQ metabolizers (defined as metabolic ratio ⩾ the antimode) was 3.5%, which approaches the lower range determined in a younger population (usually cited as 5%–9%).

The frequency distribution of the MPH S:R metabolic ratios was more continuous (Pollock et al. 1991) than reported in previous studies with younger patients, implying considerable variance in metabolic capacity that could not be predicted by age, creatinine clearance, or routine "liver profiles." This may imply that this enzyme is more sensitive to subtle environmental damage and age. The incidence of slow MPH metabolizers (S:R ratio ⩾ 0.95) (19%) in our sample of older black subjects ($n = 32$) was markedly higher than that in the elderly whites, which was 5%; this difference was significant ($p = 0.02$).

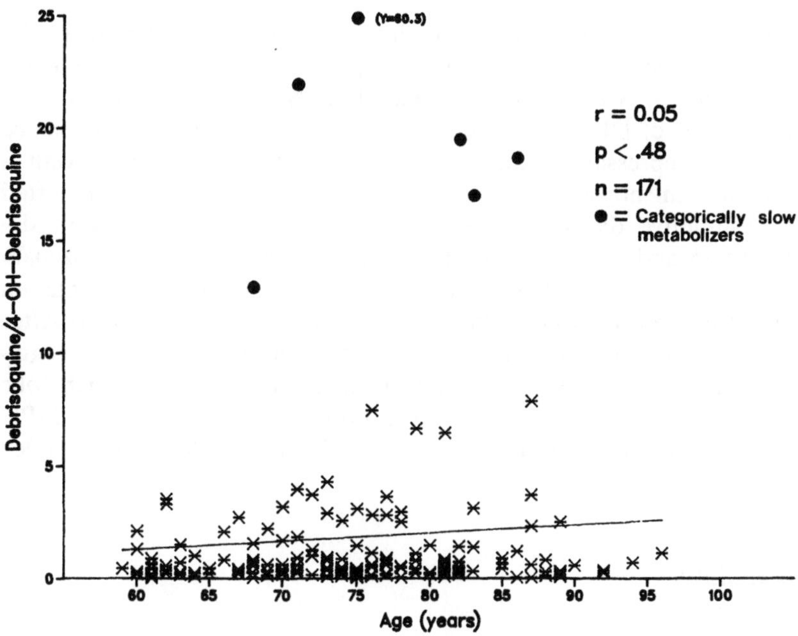

Fig. 2. Distribution of debrisoquine metabolic ratios in 171 unmedicated subjects older than age 59

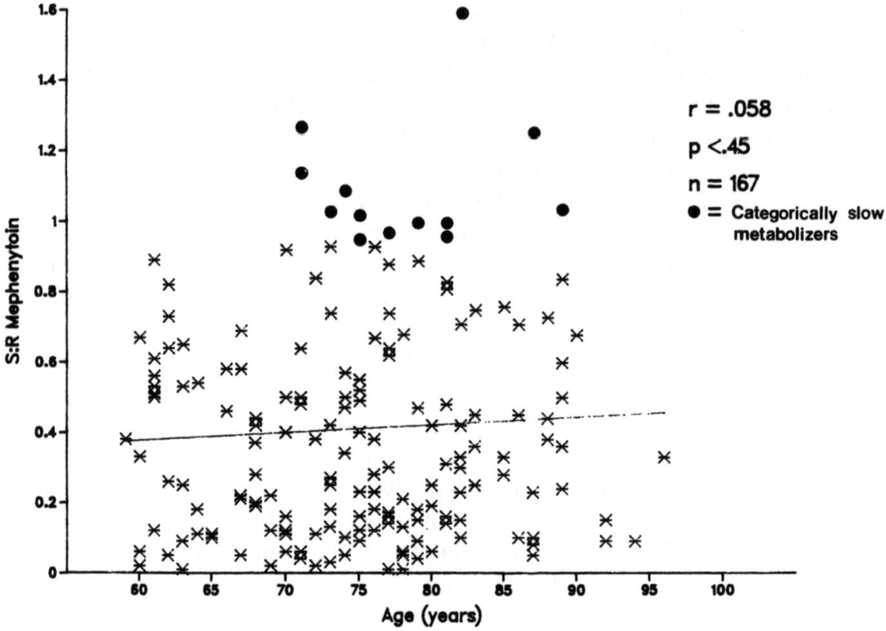

Fig. 3. Distribution of S:R mephenytoin ratios in relation to subject age

Establishing the clinical utility of drug metabolic phenotyping in the elderly will require further systematic prospective study. Nonetheless, we were impressed by two examples. An elderly lady, who was found to be a slow metabolizer of DBQ, had a history of intolerance and noncompliance with prior antidepressant treatment. She was successfully treated with a small dose of 25 mg nortriptyline. A 70 year old woman was initially admitted with a presumptive diagnosis of depression or early dementia, with significant lethargy and ataxia. She had been taking perphenazine and diazepam for several months and, as her daytime confusion and consequent agitation increased, was prescribed an additional benzodiazepine, temazepam. After 3 weeks in the hospital, following discontinuation of medications, her cognitive function showed remarkable improvement and her DBQ metabolic ratio was determined to be 1.6; she was, however, found to be a slow MPH metabolizer (S:R MPH ratio = 1.0; 4-OH-MPH hydroxylation index = 207).

4 Conclusions

A noninvasive inexpensive assessment of DBQ-MPH metabolism is well tolerated and feasible in an older population. Although the proportion of categorically slow DBQ metabolizers does not appear to increase among the unmedicated elderly, 80% of those older than age 60 are taking at least one medication and many are taking between 3 and 12 medications simultaneously (Beers and Ouslander 1989).

There has been some success achieved in genotyping poor metabolizers of DBQ by enzymatic amplification of DNA using the polymerase chain reaction (Heim and Meyer 1990). Genotyping, however, will reveal the unmedicated baseline, which may be quite different from the reality of the individual's environmentally determined capacity. Knowledge of the current metabolic ratio of a patient on several medications may someday be used to predict the possibility of a significant interaction if an additional medication is added.

Our preliminary results would suggest a need for particular caution in treating older African-Americans with medications being metabolized by *S*-MPH hydroxylase, such as diazepam. Our findings, that DBQ oxidative metabolism does not change with aging alone and that (genetic) slow DBQ metabolizers endure into old age, remaining at considerable risk for treatment with many commonly used psychotropics, suggest the importance of studying the introduction of this simple procedure as part of routine screening of the elderly. This would permit, for the first time, an examination of the risk to an older population associated with impaired oxidative drug metabolism, whether from genetic or environmental (primarily drug-induced) origin. The goal is to assess the utility of empirical indices which account for the metabolism of many psychotropics. Identification of this relationship may in turn lead to safer prescription patterns for elderly patients and fewer adverse events.

Acknowledgments. Debrisoquine and 4-hydroxydebrisoquine for use as analytical standards were obtained through the courtesy of Dr. Peter F. Sorter, Hoffmann-LaRoche, Nutley, NJ. Dr. Robert Branch, University of Pittsburgh, kindly supplied 4-OH-mephenytoin standards. We are grateful to the staff of Geriatric Health Services at the University of Pittsburgh for their assistance. This work was supported by NIMH grants K07MH104 and MH30915.

References

Beers MH, Ouslander JG (1989) Risk factors in geriatric drug prescribing. Drugs 37: 105–112

Bertilsson L, Henthorn TK, Sanz E, Tybring G, Sawe J, Villen T (1989) Importance of genetic factors in the regulation of diazepam metabolism: Relationship to S-mephenytoin, but not debrisoquin, hydroxylation phenotype. Clin Pharmacol Ther 45:348–355

Brosen K, Gram LF (1989) Clinical significance of the sparteine/debrisoquine oxidation polymorphism. Eur J Clin Pharmacol 36:537–547

Casey DE (1991) Neuroleptic drug-induced extrapyramidal syndromes and tardive dyskinesia. Schizophr Res 4:109–120
Chandler MH, Scott SR, Blouin RA (1988) Age-associated stereoselective alterations in hexobarbital metabolism. Clin Pharmacol Ther 43:436–441
Glassman AH, Carino JS, Roose SP (1984) Adverse effects of tricyclic antidepressants: focus on the elderly. In: Usdin E (ed) Frontiers in biochemical and pharmacological research in depression. Raven, New York, pp 391–398
Harrison PM, Tonkin AM, Dixon ST, McLean AJ (1986) Determination of debrisoquine and its 4-hydroxymetabolite in urine by high-performance liquid chromatography. J Chromatogr 374:204–208
Heim M, Meyer UA (1990) Genotyping of poor metabolizers of debrisoquine. Lancet 336:529–532
Herman RJ, Laverty WH (1989) Kernel density estimation: statistical power for detection of polymorphism. Clin Pharmacol Ther 45:158
Kato R, Vassanelli P, Frontino G, Chiesara E (1964) Variation in the activity of liver microsomal drug-metabolizing enzymes in rats in relation to the age. Biochem Pharmacol 13:1037–1051
Mason AS, Granacher RP (1980) Clinical handbook of antipsychotic drug therapy Brunner/Mazel, New York
Nakamura K, Goto F, Ray WA, McAllister CB, Jacqz E, Wilkinson GR (1985) Interethnic differences in genetic polymorphism of debrisoquine and mephenytoin hydroxylation between Japanese and Caucasian populations. Clin Pharmacol Ther 38:402–408
National Council on Patient Information and Education (1988) Priorities and approaches for improving prescription medicine use by older Americans. National Council on Patient Information and Education, Washington
Pollock BG, Perel JM, Reynolds CF (1990) Pharmacodynamic issues relevant to geriatric psychopharmacology. J Geriatr Psychiatry Neurol 3:221–228
Pollock BG, Perel JM, Kirshner M, Altieri LP, Yeager AL, Reynolds CF (1991) S-Mephenytoin 4-hydroxylation in older Americans. Eur J Clin Pharmacol 40:609–611
Preskorn SH, Jerkovich GS (1990) Central nervous system toxicity of tricyclic antidepressants: phenomenology, course, risk factors, and role of therapeutic drug monitoring. J Clin Psychopharmacol 10:88–95
Ray WA, Griffin MR, Schaffner W, Baugh DK, Melton LJ (1987) Psychotropic drug use and the risk of hip fracture. N Engl J Med 316:363–369
Ray WA, Griffin MR, Downey W (1989) Benzodiazepines of long and short elimination half-life and the risk of hip fracture. JAMA 262:3303–3307
Rikans LE (1989) Hepatic drug metabolism in female Fischer rats as a function of age. Drug Metab Dispos 27:225–231
Schmucker DL, Woodhouse KW, Wang RK, Wynne H, James OF, McManus M, Kremers P (1990) Effects of age and gender on in vitro properties of human liver microsomal monooxygenases. Clin Pharmacol Ther 48:365–374
Silverman BW (1981) Using kernel density estimates to investigate multimodality. J R Stat Soc 43:97–99
Skjelbo E, Brosen K, Hallas J, Gram LF (1991) The mephenytoin oxidation polymorphism is partially responsible for the N-demethylation of imipramine. Clin Pharmacol Ther 49:18–23
Tinetti ME, Speechley M, Ginter SF (1988) Risk factors for falls among elderly persons living in the community. N Engl J Med 319:1701–1707
Wedlund PJ, Aslanian WS, McAllister CB, Wilkinson GR, Branch RA (1984) Mephenytoin hydroxylation deficiency in Caucasians: frequency of a new oxidative drug metabolism polymorphism. Clin Pharmacol Ther 36:773–780
Williamson J, Chopin JM (1980) Adverse reactions to prescribed drugs in the elderly: a multicentre investigation. Age Ageing 9:73–80

Vestal RE, Norris AH, Tobin JD, Cohen BH, Shock NW, Andres R (1975) Antipyrine metabolism in man: Influence of age, alcohol, caffeine and smoking. Clin Pharmacol Ther 18:425–434

Zhang Y, Blouin RA, McNamara PJ, Steinmetz J, Wedlund PJ (1991) Limitation to the use of the urinary S-/R-mephenytoin ratio in pharmacogenetic studies. Br J Clin Pharmacol 31:350–352

Analysis of 935 Haloperidol Concentration Measurements Obtained During Routine Drug Monitoring of 134 Patients

M. Gex-Fabry[1], A.E. Balant-Gorgia[2], and L.P. Balant[1]

1 Introduction

Therapeutic drug monitoring of patients receiving antipsychotic drugs provides a valuable and ever-growing source of data about such patients. However, the inherent weakness of these data has to be recognized, since pharmacokinetic information is limited and both population characteristics and clinical data may suffer from lack of reliability. Nonetheless, the data possess advantages in terms of ethics and low cost, since their collection is part of routine clinical practice.

Monitoring of haloperidol concentration was introduced at the University Psychiatric Institutions of Geneva in 1981 and since then data have accumulated, with more than 2500 measurements in 1990. Several patients have thus been "followed" over the years, receiving haloperidol by different administration routes. The purpose of the present study was thus to analyze the information provided by drug monitoring data, with special emphasis on within-subjects variability. Although many studies and reviews have reported about a tenfold between-patients variation in haloperidol plasma level to dose ratios, within-subjects variance remains largely undocumented in a large population (Morselli et al. 1981; Shvartsburd et al. 1983; Dahl and Hals 1987).

2 Patients and Methods

2.1 Patients

The study included 134 in- and outpatients at the University Psychiatric Institutions of Geneva who received haloperidol either i.m., po, or depot. Sociodemographic characteristics and diagnoses are given in Table 1 and are

[1] Clinical Research Unit, Institutions Universitaires de Psychiatrie, 47 rue du XXXI Décembre, 1207 Geneva, Switzerland
[2] Therapeutic Drug Monitoring Unit, Institutions Universitaires de Psychiatrie, 1225 Chêne-Bourg, Switzerland

Table 1. Characteristics of the patients (n = 134)

		n	%
Mean age (years)	39 (range 20–67)		
Mean height (cm)	169 (range 145–191)		
Mean weight (kg)	68 (range 43–111)		
Sex			
Males		69	51.5
Females		65	48.5
Diagnosis			
Schizophrenia		63	47.0
Bipolar disorder, manic episode		46	34.3
Psychotic disorder, other		3	2.2
Insufficient information		22	16.4
Smoking[a]			
Yes		110	82.1
No		24	17.9
Alcohol drinking[a]			
Yes		60	44.8
No		74	55.2
Impaired renal function[a]			
Yes		1	0.7
No		133	99.3
Impaired liver function[a]			
Yes		23	17.2
No		111	82.8
Comedication[a]			
Antiparkinsonian		120	89.6
Levomepromazine		91	67.9
Other neuroleptics		13	9.7
Lithium		30	22.4
Antidepressant		1	0.7
Benzodiazepine		119	88.8
Analgesics		3	2.2
Other drugs		53	39.6

[a] Mentioned at least once on drug monitoring questionnaires.

based on information available from drug monitoring questionnaires. For each patient, plasma concentrations of haloperidol, administered either by a single or different routes, were measured 2–35 times. The attending psychiatrist was responsible for deciding whether drug monitoring was indicated, according to generally accepted guidelines, so that patient inclusion in the present study did not interfere with therapy.

2.2 Analytical Methods

Plasma concentrations of haloperidol were determined by gas-liquid chromatography with nitrogen-phosphorus selective detection, according to a method adapted from Bianchetti and Morselli (1978). The sensitivity of

Table 2. Haloperidol posology and measured concentrations

Administration route	Dose (mg)	Concentration (ng/ml)	Last dose adjustment	Last drug intake
i.m. ($n = 165$, 14.1% discarded)[a]				
Median	10	8.0	6 days	14 h
Minimum	6	2.3	4 days	11 h
Maximum	20	25.0	23 days	~24 h
po ($n = 313$, 19.7% discarded)[a]				
Median	12	5.8	8 days	14 h
Minimum	1	0.8	4 days	10 h
Maximum	50	60.2	>6 months	~24 h
Depot ($n = 336$)[a]				
Median	200	5.8	76 days	9 days
Minimum	50	0.7	4 days	4 days
Maximum	400	18.4	>1 year	57 days

[a] Data inclusion criteria are given in the text.

the method was 1 ng/ml when a 2 ml sample was used and the mean day-to-day coefficient of variation was 10%.

2.3 Haloperidol Posology and Concentrations

Raw data included 935 plasma concentration measurements determined over about 6 years of routine drug monitoring. For further analysis, data inclusion criteria were as follows: for the i.m. and po routes, the time interval since last dose adjustment was at least 4 days so that steady-state had been reached. In addition, the last drug intake had to be the day before blood samples were collected (at about 8–9 A.M.) so that trough concentrations were measured. For the depot preparation, the date of the most recent drug injection had to be known precisely. However, the last dose adjustment was often undocumented so that a steady-state condition was not warranted. A description of administered doses and measured concentrations is given in Table 2. The present study focuses on the interpretation of i.m. and po data only.

2.4 Statistical Analysis

Haloperidol clearance (Cl) and relative bioavailability (F) of the po vs i.m. forms were estimated according to the following equations:

$$Cl_{\text{average}} = \text{(dose/concentration) average i.m.}$$
$$F_{\text{average}} = Cl_{\text{average}} \text{ (concentration/dose) average po}$$

Four assumptions were made: (1) linear kinetics are followed; (2) systemic availability of the i.m. route is complete; (3) clearance does not depend on the administration route; (4) trough concentrations are used instead of average steady-state values. If the elimination half-life of haloperidol is 18 h and the time interval between drug intake and blood sampling is 12 h, the fourth assumption results in overestimation of about 20% for calculated clearance values. It must be stressed that the aim was not to establish valid pharmacokinetic parameters but rather to facilitate population description.

Statistical methods for the investigation of variability factors included components of variance analysis under a random effect model, Wilcoxon signed rank test for within-subjects factors, Spearman rank order correlation, and Kruskal-Wallis analysis of variance for between-subjects factors.

3 Results

Pharmacokinetic interpretation of the data in terms of clearance and relative bioavailability of the po form when compared to the i.m. route is given in Table 3. The concentration vs dose relationship was analyzed for 15 patients who had at least five concentration measurements for at least three different po doses. Significant differences were found between individual slopes when calculating regression lines through the origin. The average concentration increase was 0.54 ng/ml per 1 mg dose increase, with extreme values of 0.29 and 0.84 ng/ml. No significant departure from linearity could be demonstrated.

Concentration to dose ratios are given in Table 4 for patients who had at least two measurements for each of the two administration routes. Variability, measured from the maximum to minimum ratio, was 7.3 for the i.m. route, as compared to 13.0 for the po route. Coefficients of variation were 31.7% and 39.3%, respectively. Components of variance analysis revealed that between-subjects variance was 36% higher than within-subjects variance for i.m. values, but only 8% higher for po values. Since ratios exhibit significantly asymmetrical distributions, the analysis was repeated after log transformation, confirming that within-subjects variance is of the same order of magnitude as between-subjects variance for both administration routes. When considering the data in more detail, between-patients variability was

Table 3. Clearance estimates and relative bioavailability of the oral form of haloperidol

	Clearance (l/h)	Relative bioavailability
Mean	58.6	0.73
Standard deviation	20.4	0.23
Median	54.8	0.71
Minimum	25.0	0.30
Maximum	181.2	1.77
Number of measurements	165	219

Table 4. Components of variance for concentration to dose ratios

Administration route	i.m.	po
Conentration/dose (ng/ml)/(mg/day)		
Mean	0.82	0.56
Standard deviation	0.26	0.22
Median	0.79	0.51
Minimum	0.23	0.14
Maximum	1.67	1.82
Number of measurements	124	285
Number of subjects	45	83
Measurements/subject	2 to 8	2 to 9
Asymmetry of distribution (test of skewness)	$p < 0.01$	$p < 0.01$
Between-subjects variance/within-subjects variance	1.36	1.08
Between-subjects variance/within-subjects variance for logs	1.13	1.13

3.3 for the i.m. route and 4.6 for the po route, when measured as the maximum to minimum ratio of average values per patient. Within-subjects variations of twofold or more were observed in three subjects receiving i.m. haloperidol (6.7%) and 13 patients with po medication (13%). As an example, one patient had haloperidol plasma concentrations between 2.3 ng/ml and 7.3 ng/ml under the same 10 mg i.m. dose.

Factors responsible for such variability were also investigated. For each patient, average concentrations, normalized to a 10 mg daily dose, were calculated in the presence and absence of a factor and compaired pairwise in order to identify within-patients variability factors. Significantly higher po concentrations were observed when levomepromazine comedication was present (median 0.93 ng/ml difference, Wilcoxon signed rank test, $p < 0.05$). Neither smoking, drinking, lithium, benzodiazepine, or antiparkinsonian comedication had a significant influence on individual concentrations.

Correlations between the average dose-normalized concentration for a given patient and the frequency of a factor being reported as present on his or her drug monitoring questionnaire were also investigated. No effect was found for comedication. However, some increase in i.m. concentration was associated with smoking (Spearman correlation coefficient $r_s = 0.21$, $p < 0.05$), while a decrease of po levels was associated with alcohol drinking ($r_s = -0.21$, $p < 0.05$). No age effect was found, but a negative correlation was observed between body weight and i.m. concentrations ($r_s = -0.27$, $p < 0.05$). In addition, a significant sex effect was found, with median concentrations of 6.5 ng/ml in males and 8.0 ng/ml in females for the i.m. route, and 4.7 vs 5.5 for po administration (Kruskal-Wallis analysis of variance, $p < 0.05$).

4 Discussion

This study analyzes a few aspects of the information present in data collected over several years of routine haloperidol plasma level monitoring.

Recognizing that clearance values calculated on the basis of trough rather than average steady-state concentrations are expected to overestimate true values by about 20%, close agreement is found with previous work by Holley et al. (1983). They reported an average clearance of 47 l/h for six healthy volunteers who received haloperidol intravenously (range 36–69 l/h). They also calculated an average bioavailability of 65% for the po form (range 50%–88%). Other studies reporting values in the same range have been reviewed recently (Froemming et al. 1989).

The results of the present study are also in keeping with a linear relationship between daily dose and plasma concentration (Forsman and Öhman 1977; Moulin et al. 1982). However, dose dependent kinetics of haloperidol have been described at high doses (Morselli et al. 1981) and cannot be excluded from the present work, since only relatively low doses were administered.

Haloperidol, like many other neuroleptics, is characterized by important variations in steady-state plasma levels relative to administered daily dose (Bianchetti et al. 1980; Shvartsburd et al. 1983; Dahl and Hals 1987). The present study further indicates that within-subjects variability might be more important than usually thought, with variations of two- to threefold frequently observed. In comparison, between-subjects variability seems rather moderate, with three- and fivefold variations for the i.m. and po routes, respectively. Although gender, weight, smoking, alcohol drinking, and levomepromazine comedication could explain part of that variability, the magnitude of the effects was relatively small. Although contributing to kinetic variability, these factors are thus expected to play a minor role with respect to the clinical variability between patients treated with haloperidol.

The identified factors are also in keeping with those described in the literature. Similar lower levels of haloperidol in men had been reported previously by Bowers et al. (1987), while Forsman and Öhman (1977) reported that neither gender, nor body weight, nor age influenced haloperidol concentrations. However, alcoholic patients from the same study showed significantly reduced drug plasma levels. Neither anticholinergic medication nor lithium is reported to influence haloperidol concentrations, but interactions with anticonvulsants and antitubercular agents are well documented (Froemming et al. 1989). No interaction between haloperidol and levomepromazine has been described, as far as we know.

Since haloperidol is a high clearance drug, its elimination is highly influenced by hepatic blood flow and less affected by changes in protein binding or intrinsic clearance (Holley et al. 1983). Factors which may alter its bioavailability together with variations of the time interval between drug intake and blood sampling are thus of primary importance with respect to plasma level variability. For the po route, diet may be influential, although lack of compliance is more likely to play the major role. Our experience over years of haloperidol plasma level monitoring also suggests that concentration to dose ratios remain fairly constant for a majority of patients for whom compliance is ascertained. For the i.m. route, explanations for intra-individual variability are less easy to find. However, injection problems as well as discrepancies between prescription and staff practice may be invoked. The possible role of interconversion of reduced haloperidol to haloperidol is presently under investigation in our laboratories.

Acknowledgement. This study was performed in the frame of the European Concerted Action Cost B1 with financial support of the Swiss Federal Office for Education and Science.

References

Bianchetti G, Morselli PL (1978) Rapid and sensitive method for determination of haloperidol in human samples using nitrogen-phosphorus selective detection. J Chromatogr 153:203–209

Bianchetti G, Zarifian E, Poirier-Littre MF, Morselli PL, Deniker P (1980) Influence of route of administration on haloperidol plasma levels in psychotic patients. Int J Clin Pharmacol 18:324–327

Bowers MB, Swigar ME, Jatlow PI, Hoffman FJ, Goicoechea N (1987) Correlates of early neuroleptic response using a uniform haloperidol dose. Int Clin Psychopharmacol 2:255–260

Dahl SG, Hals PA (1987) Pharmacokinetic and pharmacodynamic factors causing variability in response to neuroleptic drugs. In: Dahl SG, Gram LF, Paul SM, Potter WZ (eds) Clinical pharmacology in psychiatry: selectivity in psychotropic drug action, promises or problems. Springer, Berlin Heidelberg New York, pp 266–274 (Psychopharmacology series 3)

Forsman A, Öhman R (1977) Applied pharmacokinetics of haloperidol in man. Curr Ther Res 21:396–410

Froemming JS, Francis Lam YW, Jann MW, Davis CM (1989) Pharmacokinetics of haloperidol. Clin Pharmacokinet 17:396–423

Holley FO, Magliozzi JR, Stanski DR, Lombrozo L, Hollister LE (1983) Haloperidol kinetics after oral and intravenous doses. Clin Pharmacol Ther 33:447–484

Morselli PL, Bianchetti G, Tedeschi G, Braithwaite RA (1981) Haloperidol: clinical pharmacokinetics and significance of therapeutic drug monitoring. In: Richens A, Marks V (eds) Therapeutic drug monitoring. Churchill Livingstone, New York, pp 296–306

Moulin MA, Davy JP, Debruyne D, Andersson JC, Bigot MC, Camsonne R, Poilpré E (1982) Serum level monitoring and therapeutic effect of haloperidol in schizophrenic patients. Psychopharmacology (Berl) 76:346–350

Shvartsburd A, Dekirmenjian H, Smith RC (1983) Blood levels of haloperidol in schizophrenic patients. J Clin Psychopharmacol 3:7–12

Power Analysis for Correlation of Plasma Level and Clinical Data

J.M. DAVIS and Z. WANG

1 Introduction

The purpose of this paper is to suggest a method for doing power analyses for studies which correlate plasma level versus the clinical efficacy of psychotropic drugs. We will also discuss the implications of power considerations for design and analysis of such experiments and their clinical interpretation. It has become customary for the rational planning of experimental studies, such as clinical trials, to do a power analysis to estimate the sample size required to reliably achieve a statistically significant difference. This is generally done to avoid designing a study with substantially too small a sample size to detect a difference. We suggest that the same power considerations are involved in studies designed to test the relationship between clinical efficacy and plasma levels as would apply in a clinical trial to test the efficacy of a new drug versus placebo or a new drug versus a standard drug.

In any power calculation the investigator may wish to calculate the '80% power to achieve a statistically significant difference of 0.05. These two parameters are set somewhat arbitrarily. One must define the effect size based on previous data to make any meaningful analysis for power computation. Effect size refers to the magnitude of the effect one is measuring, disregarding sample size. In the context of clinical trials comparing drug to placebo, the effect size is the drug–placebo difference when we ignore the sample size. The effect size can be the difference in the proportion of those patients who respond to drug versus those who respond to placebo. For data based on continuous measures, the effect size is often expressed in standard deviation units: mean improvement on drug minus the mean improvement on placebo divided by the appropriate standard deviation.

In power analysis there are four variables. Usually we calculate the sample size required to estimate with a given power, which is 1-p (type II error; e.g., 0.80) to a given degree of statistical significance, which is p (type I error; e.g., $p = 0.05$) to measure a phenomenon with an estimated effect size. Often the effect size is not known. The estimated effect size essentially

Illinois State Psychiatric Institute, 1153 North Lavergne, Chicago, IL 60651, USA determines the calculated sample size at the arbitrarily chosen parameter of power and significance. The problem is how to estimate the effect size.

One can estimate the effect size from previous studies. This creates an interesting paradox. If several previous studies exist, one can make a reliable estimate of power, but if enough information is available to make a reliable estimate of power, more controlled studies may not be needed. Of course, sometimes there are enough previous studies so that one can make a crude guess as to the effect size without being precise and needing more studies to verify the finding. In most cases there are conflicting data from several small studies, and the estimate of power depends on which study you picked.

For plasma level studies, effect size is usually unknown. The actual calculation of a power estimate is straightforward, and many standard statistical programs are readily available. We used the statistical program "Design," module of the "Systat" statistical package (Yale's continuity correction was used). Where a number of previous plasma level investigations have been carried out, one may estimate power from the effect size seen in that data. This said, the considerations discussed in this paper may be useful by placing such power analysis in the more general context of the effect size seen in the difference between drug versus placebo. But what if there are either no previous studies or studies are contradictory? We will restrict our discussion only to power estimates involving low plasma levels against adequate plasma levels for the targeted plasma level design but provide a method to estimate power.

We are going to calculate power analysis for a targeted plasma level study comparing low plasma levels against adequate plasma levels. In the targeted plasma level design one adjusts dose so all the patients in the adequate plasma level group have plasma levels within the therapeutic window and all the patients in the low plasma level group have low plasma levels in a predefined range. Of course, a targeted plasma level study can only be done when one has an idea of what the therapeutic window is.

We will not deal with calculating power curves where it might be predicted that high plasma levels produce a diminished therapeutic improvement. Since power function is usually monotonically increasing, power curves are not the best method to be used here.

In correlating plasma levels against therapeutic efficacy, there is measurement error in measuring the therapeutic efficacy of the drug and in measuring the plasma level. The method error in measuring the plasma levels at steady state may be principally the error of measurement of a single sample. The error of measurement of the drug-induced improvement is substantial and the major factor contributing to statistical variability in these studies. We can estimate this from the drug–placebo difference from controlled clinical trials.

2 Drug–Placebo Difference

2.1 Estimate of Drug–Placebo Difference

If there is a particularly pivotal study which for methodologic reasons can be considered excellent, one can use data from that study to estimate the effect size. (One could also pool data from several studies meeting particularly exacting criteria for methodologic excellence.) Alternately, one can pool *all* double-blind, random-assignment, controlled studies together to make an estimate of effect size. Pooling all random-assignment, double-blind studies has the advantage of eliminating bias of choice of study. These data are relatively homogeneous for the drugs considered in this paper. But if the assumption of homogeneity clearly does not hold, one must explore the reasons for this. The advantage of choosing a particularly pivotal study is that one can choose studies done in the same setting or a study of particular methodologic excellence, whose design and population is particularly appropriate for the research question. We will illustrate power analysis curves by both continuous and discontinuous methods, using both the pivotal study method and the pooled data from all studies.

For the estimation of dichotomous data, we will pool data from all random-assignment, double-blind studies, giving the proportion of patients improved with cyclic antidepressant drug or placebo (Davis et al. 1983). As an estimate of continuous data, we will use the pivotal study method and take mean improvements on drug and placebo in standard deviation units drawn from the first National Institutes of Mental Health (NIMH) double-blind study (Cole et al. 1964). Continuous measures are more statistically powerful than dichotomous measures, which lose information. Dichotomous data are more intuitively meaningful to clinicians and also allow analysis of an actual number derived from each patient (i.e., raw data, rather than a manipulation of some derived mean and standard deviation).

2.2 Drug–Placebo Difference on Percent Improved Data

We reviewed the literature of double-blind studies of antidepressants and did a meta-analysis and also calculated the effect size of imipramine, amitriptyline, fluoxetine, amoxapine, trazodone, fluvoxamine, sertraline, and paroxetine pooled together. We then combined these data to calculate an average effect size of the drug–placebo difference. All were studies in which patients were randomly assigned to drug or placebo, and the efficacy was measured in some quantitative way, such as generally a Hamilton Depression Rating Scale changed score, or a change on the Clinical Global Improvement Scale (CGI) or other global scale. Although investigators commonly reported these quantitative measures, they infrequently reported their standard deviations, so that one could not use this parameter in calculating effect size. The most common reported parameter was the percentage of patients who improved on drug and placebo. This is sometimes the percentage of patients who showed a reduction of 50% on the Hamilton Depression Rating Scale or sometimes the percentage of patients who were rated moderately improved or better. We combined the percentage of improvers from all these studies. The total sample size was 7762 patients studied in 100 investigations. Overall, 65% of patients improved with a cyclic antidepressant, in comparison to 37% with placebo, a difference of 28%, which constituted the drug–placebo difference. In a meta-analysis using the Mantel-Haenszel Test, chi squared = 500, df = 1, and $p =$

Table 1. Power to detect a drug–placebo difference based on effect size seen in pooled double-blind, random-assignment studies of cyclic antidepressants versus placebo

Sample size per group	Power	
	$\alpha = 0.05$	$\alpha = 0.01$
Power to detect a difference from a full drug effect vs placebo; drug 65%, placebo 37%		
56	0.80	0.58
60	0.83	0.63
65	0.86	0.68
70	0.89	0.76
80	0.93	0.80
90	0.96	0.85
100	0.97	0.90
Power to detect a difference from a full drug effect to 33% of full effect; drug 65%, plasma level 46%		
115	0.79	0.58
117	0.80	0.59
130	0.84	0.65
154	0.90	0.75
200	0.96	0.88
210	0.97	0.90
Power to detect a difference from a full drug effect to 50% of full effect; drug 65%, plasma level 51%		
210	0.80	0.59
275	0.90	0.75
300	0.93	0.79
303	0.93	0.80
380	0.97	0.90
Power to detect a difference from a full drug effect to 67% of full effect; drug 65%, plasma level 56%		
484	0.80	0.59
500	0.81	0.61
600	0.88	0.71
710	0.88	0.80
900	0.97	0.90

10^{-110}. This statistically significant level is vanishingly small due to the large sample size. The power of detecting a drug–placebo difference (28%) for antidepressants is not that large.

Studies done on severely ill, carefully selected inpatients with proper experimental design would undoubtedly have a greater power to detect a drug–placebo difference than the typical outpatient study. Even so, the variability of response to tricyclic drug is substantial.

If a plasma level was completely below the therapeutic window, the power of efficacy study would be identical to the power of detecting a drug more effective than placebo. The power analysis for a plasma level efficacy study is similar to a dose–response study. If a drug is given at the optimal dose or plasma level, one can calculate the optimal response rate, which sets the upper limit on response. The placebo response rate sets the lower limit. Table 1 (upper panel) is the power calculation curve for cyclic antidepressants, based on the proportion of patients responding to drug or placebo, averaging out the combined data of all the above-mentioned 100 studies of cyclic antidepressants. In order to achieve a power of 0.8, one has to have some 56-odd patients in each group (or 112 in the study). If in a plasma level study of antidepressants, those in the targeted low plasma group had essentially a completely ineffective plasma level, the power would be the same as the drug versus placebo group (upper panel, Table 1). If we make a working assumption that the low plasma level group has some therapeutic activity but not full therapeutic activity, we estimate statistical power accordingly. For example, we present in the second, third, or fourth panel of Table 1 the power curve assuming plasma levels in the low plasma level group produced 33% efficacy compared to an adequate plasma level, 50% efficacy, or 67% efficacy, respectively. For example, if we assume that the low plasma level group is one third as effective as an adequate dose, then we would estimate that 45% of the patients would improve with the low plasma level and 65% with the adequate dose, and we present the power analyses from these proportions in Table 1. If the low plasma level was 50% as efficacious as the optimal plasma level, one would need over 400 subjects, i.e., precisely 210 subjects in each group to detect a plasma level difference with a power of 80%. One would need 234 patients to detect a plasma level only a third as efficacious as the optimal plasma level for the 80% power point.

2.3 Extension of Power Calculations to New Antidepressants

It is very common to compare a new antidepressant against a standard antidepressant and find no statistically significant difference and conclude they are equivalent. If the new antidepressant were two thirds as efficacious as a standard antidepressant, sample sizes of almost 1000 patients would be needed to reliably detect a difference in an individual study. Individual studies are rarely bigger than 100 patients, seldom even as big as 200 patients, yet even if a new drug were only one third as efficacious as a standard drug, one could not reliably detect a difference unless sample sizes of over 200 patients per study were studied. If a difference of new drug versus standard drug is detected, this is clearly statistically significant and quite remarkable. The failure to detect a difference may reflect the lack of power to detect a drug–placebo difference of antidepressant drugs in typical outpatient populations. If you detect a difference, be it new drug against standard drug or drug against placebo, you are showing, despite this variability, that a difference does exist to your criteria of significance, such as the 0.05 level. If you fail to detect a difference, the failure may be due not to lack of a real difference but may just reflect the lack of the power of the clinical trial. Based on the effect size found in pooling 100 studies of cyclic antidepressants, the power to detect a difference between drug and placebo is not that large. These considerations should be taken into account in the interpretation of new drug–standard drug studies, where the new drug is found equivalent to the standard drug. It would take almost a thousand patients per study to detect that a new drug two thirds as effective as standard drug is less effective.

2.4 Drug–Placebo Difference for Maintenance Antidepressant Treatment

We identified 18 double-blind, random-assignment studies in which patients essentially with recurrent unipolar disorder were randomly assigned to drug or a placebo-controlled condition for long-term maintenance treatment to prevent relapse. Some 2225 patients were evaluated; 50% relapsed under the control conditions and 23% relapsed under drug (Chi squared = 128.2, $df = 1, p = 10^{-29}$). This allows us to calculate the power statistics under our various assumptions. It is interesting that the drug–placebo difference for maintenance medication is essentially identical to the drug–placebo difference for acute treatment. It would have been quite possible that drugs could be less efficacious in preventing a relapse than in helping the acute episode, or the methodologic problems associated with showing a prophylactic effect obscure efficacy (Table 2).

2.5 Drug–Placebo Difference for Antipsychotic Drugs

We chose as the pivotal study for the efficacy of antipsychotic drugs the first NIMH collaborative study (Cole et al. 1964). This sample included a great many patients during their first psychotic break. It was not a treatment-resistant population, but rather a population typical of first-break and newly admitted acute schizophrenics in a symptomatic episode. Since nearly 400 patients were studied, the sample size is adequate. Patients were randomly assigned to placebo, chlorpromazine, thioridazine, or fluphenazine and

Table 2. Power to detect a drug–placebo difference based on effect size seen in pooled double-blind, random-assignment studies of cyclic antidepressants versus placebo used for maintenance purposes to prevent relapse

Sample size per group	Power	
	α = 0.05	α = 0.01
Power to detect a difference from a full drug effect vs placebo; drug 50%, placebo 23%		
57	0.80	0.59
73	0.90	0.74
81	0.93	0.80
101	0.97	0.90
Power to detect a difference from a full drug effect to 33% of full effect; drug 50%, plasma level 32%		
128	0.80	0.59
167	0.90	0.74
185	0.93	0.80
232	0.97	0.90
Power to detect a difference from a full drug effect to 50% of full effect; drug 50%, plasma level 37%		
227	0.80	0.59
298	0.90	0.75
330	0.93	0.80
416	0.97	0.90
Power to detect a difference from a full drug effect to 67% of full effect; drug 50%, plasma level 41%		
507	0.80	0.59
670	0.90	0.75
743	0.93	0.80
940	0.97	0.90

treated for 6 weeks. All the antipsychotics were equally efficacious in this study, as they are in all other studies, so we pooled the three. We combined the data from the two items of the CGI. One item is a global evaluation of how much the patient has improved on the other drug, and the other item is a global evaluation of how sick the patient is. We combined both measures into a 6-point scale (see Brakel and Davis 1991). Hence, our scale was defined according to the following scale: (1) much improved and no residual symptoms present; (2) much improved with only minor residual symptoms present; (3) improved with minor symptoms still present; (4) slightly improved with moderate symptoms present; (5) no change and moderate symptoms present; or (6) worse. Patients were evaluated at 1, 3, and 6 weeks. Some patients left the study, either because of dramatic improvement or because of dramatic deterioration. Patients who were dramatically improved and thus left the hospital early were given a rating of 1, patients who dramatically deteriorated and had to be dropped from the study to receive emergency active treatment were rated as 6. This essentially uses a global rating of a clinical improvement and a semiquantitative 6-point scale, which allows computation of the mean improvement on drug and the mean improvement on placebo. Reducing this data to an endpoint dichotomous variable, improvers and nonimprovers, essentially discards part of the drug–placebo difference. The power calculations for antipsychotic drugs are based on a best-case scenario. This was a single pivotal study of carefully selected patients; even so, 88 patients would be needed for a 50% efficacious plasma level to detect a difference between the targeted groups.

Even though the drug–placebo difference for antipsychotic drugs is in a certain sense larger and more statistically reliable than the antidepressant effect of cyclic antidepressants, given some partial efficacy of an inadequate plasma level, the sample size needed to reliably show a "plasma level effect" is reasonably large (see Table 3). For example, 88 patients would be needed

Table 3. Power to detect a drug–placebo difference based on effect size seen in a pivotal study of antipsychotic drugs versus placebo (continuous data)

Sample size per group	Power	
	$\alpha = 0.05$	$\alpha = 0.01$
Power to detect a difference from a full drug effect vs placebo		
12	0.80	0.57
16	0.90	0.74
17	0.93	0.78
18	0.94	0.80
23	0.98	0.90
Power to detect a difference from a full drug effect to 33% of full effect		
25	0.80	0.57
33	0.90	0.73
38	0.93	0.80
47	0.97	0.90
Power to detect a difference from a full drug effect to 50% of full effect		
44	0.80	0.58
58	0.90	0.74
65	0.93	0.80
83	0.97	0.90
Power to detect a difference from a full drug effect to 67% of full effect		
97	0.80	0.58
130	0.90	0.74
146	0.93	0.80
184	0.97	0.90

if the low plasma level group had some partial efficacy of about 50% of the adequate plasma level group. Note also that continuous data are approximately twice as powerful as discontinuous data. We performed these power calculations on the continuous data but also dichotomized the data into responders and nonresponders and did a second power analysis (Table 4).

We pooled the results of 36 studies comparing the effects of maintenance antipsychotics versus placebo for the purpose of preventing relapse. All told, 54.6% relapsed in the placebo group, and 20.6% in the maintenance antipsychotic group, a result highly statistically significant (chi squared = 480, df = 1, $p = 10^{-108}$). We then based the meta-analysis on this effect size (see Table 5). Again, while the power to detect a drug effect is such that a reasonable sample size is required, rather large sample sizes are needed to detect differences between a full drug effect and a partial drug effect for whatever reason: inadequate dose, low plasma level, or partially but less effective antipsychotic.

Table 4. Power to detect a drug–placebo difference based on effect size seen in a pivotal study of antipsychotic drugs versus placebo (percent responders data)

Sample size per group	Power	
	$\alpha = 0.05$	$\alpha = 0.01$
Power to detect a difference from a full drug effect vs placebo		
22	0.80	0.59
27	0.90	0.74
30	0.94	0.80
37	0.98	0.90
Power to detect a difference from a full drug effect to 33% of full effect		
46	0.80	0.58
59	0.90	0.74
66	0.94	0.80
81	0.97	0.90
Power to detect a difference from a full drug effect to 50% of full effect		
78	0.80	0.58
101	0.90	0.74
113	0.93	0.80
140	0.97	0.90
Power to detect a difference from a full drug effect to 67% of full effect		
165	0.80	0.59
216	0.90	0.75
239	0.93	0.80
301	0.97	0.90

Table 5. Power to detect a drug–placebo difference based on effect size seen in 36 pooled studies of maintenance antipsychotic drugs versus placebo for prophylaxis against relapse

Sample size per group	Power	
	$\alpha = 0.05$	$\alpha = 0.01$
Power to detect a difference from a full drug effect vs placebo; drug 21%, placebo 54%		
37	0.80	0.59
47	0.90	0.74
52	0.93	0.80
64	0.97	0.90
Power to detect a difference from a full drug effect to 33% of full effect; drug 21%, plasma level 32%		
83	0.80	0.59
107	0.90	0.74
119	0.93	0.80
148	0.97	0.90
Power to detect a difference from a full drug effect to 50% of full effect; drug 21%, plasma level 38%		
146	0.80	0.59
191	0.90	0.75
211	0.93	0.80
266	0.97	0.90
Power to detect a difference from a full drug effect to 67% of full effect; drug 21%, plasma level 43%		
324	0.80	0.59
427	0.90	0.75
474	0.93	0.80
958	0.97	0.90

3 Discussion

We emphasize that we are making several important assumptions. One is, we are estimating power for the targeted plasma level study, in which patients are assigned to an adequate or an inadequate plasma level. We, therefore, base the power analysis on the drug–placebo difference, making an assumption as to what partial efficacy the inadequate plasma level group had. If we assume that the inadequate plasma level group had essentially zero plasma level, then the power calculations would be the same as the drug–placebo difference, which we have listed in Table 1, top panel. This is probably an unreasonable assumption. The dose–response curve may not be that steep. (There is insufficient data from humans to estimate the steepness of the dose–response curve in any precise way.) It probably should not be assumed to be that steep. Although below the therapeutic window, many patients may have plasma levels which do produce some, but less than optimal, beneficial effect. We make the assumption in our calculations in Tables 1 and 2 that patients have plasma levels which are on average only 50% inadequate. We assume inadequate (or 33% or 67% of an adequate plasma level) and do the power analysis. This gives a good power estimate for the type of sample sizes that would be needed under these assumptions.

3.1 A False Critique of Plasma Level Studies

Clearly, there are many patients who have adequate plasma levels yet fail to respond, and some patients with low plasma levels do respond. The lack of 100% correlation of plasma level to therapeutic efficacy leads to this variability of outcome. Because of this inherent variability, large sample sizes are required. Some of the variability in the results of empirical plasma level studies is due to the small sample sizes being studied. Plasma level studies are limited by the variability of clinical improvement per se. A negative study or one with borderline findings should be seen in the context of what reasonable expectations are in light of the variability of the therapeutic efficacy of antidepressants.

3.2 Importance of Error Reduction in Efficacy or Plasma Level Studies

It should be apparent that there are many power considerations in the design of plasma level studies since a large number of subjects are required due to the inherent variability of estimating the drug effect. Since the extremely large sample sizes required are unrealistic, meticulous attention needs to be devoted to reducing experimental error. An inpatient study assures medication compliance. If a patient is not compliant with medication, differences observed in plasma levels may relate to compliance rather than individual differences of drug metabolism. We need to increase power by improvement in methodology but also need an adequate sample size.

3.2 Power of Less Efficacious New Drugs

Exactly the same calculations would apply if we were studying a partially effective drug against a fully effective antidepressant. Assuming that a new class of antidepressants is less efficacious for depression than the standard drug, then this new class would be clearly more effective than placebo, but it would be found to be less effective that standard in small clinical trials. What sample sizes would be needed to detect a less efficacious class? It is clear that if the efficacy of the new antidepressant is reasonably close to the standard antidepressant, such as two thirds of the standard antidepressant, it would take rather large sample sizes to detect this difference.

References

Brakel SJ, Davis JM (1991) Taking harms seriously: involuntary mental patients and the right to refuse treatment. Indiana Law Rev 25(2):429–473

Cole JO, Klerman G, Goldberg S (1964) Phenothiazine treatment in acute schizophrenia: effectiveness. Arch Gen Psychiatry 10:246–261

Davis JM, Fredman DJ, Linden RD (1983) A review of the new antidepressant medications. In: Davis JM, Maas JW (eds) The affective disorders. American Psychiatric Press, Washington DC, pp 1–29

Davis JM, Janicak PG, Singla A, Sharma RP (1991) Maintenance antipsychotic medication. In: Barnes T (ed) Antipsychotic drugs and their side effects. Academic, San Diego

Davis JM, Janicak PG, Wang Z, Gibbons RD, Sharma RP (1992) The efficacy of psychotropic drugs. Psychopharmacol Bull (in press)

Subject Index

Springer-Verlag and the Environment

MIX
Papier aus verantwortungsvollen Quellen
Paper from responsible sources
FSC® C105338

If you have any concerns about our products,
you can contact us on
ProductSafety@springernature.com

In case Publisher is established outside the EU,
the EU authorized representative is:
Springer Nature Customer Service Center GmbH
Europaplatz 3, 69115 Heidelberg, Germany

Printed by Libri Plureos GmbH
in Hamburg, Germany